MYSTERY

OF THE

WHITE LIONS

CHILDREN OF THE SUN GOD

Linda Tucker

HAY HOUSE, INC.

Carlsbad, California • New York City
London • Sydney • Johannesburg
Vancouver • Hong Kong • New Delhi

Published and distributed in the United States by: Hay House, Inc.: www.hayhouse.com •
Published and distributed in Australia by: Hay House Australia Pty. Ltd.: www.hayhouse.com
.au • *Published and distributed in the United Kingdom by:* Hay House UK, Ltd.: www.hayhouse
.co.uk • *Published and distributed in the Republic of South Africa by:* Hay House SA (Pty), Ltd.:
www.hayhouse.co.za • *Distributed in Canada by:* Raincoast: www.raincoast.com • *Published in
India by:* Hay House Publishers India: www.hayhouse.co.in

Interior photos/illustrations:

Previously published by Earthyear, M&G Media, South Africa, 2001; and Npenvu Press, South
Africa, 2003.

Library of Congress Control Number: 2009943100

ISBN: 978-1-4019-2721-9

13 12 11 10   4 3 2 1
1st edition, June 2010

Printed in the United States of America

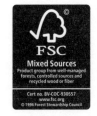

CONTENTS

FOREWORD

BY Credo Mutwa

A voice rises from the parched valleys of my ancient motherland, a lonely voice above the hills of eternal Africa, an appeal to those who do not care, to those who have no ears. A plea to those who choose to do nothing in the face of monstrous evil:

Leave the lions of Timbavati alone. Do not destroy the sacred lions of the gods of Africa. This is the book that Linda Tucker has written.

No one in their right mind would ever travel to India and massacre the white Brahmin cattle that roam the crowded streets of its cities. No one in their right mind would ever travel to Thailand and murder the rare white elephants that we find in that country. But people come to my motherland, people come to South Africa, to brutally murder the White Lions of Timbavati in the name of manliness and in the name of sport. The sacred icons of other races and nations in this world are respected, revered, and protected. But the icons of Africa are massacred with cold impunity, sometimes with the connivance of some of Africa's own children.

I understand, much to my sorrow, that there is not a single White Lion left in the wild. And I ask myself: did we win our freedom for this? This quiet devastation of our country's most sacred animals? Did we, by joining the ranks of the democratic countries of the world, also join those people who see it as their task to denude this planet of all life? I want to join Linda Tucker's appeal. I say:

Please. Leave South Africa's White Lions alone. Let them breed once more. Let them walk tall in the wilderness which is their mother.

In the past 200 years or so, the human race has lost much that is of importance in Africa. And it continues to lose much. But what is most terrible, what is most tragic, is that it does not realize what it has lost. One day, in the dark valleys of the future, people will try to turn back, people will try to investigate, to look into the past of African humankind with wide-open eyes, but they will find very little because much has been obliterated. When an animal is killed in Africa, that animal takes a large slice of African knowledge into oblivion with it. Because most of the knowledge that Africans possess is intimately intertwined with the animal life as well as the plant life of this continent.

Let this woman's plea for the preservation of the White Lions of Timbavati be heeded by this world. I pray and hope that the readers of this book will take it to their hearts, and themselves investigate many things that she here reveals. Because the diamond that you find yourself, the diamond that you discover in the red rubble of Africa, is more precious to you than the polished one that you find in the marketplace. The truth that you discover yourself is more indelible than a truth written to you or for you by someone else's pen.

Take this book to your heart, and let it guide you to even greater truths about Africa than have been here revealed.

Author's note: *The full text of Credo Mutwa's "Plea for Africa" is available on our website, www.whitelions.org.*

PREFACE

BY ADRIAN GILBERT

The story told in this book is intriguing and revealing. Few people confront lions in the wild and live to tell the tale. If they do, then their response, after thanking whatever god they believe in, is usually to make a point of avoiding crossing the paths of such dangerous animals again. Linda Tucker's experience, when she and a group of friends found their open-topped truck surrounded by roaring lions one night, is the stuff of nightmares. Yet for her, though terrifying, this proved to be an initiatory experience of the first order. Instead of forgetting all about that fateful evening and getting on with her life, she was drawn back to the bush. She had to find out more about the lions she met and the strange shamanic woman who saved her life.

From these small beginnings, and because of her determination that nothing was going to get in the way of her finding out the truth of what really happened that night, she has been drawn deeper and deeper into the mysteries of Africa. Having met Linda on a number of occasions and having witnessed the unfolding of the later part of her adventure, I can bear witness to her honesty. That she has been chosen as a vehicle through whom certain teachings are to be passed to the modern world, I am in no doubt. In spite of her being a white woman, Africa has taken her to its heart.

I believe that Linda's message from the shamans of Southern Africa is both timely and important. We may not understand, still less believe, what they have to say, but we have a duty to listen. The relationship between man and lion, hunter and hunted, is complex and far-reaching. Why else would lions figure so prominently in human art, from the ancient Sphinx of Egypt to Nelson's Column, if we had not some inkling, deep in our hearts, that these "kings of beasts" mattered? This being so, is it not a tragedy that the surviving White Lions of Timbavati are being shot for sport? Perhaps Linda's book, written from the heart, will change the perceptions of at least some of those in power and afford greater protection for these unique specimens. Maybe it is we, not them, who need to learn the lesson of natural selection and of how to protect our environment – not just for ourselves but for all of life.

INTRODUCTION

Normally, it would be a mistake for a writer to disclose the end of her story in the introduction, but this real-life story can't be spoiled. In fact, the extraordinary ending makes the beginning all the more interesting – so, prepare yourself: I'm going to tell you how this ends!

On 10 November 1991, a near-death experience changed my life forever. I was rescued from an angry pride of lions by an indigenous Shangaan medicine woman, Maria Khosa, who was also known as "the Lion Queen of Timbavati." Subsequently, I gave up my life in fashion and advertising in Europe and returned to Africa to make sense of this bizarre and miraculous intervention. I found Maria, who became my shaman teacher, and with her, I embarked on an extraordinary journey of discovery. *Mystery of the White Lions* brings together nearly a decade of research to shed light on the significance of the White Lions, believed to be the most sacred animals on the African continent.

Coming from a skeptical academic background, I was at first resistant to the wisdom Maria shared with me, but finally I succumbed to its evidential and profoundly accurate truth. And having done so, more and more secret knowledge was entrusted to me. Maria introduced me to other African medicine people from many traditions; among them was the pre-eminent high priest Baba Credo Mutwa, arguably the greatest repository of African cultural knowledge and the so-called Guardian of "*Umlando*," Africa's secret knowledge.

Most of the material in this book has never been recorded before. It was protected for centuries by the priestly initiates of Africa, who passed on hidden information in an oral tradition not accessible to the outside world. I was profoundly privileged to have portions of this guarded material – known as the "Great Knowledge" – shared with me, while some of the information came direct from lion ancestral sources.

Please join me on my journey to discover a profound mystery behind the so-called Children of the Sun God, the White Lions – the most sacred and mysterious animals alive today. But before you begin, let me remind you of Christ's words in Mark 6:4, where the Son of God speaks about being "a prophet without honor" in his home country. Tragically, nothing could be truer for these blessed Lions of Light. The Timbavati wilderness region is the only place on Earth where White Lions have been born by natural occurrence. It is also the area of their relentless persecution.

It turns out that the year – possibly the very day – of my rescue was the last occasion a White Lion was born in Timbavati, a bushveld wilderness region bordering on the Kruger National Park in South Africa. By the time this book was first published, an entire decade had all but passed without these rare animals being born on their native Timbavati soil. The reason for this tragedy has to do with the many forced removals of White Lions from their natural and spiritual homelands of the Timbavati region into zoos and circuses all over the globe, and most appallingly, into "canned hunting" operations, where they are bred in cages to be trophy hunted.

After I had spent almost ten years focusing on the importance of the White Lions and their larger connection in the world, an event occurred that made uncanny sense of Maria's teachings and my firsthand experiences. Maria had informed me that despite human attempts to destroy sacredness in nature, God's "enlightenment-bearers" would continue to manifest, and she forecasted the birth of a sacred White Lioness in a place of great symbolic significance to humanity.

Her prophecy was fulfilled just before my book first went to press: *a White Lioness was born in a place called "Bethlehem" on Christmas Day, 25 December 2000.*

This little cub was named Marah – "Mother of the Sun God" – by the African elders, who informed me that she was "the One" they had been waiting for. Her birth represented the beginning of a whole new approach to my life. From that point on, all my studies about the mythic and legendary aspects of the White Lions had to move from mere theory into concrete practice. I proceeded to campaign for legislation and embark on a very real conservation battle for the White Lions' survival and recognition. Rescuing Marah from the brutal canned-hunting camp where she was held, and returning her to roam free with her cubs in the wilds of her birthright has determined every minute of every day of my life since her sacred birth – and her legacy continues today.

Marah's arrival was the culmination of all that I had learned in my shamanic odyssey with Maria Khosa, undoubtedly the most courageous human I have ever met. Marah's birth is described in the *very last chapter of this book*. However, to understand what this White Lioness and her brethren mean for humanity in this time of ecological crisis, you need to start at the beginning.

I trust you enjoy the journey of discovery and enlightenment as much as I did.

Now, more than ever, we need to listen to the message of the lions, and act on it.

LINDA TUCKER
March 2010

AUTHOR'S NOTE

This study is interdisciplinary. In tracking the secrets of the White Lions, I was led to walk the interface between science and what I now term "sacred science." While the significance of the White Lions' appearance on Earth in our time may be understood through the supporting evidence of genetics, paleoanthropology, cave taphonomy, climatology, geology, and other scientific fields, the true inspiration derives from sacred knowledge systems. My quest into lion shamanism was not an act of blind faith, nor was it an act of blind fact. I have come to combine dualities such as faith and fact, myth and reality, and science and religion, in a meaningful, interconnected way that I hope illustrates that they should never have been separated.

The objective of this book is to deliver previously hidden information about Timbavati's unique White Lions to the public, because this information has crucial relevance for the ecological and psychological crisis in which humanity finds itself today.

It was for much the same reason that Vusamazulu Credo Mutwa broke the "Oath of Silence" that had bound him and other high shamans to a secret oral tradition. As Africa's pre-eminent "Guardian of Umlando," Mutwa understands that we live in prophetic times when it is imperative to transmit *knowledge* to humanity at large, because, simply put: *it might save the world.*

Mutwa's imperative to me was not to delay the publication of this book for any reason whatsoever. Given the urgent nature of the material, my main concern was to deliver it without delay. I have recorded events according to my best memory of their occurrence and provided factual and academic corroboration wherever possible.

Where Mutwa has asked me to record his words exactly as they were spoken, I have done so, to the word. His story of the White Lions is repeated verbatim from the original, although an extraneous section relating to Queen Numbi's son has been omitted (with Mutwa's permission).

In the various meetings described between us, I have allowed for a degree of poetic license to facilitate the flow of the narrative. That said, the final draft of this publication has been approved by Credo Mutwa himself.

1

TIMBAVATI

And I asked the people of Timbavati: "Where are your White Lions? Where are the holy Children of the Sun God?" Because that is what they are called. I never received a straight answer.
— CREDO MUTWA

Although I did not know it at the time, for me the true magic began on 10 November 1991.

It was a moonless night in the bushveld. A group of us were sitting around the campfire after the sun had set, drinking Lion lagers and exchanging stories. In the center of the reed *boma,* I remember the burning embers shooting sparks high into the darkness, like fireflies against the stars. Illuminated by the naked fire, our conversation was light and relaxed, while above our tiny group the brilliant constellations spanned Timbavati's vast horizons from east to west.

Timbavati is a name so old that today's inhabitants have forgotten its meaning. It is a landscape seemingly unchanged since our earliest ancestors roamed the earth. Traces of ancient metal-smelting sites still exist in the parched ground. And the spirit of the legendary White Lions still haunts the bushveld.

Are the White Lions History?

The White Lions were a unique strain never before recorded in zoological history, seen as simply a random mutation of the standard lion, *Panthera leo,* thrown up by chance in the Timbavati region. Yet, extraordinarily, their arrival was predicted by tribal shamans long before they made a physical appearance. The local inhabitants viewed them as the most sacred of animals and believed their appearance to be prophetic of changing times on Earth. Ever since I had first come to Timbavati, I had felt an aura hanging over the territory at the mention of the White Lions. From the awe-inspiring descriptions of the Shangaan trackers George Matabula and his brother, Jack, it seemed that these were no ordinary animals. The trackers believed the White Lions were sent as gifts from God. On the other hand, there were those who viewed them as a high-income-yielding

1

commodity. In the short time since their first reported sighting in the 1970s, they had been hunted to apparent extinction.

More elusive than the African leopard, rarer even than the legendary snow leopard of the Himalayas, as snowy white as the polar bear of the Arctic, the White Lion of Timbavati was a *rara avis* that appeared from nowhere and dissolved again without trace.

Jaws of Death

One of our group around the fire was Leonard, a game ranger and my friend since childhood, whose father owned a piece of land in Timbavati reserve. Leonard was one of the few fortunate enough to have encountered the White Lions in the wild several times on his game drives around the territory. Over many years, I had returned to visit him in Timbavati, yet I had never seen a White Lion. Now, we thought, there was no chance of seeing one, since not one White Lion had been spotted in the wild for almost a decade.

On this particular evening, as our group of friends settled down to our predinner drinks, the earth seemed to rumble in the near distance. Leonard identified this as the roar of lions to the north, near a dry riverbed called Machaton. The Machaton pride is a tawny pride of Timbavati lions that, it is believed, may still be bearing the white gene. Most of the others in the group were newcomers to the bushveld, and we listened to the primal roars with awe. Leonard explained to us that a lion does not roar when it is hunting – it would frighten off its prey. And, indeed, the rumble we had just heard was nature's most archetypally terrifying sound: a reminder of which predator, ultimately, holds the crown of the king of beasts. Then, suddenly the lions' sounds altered and became urgent and exuberant, which led Leonard to suspect that one of the Machaton lionesses, which had been heavily pregnant, had just given birth.

"Let's go!" he said on impulse.

Buoyed up by the thought of witnessing the newborn cubs, and the tantalizing, though remote, possibility of a white cub, our party of eight clambered after Leonard into the open Land Rover used for game viewing and set out into the summer night.

The Land Rover had two sunken seats in the front, behind the glass windshield, and three raised bench seats at the rear. My husband, John, and I were perched in the back, where the welded seats hung over the wheels. As we drove, the wind ruffled my hair, carrying the fresh-baked smell of the bushveld. In front of us sat my sister, Serena, beside her boyfriend, Andries, a dark, silent Afrikaner, celebrating his birthday in the peace of the bushveld. In front of them were two tourists out on their first safari. A seat secured on the hood above the left front wheel was reserved for George, our official tracker, who knew animal tracks like the palm of his own hand but tonight was off-duty. Leonard, in the driver's seat, with his petite wife beside him, swung the Land Rover off the dust road into the bushveld. The bush was Leonard's playground. He loved it with a passion, but, young and a little hot-headed, he still sought to master it.

He was our ranger, our guide; and, at the time, I trusted his bush sense. I had not yet been introduced to a more sensitive and attuned way of working with nature. All of us caught Leonard's spirit of enthusiasm as the four-wheel-drive beat a route over tall grass tufts and abandoned ant heaps into the thick blackness.

In the adrenaline rush, I remember noticing how the vehicle's headlights jerked skyward, then earthward, as the Land Rover crunched through the rough terrain. Then, all of a sudden, at the very moment we picked out the glowing amber eyes of a large lion in the darkness, there was a rasping sound, and the vehicle came to a shuddering halt.

Somebody suggested that we "get out of here" – the voice already slightly high-pitched. The lions were agitated and too close for comfort. In the flash of the headlights I glimpsed shadowy shapes and the gleam of eyes in the bush. One outline was immediately recognizable to Leonard, who knew the dominant males in the territory: Ngwazi, his eyes ablaze. Behind him, in a hideout formed by the arching roots of a wild fig tree, I caught the outline of a snarling lioness; she may have been nestled among squirming bundles of fur – the newborns. The last thought in our minds at that moment was whether or not any of them was a White Lion cub.

Leonard prepared to make a speedy exit, but then it became apparent what had brought the Land Rover to a halt in the first place. In reverse gear now, the vehicle jolted violently, a tree trunk jammed under the front axle, flinging us forward then back in our seats. I recall catching sight of the steering wheel spinning freely in Leonard's hand, before he finally explained that we couldn't move. The steering column was broken – we were stuck!

Armed with a spotlight, binoculars, and telephoto lenses, we had expected to be entertained by the animals. We had leapt into our Land Rover and ridden roughshod over the lions' territorial borders. Their cubs had just been born – yet it did not even cross our minds that the lions themselves might have been disturbed by our brutal intrusion on their sacred space. Our only thought was that the beasts were about to attack us.

Stranded and unprotected in the midst of an angry pride of lions, we waited.

Lena, Leonard's wife, was holding the only flashlight, powered by the Land Rover battery. Leonard gave the order to "cut the light" – and suddenly darkness closed in. It was 8:15 on a summer's evening. The last luminosity had faded from the horizon.

"If the battery runs flat, we'll never get out," Leonard explained matter-of-factly. It was then that I heard a rustle behind me, and cried out for light. Lena spun around, leveling the light on the bushes, and I found myself staring into the fierce eyes of another angry female. A sound to the left, and the beam was swung onto two more pairs of predatory eyes. We were surrounded.

"Cut the light, Lena." Leonard repeated his order. "You're running down the battery – we won't get the engine started again." For the first time, I detected a hint of fear in his voice.

Lena switched the spotlight off, leaving a horrible, petrified silence.

It is difficult to describe the size of a lion close-up. The tawny lions that had shown up in our flashlight were awe-inspiring. The two males, with their monumental blackened manes radiating like dark suns in our beam, were instant reminders of how puny the human species is. With the light out, the presence of the lions was stronger still. Everyone in the Land Rover stared helplessly into the pitch darkness in search of one another.

On the horizon, the lights of the camp flickered tauntingly. But it was the tracker's day off, so we could not expect help from that direction.

A sudden movement compelled Lena to switch on the light again, and I saw another fully grown lion crouched not ten meters away, eyes fiery with rage. Facing us squarely, his jaws slightly open, he contracted his belly to emit one of those earth-shuddering roars we had heard from the camp – only now we were in the middle of it. The sound began low in his belly and rose to a deafening rumble, then tapered off into a series of guttural grunts. It literally shook me to the ends of my toes. The Land Rover itself was rattling. My stomach was lurching. I thought I was going to be ill.

Leonard ordered us to keep calm. He explained that we weren't able to take the vehicle forward, and we weren't able to steer. But, he said, we could reverse straight backward to get out of danger.

Lena put the light out again, and we waited breathlessly as he turned the ignition. *Click.*

We all heard the sound, but we needed Leonard to pronounce the words for the dreadful news to sink in. Under his breath, he admitted, "Engine's dead . . ."

"Did you say dead?" That was my husband's voice. Among alarmists, John is a prize specimen, and I knew him well enough to understand what he was thinking: this night would be our last.

Yet John's ability to perceive life through a superbly dry academic wit brought an element of farce into the real-life drama.

The situation was truly absurd. One of the tourists blurted out hysterically, "We can't move; we're trapped in an open butcher's shop!"

The camp itself was probably less than a kilometer away, but between us and safety lay near-certain death. Leonard reached for the radio. It crackled, then blanked out.

"Suppose that's dead, too." John had adopted his appropriate deadpan voice again.

Leonard explained that the Land Rover was in a dip and the radio seemed unable to make contact. I sensed he was thinking hard. The radio hadn't been serviced, and in the excitement Leonard had not stopped to consider the implications. This meant that help was beyond reach. Trying to think constructively, Leonard explained that we would have a beam from the flashlight for half an hour or so before the battery died, too. The comfort drained from his words even as he was speaking them. No radio, no engine, no light, and nobody knew where we were. There were only the enraged roars that made the ground beneath us tremble and the ominous shuffles in the undergrowth as the lions moved closer. A star had risen on the eastern horizon: Sirius, glimmering an intense and unpitying red.[1]

We were frightened, and panicky, and desperate – but we each had hopes of rescue.

Someone shouted, "We're going to make a run for it!"

"Please don't," Leonard countered. "If you run, the lions will bring you down."

Someone else came up with what he thought an ingenious scheme – to form a chain and go together, slowly, like a rhino. I remember thinking this was a good plan. But Leonard tried to intervene, ordering us all to listen to him, and reminding us that lions are nocturnal predators.

Suddenly, the tide seemed to turn. One of the tourists thought he was agreeing with Leonard. "Yes, we'll never get to the camp in the dark!" he was shouting. "We'll stumble and fall!"

"Well, I'm staying right where I am," I retorted. "We're safe in the Land Rover."

The tourist shouted back at me that we were not at all safe. Our vehicle was wide open, with no protection, not even a canopy. He was panicking, standing up and waving desperately into the blackness, calling out hoarsely that it was "just as dangerous here as out there!"

Leonard demanded that he sit down at once. With his arms flailing about, the man must have been an absurdly tempting target for the predators. We were truly ridiculous and totally out of touch with the situation. We should never have been there in the first place.

Someone else had stood up and whispered fiercely that he was going to make a run for it.

"Don't do it!" someone else shouted. "Alone, you're a walking piece of meat. We must go together or not at all."

As for me, I couldn't have gone anywhere. My legs were jelly.

The situation had turned into the blackest comedy. I would have laughed, except that my stomach was aching too much from fear. Only moments before we had been city people enjoying a weekend in the bush, expecting to be entertained by the wildlife. Now we were their game.

I have never known the intensity of fear that I experienced that night – nothing since has ever approximated it. Personal fear seems magnified many times over by communal terror.

"What about firing a shot into the air . . .?" I suggested under my breath.

"The rifle has only four bullets; we may need every one of them," Leonard countered.

"Oh no!" I heard a terrified groan from John, the crouched figure by my side.

The dissension in the ranks meant that no sooner would someone make a suggestion than it would be shot down by the others. We were exhausted and confused. Squeezed into the corner on the floorboards of the Land Rover, John held the polystyrene lid of the drinks box over his head like a shield. "A drink anybody?" he proposed cheerily, playing out the farce of our situation – despite his terror. Silence.

"Anybody for a Lion lager?" Leonard quipped, adopting John's hearty tone.

The vast expanse of bushveld, teeming with unseen eyes, throbbed in silence. Somebody came up with the bright idea that we lie under the Land Rover, out of sight

– at which I heard John's ironic voice inquire who exactly was volunteering to lie on the outside?

This raised the stakes. The thought of the lions sniffing around us and hooking us out with their claws, like a cat pawing for a mouse, was too horrible to contemplate. In what remained of a beam from the precious flashlight, I could see that yet another male had begun to circle.

Reassuring us that he had his rifle, Leonard ordered us to just "sit tight." He told us we were going to be all right, but he didn't sound convincing. We could all sense that he was losing control of the situation.

"Not without the light!" somebody blurted out excitedly. "We won't even be able to see the lion before it leaps at us!"

As humans, it must be the ultimate primal terror to be eaten by a predator – and now suddenly we were living this nightmare. We had been in that fateful spot for less than 20 minutes, and I now understood the eternity of which death-row prisoners speak. What made it worse was the knowledge that Leonard's fear was well founded. If he of all people had lost his nerve, what hope was there for the rest of us?

My head was pulsating like a drum. The stars had crystallized overhead and the warmth of the African night had turned to cold sweat on our skins. We had run out of options.

Rites of Passage

Then, at the highest pitch of communal hysteria, the tenor of the drama altered.

Slowly out of the blackness a ghostly presence, which at first resembled a four-headed beast, came toward us. I was by now overcome with dizziness, and thought it must be a hallucination. In the darkness all I could see were shapes. In front was an old woman, who I later discovered was Maria Khosa, a Shangaan shaman. She carried, unbelievably, a baby on her back. Behind her followed a young African girl and, finally, a wide-eyed youth. They walked in a trancelike state, each holding on to the other.

We're saved! was my first thought. It seemed like a miracle. Rescue at last! My heart leapt, then fell as I realized there was nothing this incongruous crew could do to help us. I saw that the new arrivals simply multiplied the burden – adding stock to the butcher's block. Very slowly, step by step, they came toward us, and, still seemingly entranced, clambered into the Land Rover without a word, sitting among us like phantoms. There they stared blankly into the darkness, into the field of lions from which they had come.

I remember detecting how a new kind of silence had fallen on the scene. But my gut told me: now it's even worse. Like John, I was waiting hollowly for the end. I didn't even try to understand what these newcomers were doing here, how they had got to us. The old woman had climbed in beside Andries, with the others hunched in the seats in front of her. All I remember was the curious contrast their two silhouettes made in front of me: Andries's shoulders broad and brooding, the woman's wizened and intense.

Somewhere in my heart I must have known that what was needed was an act of pure heroism.

A moment later, in the wilderness of Africa, in that ill-fated Land Rover, Andries spoke for the first time that night. Suddenly spurred on, as if infused with an entirely new spirit, the birthday boy pushed past Maria and grabbed the wide-eyed black youth, saying, "*Kom, laat ons waai!* [Come, let's go!]"

For a moment, as Andries leapt into the night – his plan was to attempt to walk back to the camp to retrieve the other vehicle and save us all – he looked at my sister, Serena. As she had her back to me, I could not see the expression in her eyes. But I clearly remember his, fiery and determined, as he handed her the rifle and said, "*Miskien het jy dit nodig* [you might just need it]."

Andries must have assumed that the youth could show him the route back to the camp. He left Maria, and the baby and the young girl, with us. We sat frozen in the Land Rover, too stunned to speak, as the figures disappeared into the blackness. If the lions attacked, would we hear a last scream, a muffled cry, a crunch of bones? I was trying not to think. What was it like to be eaten?

Strangely, the hysteria suddenly drained out of the night. I was holding my breath and praying. Suddenly in the stillness I felt a strange calm, the likes of which I had never experienced before. There was no way of telling exactly where each of the predators had positioned itself. They had fallen silent. I was hoping the others were not also thinking of Leonard's words – "No lion roars when stalking its prey."

Andries walked through the lion-infested darkness and back to camp unharmed. He collected the other vehicle and returned to rescue the rest of us.

That night, as we all lay in bed rigid with unspent adrenaline, Ngwazi, the dominant male lion, padded straight through our bush camp, as if to reinforce his sovereignty. Leonard discovered his spoor in the sand the next day. The rest of us awoke barely able to move a muscle – apart from Andries, who looked as fresh as an impala lily.

It is said that a cat has nine lives. If the same were true of humans, I have no doubt that everyone in that Land Rover would have lost a life that moonless night. Certainly, each one of us viewed mortality in an entirely new light from that day on.

Serena ended up marrying Andries, the lionhearted hero of the day. Of course, Andries was heroic. He has been nicknamed "the Hero" ever since, and this tale not only formed the substance of the speech that John delivered at Serena and Andries's wedding but also provided spellbinding conversation for many a dinner party to come. Which only serves to show how out of touch we all were with the other hero of the piece: Maria, the *sangoma* or medicine woman, who appeared to have calmed the enraged lions and walked through their ranks to reach us.

My life has never been the same. I had visited Timbavati many times prior to this incident, but from that day forward the place took on a new electricity. The experience was so foreign to my everyday perception of reality that I made no attempt to analyze it. Amazingly, it was a full three years later, after I had suffered a period of protracted illness that forced me to re-examine my entire value system, that I was finally prepared to consider the implications of Maria's courageous act.

In 1994, with new purpose, I returned to Timbavati. I felt ready to face the medicine woman and hear her side of the story. Perhaps I had simply not been prepared to know the truth before.

2

MARIA, LION QUEEN OF TIMBAVATI

Do not let Maria die alone. . . . So many healers have died without the world understanding.
– CREDO MUTWA

It turned out that 1991, the year of my near-death experience, was the same year a white cub was born in Timbavati. Sadly, it disappeared soon after, and no White Lion has been seen there since.

Three years after its appearance, I returned to the site of our encounter with the Timbavati lions. It had been one of my favorite retreats since childhood, and I had continued to make regular return visits to Timbavati in the intervening period. Yet this time was different. Something had shifted in my own consciousness. In the meantime, my life had carried on as normal. The experience with Maria and the lions had been so unusual that I had not known how to integrate it into everyday reality. Then, one day, all of a sudden, everything came to a standstill. In the midst of the hectic pace of working life, it suddenly felt as if I had pressed the buttons on a video machine. Stop. Rewind.

What was that all about?

Coming from an academic background, I was used to explaining things rationally. I had no religious belief by which to account for otherworldly phenomena or "miracles." Yet circumstances finally conspired to force me into a new way of seeing. I had been living in London, working in a frenzied advertising environment. After a period of intense, high-stress activity, I suffered what is routinely called "burnout." I resigned, feeling utterly exhausted. In the months of recuperation that followed, I inevitably began to consider the nature of reality and virtual reality, truth, and illusion. I also began to question my role in the creation of false images, in branding and mass-marketing strategies that relied on psychological manipulation of the population for material gain. I was plagued by questions about the Timbavati lion encounter, particularly the dramatic rescue by Maria the *sangoma* – a shaman. It occurred to me for the first time that not only had these questions remained unanswered, but that they had never been properly asked.

Returning to Timbavati, I resolved to open myself to the answers I sought. In retrospect, this change in attitude represented my first means of entry into Maria's world. For one who had had no dealings with alternative forms of consciousness; who had never before encountered a psychic, a diviner, or a shaman; who had not so much as had her palm read by a gypsy at a country fair, this was new. Although I sensed that what Maria represented might shake the foundations of the comfortable reality I inhabited, I knew I could no longer continue living in a state of blithe ignorance.

As night fell back in Timbavati, I walked up the dry sand path to the reeded *boma* where Leonard stood in his khakis, beer in hand, exchanging pleasantries with a couple of newly arrived guests. Instead of joining the group around the campfire, I lingered in the shadows outside the circle of light, listening to the glug-glug-glug of the nightjars, like water poured from a jug. All around me the highly vocal yet harmonious African darkness pressed in. It was hard to believe that only a day before I had been in London, embroiled in the throb of the city.

At the time of the incident with the lions in 1991, Leonard had been living in a primitive camp house in the middle of the wilderness. Since then, he had set up a commercial game lodge that could accommodate 16 guests, with a staff of around 20. Maria, the medicine woman or *sangoma*, was one of the staff members. One of the damaging consequences of old-style South African politics is that traditional systems, which once supported tribal healers at the very heart of the community, have broken down. Despite the lowering of her status to that of a housemaid, Maria was grateful for the income. She was too old for menial work but Leonard had found her a token position. I suspected that he, too, felt he owed her something.

Leonard, nevertheless, was a pragmatist. He was concerned with the practicalities of running a successful operation – the training of the rangers and trackers, the building of camp accommodation, the feeding of guests, the servicing of Land Rovers. Yet, over the years, he had grown to respect Maria's subtle bushcraft. He now consulted her before making any important decision in camp. He had noticed how people from all over the region came to Maria with their ailments, so when he himself got ill he consulted her, too. He confided in me that there had been critical times when he wished he had consulted her earlier, such as the period when he desperately needed to find water. Timbavati is a dry land of dense bushveld with riverbeds that stand empty all year, apart from a couple of days when they flash flood after the rains. Water is a desperately scarce commodity. After drilling a dozen dry boreholes, Leonard eventually called upon Maria's water-divining powers. The site the *sangoma* went on to identify – a needle in the haystack of Timbavati's 50,000-hectare territory – turned out to be where the drillers finally hit water.

On learning of my intention to meet Maria again, Leonard warned me that she spoke no English, only a mixture of pidgin Afrikaans and Shangaan, so I would need to take along a local translator. This was arranged, and together with the Shangaan intermediary I walked to Maria's living quarters with some trepidation. Apart from Leonard's encouraging anecdotes, I had no idea what to expect.

I had always thought *sangomas* were relics of primitive superstition. I had assumed they were outmoded products of tribal Africa who had the gullible and uneducated in their thrall, and whose power was illusory. This view, I would come to learn, was hopelessly misinformed.

I had also imagined a traditional mud-baked *rondavel* bedecked with indications of Maria's regal status; instead, she now lived in barrackslike quarters with the other staff. On arrival, I found her poised in the concrete doorway, barefoot, a broad-shouldered figure swathed in bold fabrics, with simple colored-glass beads around her ankles. Other strings of beads ran from her right shoulder across her chest to her waist. Seeing us approach from a distance, she stood unmoving until we drew near, then exchanged formal greetings with the interpreter.

From Shangaan rangers and trackers, I had learned that people traveled great distances in order to receive healing from Maria, and I was told that she was known throughout the region as Maria, Mother of Lions, Lion Queen of Timbavati. For this reason, it surprised me to find her in such diminished and spartan circumstances. She lived in simple concrete barracks. It was plain, however, from the interpreter's deferential attitude, that he held the *sangoma* in the highest regard. He told her that I had come to see her, and it seemed she remembered me. She acknowledged me with an impassive nod.

"Please explain to Maria I would like to talk to her about that night several years ago when she came to our rescue," I instructed the interpreter.

Maria had a slightly quizzical expression on her face when he explained my purpose. Shrugging her shoulders, she gestured to the grass mats at the fireside. There we sat down.

Maria must have been in her seventies, yet she gave out a strong sense of power, almost youthfulness. She had one blind eye: the translator explained that a cobra had spat in it when she was a child. It struck me, however, that it is not merely convention that "seers" tend to have restricted eyesight in the normal sense – symbolically, they have the power to see elsewhere. The clouded retina of Maria's blind eye had changed from black to murky powder blue, but it still seemed to see, not outwardly, but into some inner region.

My first thought, on encountering her again, was a sense of her belonging to this precise location on the globe. I could not immediately put it into words, but I was reminded of this quality when I finally came to meet the high shaman of Africa, Credo Mutwa, who identified it succinctly: "Maria has guardianship in Timbavati. Sanctity. She should never leave that place."

As Maria waited in silence, I thought it best to get straight to the point. I told the interpreter that I wanted to know why Maria had walked through the darkness, through the angry pride of lions, to rescue a clutch of unfamiliar people. Why risk not only her life, but that of three others, including her infant grandchild, for the safety of strangers? How did she know she would not be eaten alive?

I watched as my message was transmitted. Maria listened, then gave a brief snort. Her expression darkened as if a shutter had passed down between us. Yet it seemed that communication had been established. I sensed a tacit connection.

I rephrased my question, hoping that the interpreter would do the same in his translation. "Ask Maria to think back to that night when we were stuck in the middle of the lion pride – why did she come to rescue us?"

He put my question to her and she shrugged again, offering a curt response, as if the answer were obvious. "She says you were calling; you needed help."

"I see," I said, unexpectedly touched again by her selflessness. "But now ask Maria how she knew it was safe to come and rescue us."

"She says she is never afraid of lions."

"Never?" I asked.

"She says when she hears the lions roar, she feels happy."

"But lions are dangerous . . ." I stated the obvious.

Again, I felt her reluctance to talk. She made a sweeping movement with her arm as she spoke, and her expression was brusque and dismissive.

"She says if there was a lion sitting here," the interpreter gestured dramatically to the clump of mopane trees right beside us that Maria had indicated a moment earlier, "she would not be afraid."

"Really?" I responded, scrutinizing Maria closely now to see if this was a straight answer. "Ask her if this is really true."

Unexpectedly, she gave a sparkly laugh in response to my query. And I was struck again by her unlikely fresh-faced look. Her cheeks were full and round, despite the web of fine lines that etched them. Engraved more deeply in her skin, beneath the wrinkles, I detected what appeared to be tattooed symbols: a cluster of three circles in deep blue. These were discernible on both her left and right cheeks, and again on her forehead. Her eyes were downcast as she spoke but when she lifted them both eyes were bright – almost luminous. It struck me as mildly appropriate that her blind eye's opalescence resembled the surface of a crystal ball.

"She says she can speak to lions," the translator responded. "She is not afraid – even when they are close by. They won't get up, but they will twist their ears – and then she knows they are listening to her." This explanation made sense of Maria's gesture of twisting both hands, and it conjured a curious visual image of lions lounging in the grass, lazily listening to the medicine woman as she chatted to them.

"You mean she actually talks to the lions?" I repeated, trying not to appear incredulous. I was still unsure whether she was playing games with me.

"Yes. She says yes, and they talk back to her. They say, '*Famba kahle*, Maria [Go well, Maria].'"

"So is that what happened on that night when she came to rescue us?" I asked. "Did she somehow communicate with the lions? Why didn't they harm her?"

After consulting with Maria, he translated once more. "She communicated with the ancestors. When she heard you calling she took some snuff[1] and spoke to the ancestors. They spoke to the lions to let her through safely . . ."

So the "ancestors" granted her safe passage. That's how she knew it was safe to venture through the lions. I tried to visualize this strange sequence of events.

"Is that why she took the baby along?" I added.

"She says she took the baby because she understood that there was nothing to fear."

"As a symbol of faith?" I mused. That was precisely how it had seemed at the time. The incongruity of carrying an infant through the darkness into the jaws of death could only be an act of blind faith. "So she did not speak to the lions directly?" I reiterated to the interpreter.

I was still under the misapprehension that the ancestors and the lions were separate entities. Only much later would I understand that, for lion shamans such as Maria, only a fine veil separates the ancestral figures from real lions.

There were times when Maria's impassive face appeared to place a barrier against me, and other times when her countenance radiantly opened up. Now she was answering at length, with expressive hand movements, emphatic and graceful. It felt like a breakthrough – but I was still frustrated at how much I was missing in translation.

"No, she did not speak to the lions themselves," came the answer. "She went into *twasa* . . ."

"*Twasa?*" I asked.

The elaborate explanations that followed did little to satisfy my attempts to understand. I gathered that *twasa* was a state of dreaming, a kind of self-induced trance which shamans entered to gain access to higher powers. In this state, Maria had spoken to her dead father and her dead grandfather, and they had calmed the lions. Her ancestors, on her behalf, had spoken to the lions.

"Tell me what Maria is saying now," I persisted, frustrated at my inability to translate the experience.

Maria's language had a rhythmic, almost mesmerizing quality, both melodious and emphatic. A word that I would hear time and again was *matimba,* pronounced "Mah-teembah!" – with great emphasis. In translation, the closest approximation was "power." Overhearing the translator relaying this to me, Maria soon picked up on the English equivalent and drew on it in her subsequent descriptions – only, in her usage it became "Pow-wah!"

She also applied the Afrikaans word *sterk,* meaning "strong" or "powerful," in her own descriptive manner: "Ster-aa-kah!"

"*Ngala moya . . . sterk!* [The spirit in the lion is good and powerful!]" she indicated, making a power sign with her hand – the tips of her fingers clenched – in response to my question of why she did not fear them. "*Ngala yina matimba yinga hi pfuna* [The lion has power and can help]," she went on to explain.

This was the first time I noticed the concept of lion as helper or guardian. Initially, it struck me as so incongruous that I did not pursue it further. "So how did she speak to the ancestors?" I ventured instead, trying not to appear baffled.

"The ancestors spoke to her through the bones," said the translator.

At least this connection was familiar. These were the bones of divination – the means by which African shamans divine the causes of illness and foretell the future. On that particular night, when Maria had heard distant screaming of human voices, I wanted to know what she had felt. What had the bones told her?

In answer to my question, Maria emptied her basket of bones into her hands, clasped them in her grip, tapped them rhythmically against the grass mat beside her, then cast them out before her. I understood from the interpreter that she was replicating the patterning of the bones that had occurred on that night three years earlier.

Among Maria's relics were two bones that immediately caught my eye. They turned out to be bones from felines, both of which distinctly resembled the animal from which they originated. From one angle, the profile of the bones evoked a lion, or lioness rather, with her long back extended like the Sphinx – except that, resting on her paws, she seemed ready to pounce. From another angle, the same bone resembled a reclining lioness, stretched out on her back, paws in the air. I gathered from the translations that the recumbent lioness symbolized safety and security, while the primed lioness was an omen of impending danger. If both feline bones fell on their backs when Maria threw the bones, it was a particularly propitious sign; if they both landed in a crouch, they portended calamity.

Yet this in itself was too simple an explanation. For a start, I was beginning to learn that the concepts of danger and power were virtually synonymous in the lore of Maria.

In response to my question about what the bones had told her on that night of rescue, the picture in the newly cast bones showed the two lion bones standing like sentinels on either side of what appeared to be a long passage through the other scattered relics. It amazed me to see how they offered a perfect symbolic picture of Maria's safe passage through the Timbavati lions, with the ancestral lion bones themselves apparently standing guard.

I discovered that my training in ancient symbolism made it relatively easy to follow and understand Maria's interpretations, since symbolic language is surprisingly consistent across the centuries and around the globe.

Maria threw the bones again to illustrate what had happened after her arrival at the scene. Now the smaller feline bone lay on its back and the big one attached itself to another piece, which turned out to be the bone of a baboon. The baboon bone was distinctly phallic, therefore symbolic of the male – in this case, representative of Andries, my brother-in-law. Beside it, the lion bone had now fallen in its rampant position, perfectly illustrating the heroic leonine power that Andries displayed that night. In confronting the lions, he had acted as the lionhearted hero.

Increasingly, I detected the subtlety with which this system of divination operated. Every position, every nuance, every relationship between the bones counted. The composite picture was laid out on the mat as if one were being shown a photographic scrapbook of one's past – or future. It was a system – a cogent, coherent, and consistent means of symbolizing reality. Ultimately, too, it was accountable. It could be referred to, much as one would consult a reference book. The message was clear and unambiguous and, most remarkable of all, it appeared to be repeatable. Consulting Maria once more about that night of our rescue, I saw in the array of bones how the two lion bones had resumed their previous guarding position. This astounded me.

The assorted bones were burnished by constant contact with Maria's hands. From what I could ascertain, the bones themselves were believed to carry the energy of their handler. I later determined that these were the very objects she had used since her initiation as a young girl – which I guessed must have been some 60 or so years back. Trying to fix a clear date for her initial possession of the bones, however, gave me my first indication that Maria's sense of time might be different from my own.

"Maria says she is not educated, she does not know how old she is," the translator conveyed her words to me.

"But surely she knows when and where she first found the bones?"

"She says they date back to the time of *twasa,* when the bones were given to her by her ancestors."

So *twasa* was not only a state of consciousness by which the *sangoma* broke through to the ancestral realm, it also appeared to be a moment in time when the *sangoma* first gained the symbolic tools – the set of bones. These were "gifts from *twasa,*" handed over to Maria by her great-grandfather, after his death, who then used them as a symbolic means to communicate with her from the realm of the spirits. I later learned that *twasa* was associated with the characteristic "illness" from which shamans suffer as a critical part of their initiation into the higher realms. Shamans do not choose their profession; rather, they are chosen by the spirit world, and thus become "the chosen ones."

Sitting at a right angle to Maria, I noticed on a number of occasions when the bones were thrown that one particular relic rolled off the mat in my direction, and asked Maria whether this had significance.

"Yes. Maria says, yes," came the interpreter's reply. "Big, big importance."

I waited for the answer, but none was forthcoming.

That the bones should be drawn in my direction remained a curiosity. Just as they appeared to contain Maria's energy and resonances of lion energy, I now sensed my own energy was coming into play. I had to accept, however, that I was not yet deemed fit to know the reason for this. As time went on, I grew to associate closely with those two burnished bones. Taken from the forepaw (metacarpals) of a lion, they contained symbolic lion-force.[2] In symbolic systems, the part signifies the whole. The same applied to the other bones. The interpreter explained that each came from a different animal. With time, I would come to pick out the differences, identify the animal from which each bone originated and appreciate some of the array of symbolic meanings attached to each piece. But from as early as this first encounter with Maria, the lion bones sprang out at me from the rest of the relics – illustrating clearly in symbolic language what I was struggling to understand through verbal translations.

"So those were ordinary lions she spoke to that night?" I returned to my central question, now that the picture was laid out before me on the mat.

I watched Maria laugh as my question was put to her.

"She says yes, they are ordinary lions, but no, they are not ordinary lions."

"Then ask Maria what makes those lions special."

At this, Maria cocked her head, and looked up at me with that same laughter in her eyes. "She says they are lions that come from God."

"Lions from God . . ." I mused. The more I learned from Maria, the more her perception of reality fascinated me. Certainly, for me, a mystique had always surrounded the idea of Timbavati's unique White Lions. "Ask Maria what she knows about the White Lions, then. What do they mean to her?"

"She says that is the bone from a White Lion," he explained, pointing to the larger of the two feline bones that had first caught my eye.

"Where did she get this White Lion bone? Did she herself actually see these lions?" I asked.

"Maria says the man who knows the story of the White Lions is Mutwa."

This was the first mention of Credo Mutwa, the man who would later become the key to unfolding the extraordinary mystery of the White Lions of Timbavati. My immediate thought, however, was that Maria was attempting to brush me off, and I was determined not to give up so easily.

"Maria has a White Lion bone in her collection. I want to know if she has actually seen the White Lions."

"She grew up with them. She says to tell you that she still sees them."

"But they are extinct," I pointed out.

"No. Maria says not here. She says the White Lions come to visit her in her dreams."

"Oh, I see; not in real life, only in dreams . . ." I responded, disappointed, as yet unaware of how critical the dreamworld was in the *sangoma*'s divinatory repertoire.

"What about the real White Lions that existed here in Timbavati until recently?" I persisted, despite sensing a resistance to this question. "Everybody knows that Maria has lived in Timbavati all her life. Many generations of her family have lived in this region. What does she know about the White Lions?"

The interpreter put the question at some length now, apparently repeating it several times. When he returned with an answer, I was frustrated to hear how brief it was.

"She says they are very dangerous. All lions are dangerous, but the white ones always kept to themselves. They were apart; they were the most feared."

"Is that why they were killed – because people feared them?"

"No, no," the translator protested, visibly reluctant to even put such a sacrilegious question to Maria. "Never, never kill a White Lion . . .!"

Clearly there was no correlation between any real threat and the perceived danger the White Lions posed. I could not miss the signal that this was critically important. I now gathered that *danger* should be interpreted as "power." That all-important word *matimba* appeared repeatedly in Maria's descriptions of the White Lions, but in translation came across inadequately as "dangerous." When I asked whether these dangerous animals were good or bad, Maria's answer was emphatic: "Good."

"If you harm the White Lions," the translator relayed her words, "you harm the land; if you kill the White Lions, you kill the land."

After it was first voiced, I returned to this point again, and then a third time – because it did not immediately make sense. I hoped for elaboration, yet the response remained the same.

"Maria says she cannot say it more clearly," the interpreter finally concluded, "*Loko u dlaya ngala yo basa u dlaya tiko* [If you kill a White Lion, you kill the world]." There was no further explanation.

I observed that Maria was focusing into the distance now, and could tell from her remote stoical expression that this critical point really should have been obvious to me. But it was only later that I began to understand how radiantly clear Maria's symbolic logic was, even at the most basic ecological level. Most obviously, the lion is the top of the food chain, the king of the beasts. Destroy the king, and his subjects are at risk. Disturb the balance of power, and each link in the food chain falls apart. But, at the time, the lion–earth connection appeared to be an entirely new and difficult concept to appreciate.

Maria went on to describe the harm that comes to those who hurt a White Lion in any way, recounting particular examples of bad luck that had come the way of individuals, and the families of individuals, who had White Lion blood on their hands. The White Lions, though dangerous, are not perceived as threats, but rather revered as supreme protectors of the land, sacred guardians of our earth.

"She says that the land belongs to them – they are guardians of Timbavati."

"Timbavati . . .?" I seized the opportunity to ask a question I had long wondered about. "Can Maria tell me what that name means?"

"Timba-vaati." Maria mouthed the words contemplatively before responding that the name itself was much older than current Shangaan usage. Again, she referred me to the shaman Credo Mutwa, explaining that he alone had the answer.

This perplexed me. "So Maria herself does not know the meaning of the place where she has always lived?"

At my observation, Maria's expression lightened with humor, and she retorted that Timbavati meant "the river that never runs dry." This seemed like a curious name for a region made up entirely of empty watercourses and arid sodic deposits. "She says it means 'river of stars,'" the interpreter continued.

It seemed she was referring to the Milky Way, which, come to think of it, never did run dry in the manner of the Timbavati watercourses.

"She says it is the river the White Lions came from." Now she had lost me. The fire was shining in Maria's cloudy eye. She was looking straight at me, so that I felt the force of her communication but could not identify it.

"Ask Maria to please explain further," I instructed the interpreter. "I'm no longer following..."

After listening to my translated words, Maria made a curt, sweeping gesture to the sky above us. Then she and the translator conferred. She repeated the gesture, and they talked more. Clearly he was having difficulty with her message here. He went on to translate for me, but I could not make out her meaning. The translation went something like this: "Maria says that her ancestors have told her that a long time ago, when the river was in the sky, a great many people died. When the river is in this position again, the same will befall human beings."

This was not very intelligible, although it had an ominous end-of-the-world ring about it.

For a moment, it seemed, time stood still. I could hear the gurgle of a nightjar and the long drawn-out *who-oop*s of the hyenas, beginning low and rising to a high-pitched cadence, then trailing off into a low moaning. Above us, the clarity of the night was spangled with what looked like a fine watercourse of droplets: the Milky Way, eternal "river" arching above Timbavati's dry plains, which gave rise to the mysterious legends of White Lions. Out here, under the brilliance of the night sky, I began to put humanity's trivial pursuits in cosmological perspective.

Maria sat in front of me, her head slightly cocked to one side, as if listening to something in the far distance. I sensed it was time to go.

I had come with a clear purpose in mind: to find out what had motivated this woman to save us from the lions on that dark night. It was a personal question, and I had expected a personal answer. Upon leaving the shaman's powerful presence, I had the first hints that Maria's perspective on lions was about to pave the way for my future. The Lion Queen of Timbavati seemed to challenge my familiar reality and shift my personal question into a more primal, archetypal way of seeing. But I had no idea, then, that Maria and all that she represented would ultimately lead me back to the very origins of humankind.

3

LIONS OF GOD: PEOPLE OF LION IDENTITY

The lion is the sacred totem of my family. . . . Lions being my family gods on my grandfather's side,
I must protect them. . . .
— CREDO MUTWA

After this first visit, I returned to Maria many times. I also began to search South African libraries for information on the subject of shamanism, in particular its curious lion–human culture. I imagined that I might understand Maria's story better by gathering background information. In this way, I hoped that eventually I might come closer to comprehending what powers African shamans possessed that enabled them to convert humankind's archetypal adversary – the lion – into our most powerful ally.

Shamanism, associated with the healer (or medicine man/woman), represents a long tradition of primitive, instinctual magic found on all five continents. It is a worldwide phenomenon which stretches back into humanity's distant past. Along with the rulers in traditional communities, shamans are the most powerful figures. They are viewed by their communities as intermediaries between this world and the spirit world, and their power lies in the connection between the two. They are also viewed in terms of animal incarnations, as a direct result of the shaman's respect and affinity with wildlife. Their close communication with species other than their own leads to apparently superhuman powers, of the kind I had witnessed in Maria. Their ability to conjure up animal spirits, or to pacify real-life ferocious predators such as lions, appears to represent, in a true and positive sense, the first "lion taming."

While others believe that shamans have the wild beasts at their service or their command, I was beginning to understand from Maria that the true power of the shaman lay not in dominance, but in the ability to work in harmony with nature's own laws.

It is now also generally understood that Stone Age cave art was executed by shamans after receiving wisdom in a state of self-induced trance. Many paintings relate to a process that anthropologists call "hunting magic" – symbolic representations of the hunt painted in a bid to create magical success in the actual hunt.[1] Certain shaman-hunters are also believed capable of magically entering the minds of dangerous predators, or bringing down their prey through concentrated will alone. While these unusual beliefs may seem simpleminded, in time I would come to see that they represent an infinitely more sophisticated process.

In describing Paleolithic cave paintings, scholars generally use the term *therianthropic* to describe part-human, part-animal forms. But this term can also be used to describe the part-human, part-animal consciousness that characterizes shamanism today.[2] Gradually, I became aware that, according to Maria's mode of consciousness, my questions as to whether it was her ancestors or the lions themselves who assisted her actions were simply nonsensical. In the therianthropic view, lion and human cannot be separated in terms of our regular understanding of things. Maria acted with the consciousness of a lionhearted woman.

I had come to this lion priestess hoping for clear answers as to what had inspired her act of selfless courage, but gradually it dawned on me that Maria had no objectivity with respect to herself. She did not stop to question or analyze her actions; that is why she had behaved as she had that night. Only once I understood this did I come to see what motivated her. Her bravery was an act of pure, unquestioning spiritual attunement to her natural environment; in this fine-tuned action lay her remarkable power.

One of the primary difficulties that stood between Maria and me was the translation process. There were numerous occasions when she gave a full dramatic explanation to my question – but the translator returned with a one-liner. Even more frustrating were the times when she provided a succinct explanation, which the translator went on to expound upon with his own elaborate version. But the translation difficulties went deeper still. Increasingly, I became aware that I was dealing with a different perception of reality.

While perfectly in tune with the present moment, Maria's action also appeared to spring from something much older – from ancestral attunement to a tradition that informed the continent of her birth. In Africa there are two complementary legacies that draw their inspiration from the awesome powers of the lion. The one is lion heroism, the other is lion shamanism.

In some African traditions, young men are initiated into manhood through lion combat. In this way they become lion heroes. In direct contrast, African lion shamans do not slay their leonine avatar; instead, they befriend it, recognizing that the lion is not their enemy but, in fact, their guardian spirit.

Years before she had accepted employment with Leonard, when she was living off the land, Maria said she would, during times of drought or duress, gain assistance from the Timbavati lions. She explained that she did so by leaving an offering overnight – a jug of home-brewed beer, or bread on a plate, at a strategic site for the ancestors – and then asking for their help in providing meat. The next day, once the lions had made a kill, she would go out into the veld and cut herself a portion from the carcass, right under the cats' watchful eyes.

This reminded me of a strange incident I had witnessed some years back and never understood. On one of our game drives we had encountered a group of Shangaan, unarmed and on foot. This in itself was highly unusual for a game area dense with predators. More surprisingly, they were heading directly toward a lion kill. As we drove a little farther, we discovered several lions in the process of taking their fill of an impala that they had brought down. We then watched in astonishment as the people on foot walked directly toward the lions, beating on drums and singing what appeared to be praise songs, at which the predators moved off and the humans proceeded to take a share of the food. On investigating this incident now, I learned that these people had been sent on this expedition by Maria herself, who had instructed them to get meat from the lions – informing them that they were safe because they had her ancestral protection. When this practice was discovered by the conservation authorities, it was labeled "carcass robbing," and they forbade it. To my mind, the authorities had it all wrong. It was clear to me that far from robbing the lions of their food, this interchange represented an extraordinary act of mutual respect between the Lion Queen of Timbavati and the king of the beasts. This was further indication of Maria's power and her reputation in the region.

Similarly, it occurred to me, the same process of empowerment and trust was at work with the youth and the young girl who had accompanied Maria into the darkness that night of our rescue. While the baby had no choice in the matter, the other two had every reason not to accompany the old woman into the face of such danger. Yet they must equally have chosen to risk their lives on that night, in complete faith that Maria, Lion Mother, knew what she was doing.

Through my research I now knew that Maria fit into a long and majestic tradition. From all over Africa, there are fairly well-documented reports of a reciprocal arrangement, an honored contract, that once existed between humans and lions. Eyewitness accounts detail how lions were included in the harvest rituals and were directly associated with the earth from which humans drew their subsistence. These stories grounded Maria's allusion to the lion as guardian of the earth.

Throughout the continent, there are also numerous accounts of trained lions protecting tribespeople from marauding enemies. The basis of the tribes' welfare and livelihood – providing food and protection – is linked to their companionable lions. I also learned that one of Africa's founding myths is that the souls of great heroes and kings become lions after death.[3]

Although this material did not help explain interspecies communication between African priests and African lions, it did give some credibility to what I had considered some of Maria's less credible utterances.

One evening, Maria told me the story of the great king Magigwana and his prize warrior, Girivana. Magigwana was the mightiest of warriors, who slew many enemies in a fierce battle for supremacy after hiding in a tree trunk in ambush. When he died, his spirit lived on as a lion. Girivana, King Magigwana's neighbor, had his very own pride of lions living in his *kraal*. When he was attacked, the warrior unleashed his warrior-lions, which made quick work of the enemy. When he died, he too became a lion. At the time I found this a compelling notion, if hardly believable.

These "lions" survived to this day, Maria informed me, although Magigwana and Girivana themselves died (as men) a long time ago. While lions in the wild enjoy less than 20 years' lifespan under normal conditions, the spirits of great kings are believed to reincarnate from father to cub unceasingly through the lion lineage. Maria also explained that, if one were to pass the place where spirits took on lion form, one would need to perform a ritual involving the placement of leaves and an offering of sanctified food, or else be devoured. It was not that they were bad lions, she emphasized at my insistent questioning, but that they were powerful lions, and so commanded the highest respect.

It turned out that Maria herself was directly related to these heroic lion figures, although not by blood. Her husband was the brother of Chief Kapama, the direct descendant of Magigwana. In old Africa, a close association exists between lion priests and lion warrior-chiefs, with the chiefs taking their advice from the shamans who speak on behalf of the ancestors.[4] It appears that this close association may result in the chief himself sometimes combining the qualities of lion shamanism and lion heroism, with displays of prowess and courage in battle, as well as powers of prophecy and enlightenment in peacetime. In Maria's case, she was descended from a priestly caste of lion shamans, and she married into a royal line of lion chiefs.

Significantly, not all chiefs become lions in death – only the greatest of the great. When I asked about Chief Kapama, the former chief of the region, Maria answered that unfortunately he had not achieved lion status. With respect to famous chiefs such as Shaka, Dingane, or Dinizulu, Maria responded that she did not know the answer, and that I would need to ask the Zulu *sangomas* from that region to determine this.

The finest of veils appeared to separate Maria from both the lions and the ancestral forces. Maria had requested safe passage from the ancestors, yet it was the lions that allowed her to walk unharmed through their ranks. She had left beer for the ancestors, yet again it was the lions that provided her with meat in exchange. While she was able to communicate with the ancestors and hear their answers, she could equally exchange greetings with the Timbavati lions. *Sangomas* tend to speak in riddles. Only now was I beginning to make sense of Maria's paradoxical response to my question about the Timbavati lions: "Yes, they are ordinary lions, but no, they are not ordinary lions."

On one unusual occasion, I had the opportunity to accompany Maria to visit members of her family, some 60 kilometers away. Among them was the daughter of Maria's brother-in-law, Sarah Khosa, another *sangoma* of note in the territory. There was also an intensely good-looking man called Axon Kapama Khosa, the eldest son of Chief Kapama. He would act as interpreter on this occasion.

Although most of the conversation was conducted in Shangaan, it was apparent that the family was asking how Maria and I had come to meet, and Maria was responding with a full account of what occurred on that mysterious night with the Timbavati lions.

Curiously, it was also soon clear that she was making light of the incident. That youthful glow I had come to anticipate in her shone through as she recounted the story. In contrast to her lighthearted manner, everyone else was awestruck in response. Feeling the communal electricity, as the rapt listeners uttered appreciative "Shoohs!" and "Haahs!" and "Hawus!" in waves of unison, I was anxious to know exactly what she was saying, and asked Axon to translate.

"She said she walked through the veld in the dark, without a flashlight," Axon translated.

Another whistle of amazement went through the audience. Maria was laughing joyously as she spoke, while the others were visibly caught in the grip of her story.

"This is unbelievable! It's amazing!" said Axon, shaking his head.

"What did she say?" I asked eagerly.

The chief's son was transfixed again as Maria continued, and made no attempt to translate. "Amazing . . ." he commented, shaking his head again.

Eventually, I gave up trying to extract snippets of translation while Maria's version of the story was in progress, since Axon himself was so engrossed that I dared not interrupt. Instead, I observed Maria's cool yet animated gestures, her occasional uproarious laughter, and the scintillated responses of her audience. Watching the admiration in the eyes of her listeners, I thought about the majestic lion heroines from world mythology who kept declaring themselves in my research. Rather than depicted in arm-to-arm combat with lions in the male heroic tradition, female deities such as Atamgatis and Cybele from classical mythology are shown astride lions, while the Great Mother of Asia Minor, Rhea, goddess of the earth and wild beasts, is inevitably represented with lions

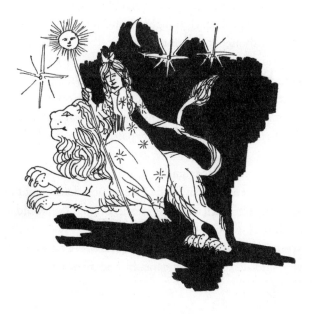

Lion-taming earth goddesses are associated with attunement rather than conflict with the lion.

at her side, seated upon lions, or in a lion-drawn chariot. The Japanese personification of ultimate wisdom and the mother of enlightenment, Monjubosatsu, rides the back of a lion. Similarly, the Germanic goddess Freyja, head of the Valkyries, is depicted astride a great cat, while her Babylonian counterpart, the goddess Ishtar, rides mighty lions, betokening her feline potency.[5] Across the continents and the ages, this portrayal of female leonine figures is consistent.

Unlike the lion-hero tradition associated with the initiation into manhood, each female deity reveals how the physical domination of lions and the befriending of the beast is one and the same expression. This is well illustrated in the tarot card entitled "Strength," which depicts a female (rather than a male) figure in command of a lion – not through slaying the beast but through working in unison with its power.

Watching Maria in the atmosphere of the darkened *rondavel*, Timbavati's own Lion Queen began to take on the aspect of one of these mythological lion heroines. For the first time in my presence, Maria was in full Shangaan *sangoma* dress, draped in vivid fabrics, overlaid by an ornately beaded skirt with feathered pompoms. Against the bright colors of her garb her face and limbs were ebony, and an electric current seemed to charge though them as she relayed her account. Before long, she brought the story to a tidy close.

"What did she say, Axon?" I insisted. "Please repeat for me."

"She said she could hear from the shouting that the people were in the same place where the lions were snarling."

"True!" I observed. "And then what did she say?"

"She said that she spoke to the ancestors and then she just walked – *famba, famba, famba* – she remembers nothing."

That Maria had no recollection of the walk itself confirmed my sense that she had been in an altered state when she performed the seemingly miraculous act.

"But when she was telling the story," I probed, "I thought I heard Maria mention the names Magigwana and Girivana..." Although my instinct anticipated the answer, when it came, I felt the hairs on my neck stand on end.

"Those are the names of the ancestors that she spoke to..." Axon replied.

So Maria's ancestral spirits were the very same humans who had taken on lion status after death. These lion-humans communicated with her from the ancestral realm using the bones of divination as their tools, and had secured her safe passage through the lions on that fateful night.

"And after that, what did she say?" I asked expectantly.

"She said that when she arrived at the Land Rover, the man Leonard was shouting at her to climb in. He was so angry that she had walked; he was afraid that she would be eaten in front of all the guests."

I laughed. "Well, wouldn't you yourself be frightened of being eaten?" I asked Axon.

"Me? Yes! But Maria said no – she said that by that time she had made friends with the lions."

"Made friends" – it was a delightful term. I knew by now that Maria's friendly affiliation with the lions of Timbavati was no obscure cultish notion. Lion priesthood went hand in hand with lion heroism as a defining principle underlying African culture.

Lion Priests and Lion Heroes

Although now virtually an extinct phenomenon, feline–human interaction of the kind I had witnessed in Maria not only survives in Africa but has been documented on all continents. A magnificent recent example of tiger shamanism in action in Asia is described by the South African writer Laurens van der Post. In a lecture delivered in South Africa many years after the event, van der Post recalled his own close encounter with a predatory feline. It occurred during World War II, when van der Post had the good fortune to meet some of the indigenous inhabitants of Java, the Badoeis. He was on a military patrol one morning. With only a Badoeis guide, he was walking through a narrow track in the jungle, tall bamboo on either side obstructing any means of escape, when he came face to face with a tiger. Van der Post described how the tiger walked slowly toward them down this path, stopped, glared, and then snarled angrily. He thought, Well, *we've had it*. Then, amazingly, the Badoeis – who was in front of him – went down on his knees in an attitude of grateful prayer – and began praying rhythmically to the tiger. Van der Post could not understand the language, apart from the repeated phrase *Tuan Tiger* (Lord Tiger). He watched, mesmerized, as the tiger gradually grew quiet and his tail stopped thrashing. First the snarl and then the look of aggression left the tiger's face, which became "filled with light." Van der Post went so far as to recount a moment when "the ghost of what I can only describe as a smile flickered over the tiger's face," and the great cat turned tail and padded back along the route from which he had come.

Van der Post was led to conclude, after surviving his revelatory death-defying experience, that this encounter was an illustration of how "it is possible out of a true wilderness awareness to communicate with animals and get a mutual recognition of kinship . . ." He concluded that he would never forget "the first great lesson from the Badoeis . . . an awareness that encloses and protects people as helpless as the two of us were that morning in the face of the tiger, more effectively than any contrived armour can."[6]

This communication that saved van der Post's life approximates a telepathic connection, or mind-call, of which the highest lion priesthood are capable. It goes beyond simple communication to entering the minds of wild animals, which then act at their command.

This was an astonishing story, yet it harmonized with my own experience and with other documented material I had begun to uncover. I would have reason to recall van der Post's description of the tiger's face becoming "filled with light" when I uncovered the phenomenon of the great cats as symbols of enlightenment-bearers across the globe.

Virtually all the world's spiritually evolved leaders, both Eastern and Western, have been endowed with leonine identities. In all world cultures, there are references to the "Enlightened Ones" or the "Shining Ones": luminous leonine figures bringing the civilizing principles of love, light, and truth to humanity, whom Mutwa calls the *Abangafi Bapakade*.[7]

Our Christian saints, such as Saint Jerome with his companionable lion, and Saint Mark, whose famous winged lion peers down on humanity from on high in Venice's St Mark's Square, are transcendent figures whose enlightened message is directly associated with lions. The Gospel of Saint Mark beneath the paw of Saint Mark's winged lion is the symbol of culture and learning, offering humankind principles of law and civilization. Similarly, the Sphinx of ancient Egypt is said to guard a secret store of knowledge known as the Hall of Records, just as the emblem of the gryphon, winged lion of heraldry, is the mythical animal that guards sacred knowledge. While Christ was the lion of Judah, king of kings, Krishna was a lion among wild animals; Muhammad's son-in-law, Ali, beloved of the Shi'ites, was lion of Allah; and Buddha was the lion of the Shakyas. Buddha is said to have had a pet lion, endowed with miraculous powers. Upon the prophet's death, he is described as lying down in the manner of a lion.[8] Vishnu takes on the lion-man incarnation in the form of the avatar Nara-simha,[9] and in his leonine form brings qualities of enlightenment and courage to the ignorant.

The thought of felines showing qualities of magnanimity and protection – even enlightenment – was curiously uplifting. Respectful communication, in this case, prayer, proved the key to preservation. According to van der Post, the feline priest was "protected" from the jaws of death not by "contrived armour" in the manner of the feline hero, but through mutual respect which provided spiritual armament.

While such an approach to predators was absolutely beyond my personal understanding at the time of my own brush with death, contact with lion shamans such as Maria gradually introduced me to a different way of seeing, which would ultimately become second nature.

Lion Guardian

After my reunion with Maria, one strangely symbolic event followed another. For example, I began suffering from recurring nightmares in which a lion appeared and roared directly into my face – not a meter away, but right in front of me: open-jawed, face-to-face. Each time this happened, I would jerk myself awake with a terrified scream and lie in bed, shaken and sleepless, my heart pounding. It was natural to suppose that this dream was prompted by my research into lion symbolism, but there was nothing remotely academic about the awesome reality of the dream experience. With gruesome horror I lived it, and relived it, every time it recurred.

Finally, having resolved to ask Maria about these nightmares, I received a surprising response. She nodded slowly as the question was put to her and told the interpreter that this was a very good sign. Pointing to the horizon, she explained that my lion ancestor had come to greet me at last – he was no longer in the distance but had finally arrived, as my closest friend. I stressed that this was no friendly dream – it was nothing short of terrifying. She smiled with a knowing expression, and responded that my lion guardian had arrived as my teacher; he was inviting me to exchange power with him – *"chicha matimba ni nghala"* – reverse his energy, and become a lion.

Clearly, a powerful psychic process was indicated here – one that I was only beginning to understand. *Psychic* generally means "concerned with processes and phenomena that seem to be outside physical or natural laws." But the word *psyche* also refers to "the human soul."[10] This would become a very important connection for my understanding of human–animal relations, and has specific relevance for the relationship between humans and lions.

Psychologists recognize that dream states may serve as critically significant sources of wisdom. They have always been treated as such by shamans the world over; only, shamans go further and use dreams and other consciousness-altering states, such as meditation or trance, to access different realities.

With my own nights disturbed by lion visions, I was led to recall how Maria referred to dreams of the legendary White Lions in the same breath as she spoke of lions of flesh and blood, virtually as if the two were indistinguishable. Incorporating truths from the dream world into the physical world is one art of the shaman. On the question of lion dreams, I knew personally of another academic skeptic who unexpectedly made contact with a lion in a dream state. Lecturer, radio talk-show host, and author Kate Turkington described this experience in 1997 in her book *There Is More to Life Than Surface*, explaining how under the guidance of a shaman in Peru she was taken through a meditation program that ended in her "connecting" with her "power animal." She discovered this animal to be a golden lioness, which greeted her lovingly in her vision, curling her lion's tail around Turkington's legs, before departing once more. The interesting follow-up to this psychic experience came when Turkington returned to South Africa, where she met up with "lion man" Gareth Patterson. Patterson took over the care of George Adamson's lions, of *Born Free* fame, after Adamson was murdered. As with George Adamson and his wife, Joy, both of whom met untimely deaths, tragedy also struck their lions, Furaha and Batian. Both were killed by humans after being released into the wild by Gareth Patterson.

When I was introduced to Patterson in 1998, he described to me how his lioness, Furaha, had the peculiar characteristic of curling her tail affectionately around his legs. When he heard of Kate Turkington's "meeting" with a lion spirit guide in Peru, he considered this an amazing coincidence, convinced that it was the soul of his dead lioness making contact with the physical world once again. Patterson later confided in me that he himself had experienced psychic moments with his lions, although he had hesitated to recount this in his various published books. Patterson's recent book, however, *With My Soul Amongst Lions,* has begun to make the connection between humankind and the king of the beasts at a soul level.[11]

These firsthand accounts of psychic experiences with lions helped clarify why shamans consider sacred felines so powerful that the act of "dreaming them" alone can bring about physiological changes in humans.[12] Lion shamans are believed able to grow hair and physically take on the identity of lions, and even mix with real lion prides in this state.

Were-Lions

My research had unearthed an extraordinary notion of which I had no former knowledge: there was a commonly held belief in old Africa that the most powerful shamans were able to take on lion identity, and may even have gone on hunting missions with ordinary lions, before returning and assuming their human form again. I wondered whether there was a real equivalent for what was referred to in these tales. Why should the notion of astral travel and the assumption of lion identity be connected? Was this phenomenon real and physical, or did it only exist in the imaginations of so-called primitive people the world over? What was the truth behind the mythology?

I realized that what we were talking about here was a notion of were-lions. *Were* comes from the Old English word *wer,* meaning "man," hence human-lions. Did humans actually transform into lions, or was it rather a ceremonial act?

While these accounts of human-lions were bizarre, to say the least, there was much to suggest that they once represented a widespread belief across old Africa. The term that is often used for a shaman who exercises these powers is *Lion of God.*

When I asked Maria whether she herself had the power to take on the form of a lion, she replied that she used the power of the lion – *matimba* – in her work as a healer. Clearly, the notion of assuming lion identity was perfectly comprehensible to her. "*Va sangoma lava chichaka kuva tinghala*" was her phrase for a *sangoma* who takes on lion form. The word *chichaka* was one I would hear time and again associated with change, evolution, or transformation. As time went on, I learned that the shape-shifting notion of human-into-lion is best described as "assumption." The shaman takes on, or "assumes," the identity of the animal. But just how this might be effected remained unclear. Was I really supposed to believe that certain shamans could grow claws and manes and tails?

Observing Maria closely as she threw the bones of divination in our encounters together, I pondered over my research into the ancient culture of the lion incarnations. That Maria was a lionhearted woman was not in dispute – the vision of her walking silently through the midst of the Timbavati pride will live with me always – but could she really become a lioness?

I concluded that she could not, and let the matter rest there. Rather, what was referred to was some kind of psychological power in which an individual takes on lion-type traits: courage, truth, wisdom, magnanimity, and protection. This seemed a fair enough résumé. It was only after further research that I began to sense how inadequate it was.

Through my personal experience of rescue at the hands of this extraordinary lion-woman, I had come to see lion shamanism as a force of healing and enlightenment. Unfortunately, there is a fair amount of documentation to suggest that lion–human interchange can be applied to heinous deeds such as murder and cannibalism. As with all power, it seems, lion power can be wisely used or dangerously abused.

When I confronted Maria about some of the disturbing accounts I had seen documented in my research into lion shamanism, including gruesome incidents still reported in today's newspapers, Maria listened gravely.[13] She confirmed that there were evil *sangomas* – witch doctors or sorcerers – who could enter a lion and use it for dark purposes, such as murder. Her term for these harmful witch doctors was *rigedle.* Some were capable of assuming the form of a lion, she said; others simply made tracks in the ground to resemble the real lions' pugmarks as a cover for their misdemeanors.

While these forces of darkness have always existed in Africa, I now realized there were opposite and equally powerful forces of light ranged against them. These are the unsung heroes and heroines of our day – healing agents for good on Earth – a priestly caste of tribal shamans operating at a level that most of us cannot begin to comprehend, and of which we are completely oblivious. Understanding this distinction is critical. The terms *healers, medicine men,* or *medicine woman* more accurately describe shamans working with forces of light, while *sorcerers* or *witch doctors* suggest shamans working with forces of darkness.

While the term Maria herself had used, *Lions of God,* recurs in documented accounts of humans who can assume the identity of lions, it may only be applied to shamans working with forces of light.[14]

The existence of dark forces explained why Maria carried amulets for protection, emulating many of the heroic goddesses from world mythology. The Asiatic goddess Ishtar, for instance, while standing in a warlike posture on a lion and armed with a bow and arrows, also wears a star or sun on her helmet as an amulet talisman for protection.

Although Maria's appearance was generally unadorned, every aspect of her simple attire had symbolic meaning. Apart from the single strand of threaded seed pods that ringed her wrists and ankles and denoted her status as *sangoma,* other meaningful accessories had to do with employing powers of light against powers of darkness. On one string of beads across her shoulders hung desiccated strips that resembled cured leather but turned out to be roots from trees. Each of these roots came from a different tree, the names of which were unfamiliar to the translator and so could not be conveyed to me. But the purpose of the threaded strips, I discovered, was protection against bad spirits or witch doctors who used dark powers. Similarly, in the center of the string of roots that crossed Maria's heart was a knotted pod ending in a sharp ivory point. This, I learned, was a crocodile tooth containing *muti,* or medicine, which equally had powers of protection. Maria told me she removed these amulets before bed, laying them under her pillow to ensure her safety.

Son of the Sun

On one occasion, Maria was wearing a new necklace, hung with masklike beads that were carved and painted. Upon my inquiry, she told me that this was a "power gift" from Credo Mutwa, and she always kept it above her head when she slept. She told me that she needed it today, but would not say why.

"This man, Mutwa, that you talk about with such respect, Maria," I said. "Who is he?"

"Maria says Mutwa is the most powerful lion *sangoma* – *Inyanga ya Nghala*," the interpreter explained, "but not one who kills people." Again, I felt the mixed surge of fascination and trepidation at the potency of this information. Maria informed me that it was time I met Mutwa. Although I still had little idea who Credo Mutwa was, I had learned in the meantime that his name was widely known in South Africa, and that he was often in the public eye. I told her that I would arrange to meet him, little knowing what efforts I would have to go to to fulfill this promise.

"He is a son of God," Maria's translated words were conveyed to me. "He is a son of the sun. He knows the story of the Lions of God . . ."

What greater accolade could one hope for? I wondered. Although the South African establishment has tended to dismiss Mutwa's words as the melodramatic utterances of a self-proclaimed soothsayer, the more Maria told me about this great lion shaman, the more I suspected he might be worthy of the high regard in which she held him. If there was one man in Africa I wished to meet above all others, it had to be Credo Mutwa.

4

LION PRIEST OF AFRICA

Because we are stars, we must walk the sky.
— TRADITIONAL SONG OF BUSHMEN LION SHAMANS[1]

Almost two years after my first efforts to contact Credo Mutwa, I finally met the lion sage early in 1996. Through clues that Maria had given, I had learned of Africa's Great Tradition, known as *Umlando* ("the Great Knowledge"): a tradition of oral history, fiercely guarded through the ages, which remains intact within the memories of an élite band of initiates. The highest-ranking shamans are known as Sanusis. Of these, a select few are entrusted as tribal storytellers, and honored as the so-called Guardians of the Umlando. Credo Mutwa was such a guardian, the only guardian known to have broken with tradition and reveal secrets from the oral records. In my endeavors to track this extraordinary man, I soon learned that he himself was "guarded" – at an everyday level, at least, by a barrage of minders and keepers, who apparently wanted to protect him from the outside world.

Guardian of Umlando

Dispossessed of his own land, Credo Mutwa was ever on the move without any fixed abode. I also got the impression that he was not adept in dealing with daily practicalities. People who maintained they were taking care of him, shielding him from worldly considerations were, it was finally apparent to me, instead intent on caging him up. None of the messages that I had left with these people had reached him. I was no closer to getting through to him than when I began, after leads from Maria. The contact numbers I had accumulated for various individuals claiming to know him had all led nowhere. My only option now was to identify a direct route to the High Shaman himself.

My opportunity came unexpectedly one weekend, when I phoned one of those numbers that had been unhelpful in the past. Credo Mutwa himself was at the other end of the line! I learned later that he just happened to be in Johannesburg's township suburb of Soweto and, with the owner of the phone out of the room for the moment, had uncharacteristically answered when the phone rang. I explained how long I had endeavored to reach him. To my relief, he agreed to meet the following day, although not without a trace of wariness creeping into his voice.

This encounter was so long-awaited; yet, as the moment of our meeting approached, I felt a gnawing sense of trepidation. I had seen pictures of the ceremonial *rondavel* built by Mutwa in the Northern Province, which is now called Limpopo. The walls of the *rondavel* had been strikingly painted with symbolic motifs by the medicine man himself, and the gates had been adorned with larger-than-life mud figures of lion ancestors. If Mutwa was the great lion shaman I had been led to believe, it was in such a context that I expected to find him. But the actual setting for our encounter was not what I had anticipated. I was disoriented and apprehensive, as a white South African, to have to venture into the black township of Soweto, the site of so many riots in the days of apartheid. Approaching the ordinary Soweto house, one of thousands of similar boxes lining the dust road, I wondered what I should say on greeting. I realized now that I had no idea what the correct form was: what title to use, whether or not to shake Mutwa's hand.

I found the street number outside a prefabricated house identical to the others. A dusty path led up to the front door. I knocked, and the door was opened by a striking black woman with her hair in beaded braids. She let me in without comment.

"*uBaba?*" she called, using the African term for *Father* or *Patriarch*, and Credo Mutwa appeared from an adjoining room. He was a monumental man with gray hair and thick spectacles.

The woman seated herself on a bench in the corner, where she continued to sew colored glass beads onto a traditional rag doll. Beside her sat another large black woman, who patiently did the same, without acknowledging my presence. They seemed to reflect Mutwa's own aversion to visitors.

Credo Mutwa and I stood in the center of the room. I knew from my research that African handshakes are imbued with far more meaning than the Western custom of grasping hands. For instance, one never lays a hand upon an elder without invitation. So I did not extend my hand when meeting him, and simply introduced myself.

I addressed him as Mr Mutwa, but after a few occasions of my using this title, he corrected me: "Just call me Credo, ma'am."

"Then please," I responded, "call me Linda." But I would notice he returned time and again to the formality of *ma'am* in addressing me.

My first impression of Credo Mutwa – apart from his unexpectedly mammoth proportions – was of a curiously androgynous quality. Not in the modern sense of fashionable cross-dressing, but in some very ancient, unfamiliar sense. He made me think of Tiresias, the blind seer of classical mythology in which both sexes meet. I had the uncanny feeling that I was speaking to a male and a female at one and the same time.

He was wearing what appeared to be a voluminous denim smock, over which was tied a thick leather apron with no seams, resembling an entire animal skin. He began by excusing his "workman's clothes" – and I felt I had interrupted something important.

"Maria Khosa sends you her greetings," I informed him.

"Thank you, ma'am, thank you." Despite his overwhelmingly powerful presence, he had a humble manner.

Having seated himself, he now rested his large hands almost demurely in his lap. Looking at these gentle hands, I remembered how Maria had described the secret handshake of the High Shamans – the "handshake of power." Gesturing herself, she had relied on the Shangaan interpreter to explain how one shaman extends his right hand with palm up and fingers clawed. The other then grasps it with palm down and fingers also clawed. The two sets of fingers hook, and a brisk pull is given. Then they disengage.[2]

"How can I help you, ma'am?" Mutwa asked, as if he sensed the urgency of the questions I concealed.

"The White Lions of Timbavati, Credo. I need to know about them. Maria tells me you are the one person alive who knows the story of their origins."

"That is not true, ma'am. There are many in our ranks who know the story, but they are sworn to secrecy. It is only I who have been fool enough to speak of such things."

For all his humility and deference, I could not for a moment forget that I was in the presence of an immensely powerful man, the man many considered to be the most powerful shaman in Africa. But he had an air of one burdened with suffering.

Maria had warned me that Credo Mutwa had broken the blood oath that bound initiates to their secret oral tradition. In doing so, he had brought upon himself a lifetime of ill fortune. As I grew to know him better, I would learn that his personal story sprang from a series of desperately tragic episodes. From the moment – some four decades ago – when he began committing the "ancient memory" to writing, he was labeled Vusamazulu, "the Outcast." What followed was one appalling tragedy after another, among them the cold-blooded murder of his son – the heir to his shamanic tradition.

Taking a deep breath, I contemplated how I might best phrase my next question.

I had come to listen, to find out for myself what Credo Mutwa knew. Now in his presence for the first time, I detected, beyond the physical suffering, a keen sense of metaphysical burden: the burden of knowledge. What was this "Great Knowledge" of which he spoke? What was so important that he was prepared to sacrifice his life to its delivery?

If Mutwa was all Maria believed him to be, I did not expect to find a ready answer.

Custodian of the Sacred Relics

Maria had revealed that Mutwa was the custodian of some of the holiest artifacts of the African continent. Mutwa would, over time, show me more than 50 items in his possession – great pieces of copper, bronze, verdite, and crystal, some once belonging to the mightiest of kings, some inscribed with cryptic symbols, many dating from a time when, Credo Mutwa says, an ancient seafaring civilization, neither of African birth nor of African race, came to African shores.[3]

Yet, as Maria had explained through our Shangaan interpreter, it was Mutwa's belief that their living powers should not be held captive in glass boxes in museums and other places of curiosity. Without a successor, his duty as a "custodian of the sacred relics" was to bury these precious artifacts before he died.

None of these sacred objects was on show in the bleak Soweto room. The space was so inhospitably barren that it formed the starkest of contrasts to the rich living treasure that Mutwa himself seemed to embody.

Aware that I was imposing on his time, yet not sure how best to proceed, I sat in tense silence for a while.

Finally, in an attempt to establish my credibility, I decided to recount the story of how Maria had rescued us from angry lions on that unforgettable night in the bushveld. This was the right tack and, although he seemed to fix his stare, I could tell I had his full attention.

He nodded slowly as I spoke, as if none of it surprised him. But when I came to the detail of how Maria had brought the baby with her in the pitch night, through the angry field of lions, I heard him draw a sudden breath. I could see that even he was impressed by Maria's courageous act.

"Do not let Maria die alone," was his comment when I came to the end of my story.

"Do you mean I must not let her action go unacknowledged?"

"Yes, ma'am. So many healers have died without the world understanding."

"I see . . ."

"Maria should never leave the land of Timbavati," Credo continued. "There she has guardianship."

Here, once more, was this idea of guardianship. Did he mean that the lions were her ancestral guardians, as Maria had more than once intimated? Maria was born in the vicinity of Timbavati, like generations of her own family before her, and raised in the untamed African bushveld. She, more than any, would have been aware of the real dangers that lions posed. I needed to understand how she and others of her kind had achieved this command over the king of beasts.

"I want to know, Credo, what supernatural quality shamans possess which enables them to enter the minds of lions," I ventured.

"There is nothing supernatural. Everything is natural," he responded. "You in the West say that man has five senses. This is not true. In fact, the human being possesses 12 senses. One of these senses is the ability to move out of one's body at will and enter another space. It is not supernatural. It is a natural thing."

"Yet the rest of us are not capable . . ."

Mutwa smiled. "Man possesses the ability to influence not only animals but inanimate objects, also."

The shaman seemed to imply that we all had the potential to access these "God-given talents." He went on to explain that most of us have experienced glimpses of these alternative senses, particularly in moments of crisis. At such moments, our perception of time changes. We suddenly become aware of strange coincidences, or premonitions, or exhibit the uncanny ability to control objects in our territory.

Mutwa told me that he had intimations of extrasensory powers long before he became a shaman, even as a wayward youth in Sophiatown in the 1930s, where he fell among criminals. He discovered he was able to control the throw of dice when gambling on the streets – much to the chagrin of fellow gamblers. But, he added, this unexpected gift worked only when he was in trouble, and in need of an urgent resolution to a tricky situation. He could not summon it at will. The harnessing of power, I gathered, was the harvest of a dedicated and often agonizing journey into shamanism.

I ventured to ask how one might access those powers beyond the five senses.

"We may not talk of such things as power," he told me. Although polite, he made it clear that he would not be pressed on how the lion shaman achieved the gifts which to other mortals appeared supernatural. At this moment, and many others in our first encounter, I was aware of attempting to hear things that were not intended for my ears, and I castigated myself for treading so carelessly.

"There are those things, ma'am, of which we may not speak. Even I, who have broken many taboos – to my detriment – even I will not tell, or should I say cannot tell, of certain things. Our people believe that those who hand over great secrets to the common people will be cursed forever. You will understand, ma'am?"

Behind his thick glasses he did not appear to be looking out. Like Maria, his consciousness seemed to reside in some inner region of the mind. Speaking slowly and rhythmically, he seemed short of breath and – although this was hard for me to appreciate fully – it struck me that here was a man waiting for death. I resisted pursuing the subject.

Over the course of our discussion, however, I began to get my first intimations of the processes involved in acquiring these extrasensory perceptions. Mutwa explained that much of our modern technology – television sets, computer screens, cellular phones – interfered with heightened natural abilities. Even seasoned shamans would lose these arts, he said, if they were brought too regularly into close contact with such technologies. I thought of Maria, under the clear night skies of Timbavati, the keenness of her senses attuned to the rhythms and sounds of the bushveld enveloping her on all four horizons.

Clearly, these heightened senses had to do with concentrated will. Mutwa went on to describe how the use of the sacred drum in shamanic ritual also served to concentrate the mind to a focal point. The drumming ensured that nothing broke the power of concentration. His description of this process made me think of a magnifying glass concentrating the power of the mind like a beam of sunlight until the intensity ignites the object on which it focuses. Could the concentrated powers of the mind act on inanimate objects in much the same way?

I pressed him. "I need to know, Credo, how could Maria have taken that risk in order to bring us to safety?"

"The lions brought you to safety. Maria communicated with them. You think that the lions were threatening you. In fact, they were guarding you. Just as you think you look after your domestic cat. You think that you tame it, that you feed it, that you take care of it. What you do not realize is that it is taking care of you."

In that moment his words somehow made sense, although I would have had difficulty explaining this. They seemed to spring from an understanding of the relationship between all things. Our mistake is to believe that we are separate and different from everything else on the planet. From Maria I had already begun to understand how shamans could somehow penetrate the boundaries that we think separate us from other living creatures.

"So she communicated with the lions," I repeated his words out loud.

"That is the greatest art, ma'am, since the lion is the king of the beasts," he explained. "But we humans can communicate with all the animals, and with plants, also."

I tried to suppress my incredulity.

"You know, ma'am, today's wildlife statistics tell us that hippos are the biggest killers in Africa. This should not be the case. When I grew up, ma'am, there was a drought and our mothers used to do their washing in the river, which they shared with the hippos. Not a single woman was wounded by hippos."

"And now we have lost our communication with nature," I observed.

"Much to our regret." A protracted silence ensued.

"It was from my grandfather that I learned how to communicate with animals, whether domestic or wild, and to communicate with plants, both edible and poisonous," Mutwa continued. "Do you know ma'am, that in our ancient culture our people used to sing to their corn in gratitude for its producing food?"

I suspect that I was staring, unable to reconcile this with my Western upbringing.

"I see you smile, ma'am. It is not an easy thing for you in this day and age to understand. I myself had trouble learning this lesson, but it is one that I shall never forget.

"You see, I had a very fierce teacher, who was my grandfather, and many strong and fierce-willed teachers after that in all the corners of Africa."

I had learned through my research that Credo Mutwa was the grandson of a Zulu shaman-warrior, Ziko Shezi, who survived the Zulu Wars and the final bloody battle of Ulundi. Maria had explained to me that Mutwa's grandfather was a traditional healer in the days of King Dingane; he attended to the king himself, and was a High Sanusi, custodian of relics of the tribe and guardian of tribal history (Umlando), a position that, after his death, was endowed upon young Mutwa.

"When I was a small child, ma'am, I served as my grandfather's attendant, and was allowed to carry his medicine bags," Mutwa explained. "In that way I shared a few of his forbidden secrets. But then I was taken away and did not see him again for many, many years. In all that time, I did not know of the things that the great healers do."

His eyes were downcast as he spoke, the thickened lenses giving an oddly distorting aspect.

"It was my grandfather, ma'am, who was the only person capable of curing me when I was struck down by an incurable sickness which kept me bedridden and unconscious for three years right here in Soweto. It was during this time that I had many terrifying visions, ma'am, some of which we *sangomas* call the 'sacred dreams' that occur before you become a *sangoma*. I had the vision of the earth stretched out like a lion skin pegged at all four corners – north, south, east, and west – with the four lion brothers tearing at it in four directions. We call this dream 'the Sacred Dream of End Time,' ma'am, *Ndelo Ntulo*. In our tradition we believe, ma'am, that the universe is sustained by four great forces and in the center is the fifth power, *Nxaka-Nxaka*, meaning 'confusion' or 'chaos.' From this power comes order and from order again comes chaos – and so on for all eternity."

He paused, and looked up momentarily.

"There is a stone ornament made out of a round stone with four holes and one hole in the center, which resembles a big button, ma'am, which our Sanusis use in their sacred rituals during the time of the equinoxes to simulate the workings of the universe – but that is another story. After the process of healing, ma'am, my grandfather showed me how to control my powers of perception, and how to sharpen my senses and make them more accurate – like the arrow from a hunter's bow.[4] He taught me the art of rhythm, and the secret art of joining my consciousness to the great gods of the unseen world. He taught me not to fear them, but to work with them as helpful guides who would sharpen and broaden my perception, not only of this world, but of the whole cosmos."

I was listening to Mutwa's every word, but at the same time burned to ask him other, more direct, questions related to my own experiences. We had not even ventured onto the question of Timbavati and its White Lions. Mutwa proceeded to tell me more about his grandfather in the slow, unfolding manner of the fireside tale: a storytelling technique to which I was as yet unaccustomed. I would have to learn that Mutwa would address my questions in good time. In the meantime, the stories he was recounting, of his formative experiences with his grandfather, had their own peculiar magic.

"At first I could not understand how the spirit of the Star Gods lived in everything," Mutwa continued. "I was very stupid in those days.

"When I first asked my grandfather how it was that everyone and everything had God within them, he had trouble controlling his Zulu temper. He took me outside our *rondavel* in anger and showed me his favorite tree, a tall, fruit-bearing fig tree which he had planted when he was a young man. He demanded what I thought this tree was. I told him: 'A tree, Grandfather.'

"Then my grandfather struck me across my face, and told me: 'This is not a tree, you little dog, this is a person.'"

Mutwa noticed my amused surprise.

"I see you laugh, ma'am. Well, I might have laughed, too – if I had not felt the weight of my grandfather's wrath. He told me that in the days when he himself was a child in old Africa, and in the centuries before – in the time of our Zulu ancestors – trees were not called 'trees' but 'growing people.'

"I had seen him standing beside this tree at certain times. I had watched him touch the bark of the tree, and once I had seen him perform a ritual in which he had taken the snuff out of his own snuff horn and poured it at the foot of the tree. My grandfather asked me fiercely what I thought he was doing. Did I really think he was worshipping the tree? 'No, Grandfather,' I said.

"Again, he gave me an angry blow and said: 'I *was* worshipping that tree, you ignorant youth! I was talking to it, and I was sharing my snuff with it. I often talk to it and sing to it and share my good news with it. I honor it and thank it for the plump figs that it offers us, because I believe that it is a person. Do you understand now?'

"I said, 'Yes, Grandfather!'

"But I did not understand at all and he knew. 'You understand nothing,' he told me that day.

"Well, ma'am," Mutwa concluded with a sense of *gravitas*, "it would take me a very long time to learn the earth-shaking knowledge that my grandfather was endowing me with, but soon I began to drink his teachings; because I have a thirst, ma'am, an insane curiosity to know as much as possible, which has been with me ever since I can remember. It is this thirst that has been my downfall – but I could do nothing other than drink in the knowledge."

Rather than comment on matters of which I had no understanding, I remained silent, sensing that he was leading up to address my question about the powerful connection that existed between shamans like Maria and lions.

"At first, I did not fully understand my grandfather's words," he continued, "but I would have reason to call upon them many times in my life.

"It was from my grandfather that I learned the first lesson of the lion shaman: that of overcoming fear. Much of the violence and stupid activity in our world is because people are still enslaved to this thing called fear and have not come to see the connection between all things." Mutwa paused. "There was the occasion, ma'am, when I met a man-eating lion."

Now I could not help myself. "Man-eating?" I repeated, a touch nervously.

"Yes, ma'am. It was when I was in Kenya as a young man, working in a game reserve as a guard for tourists on safari. I was erecting a tent for the camp when suddenly the whole thing crashed down upon me, and I was pinned to the ground by something very heavy. There was dust all around, and I could see nothing for several moments until suddenly from under the tangle of canvas I beheld the most fearsome face I had ever seen in my life. It was a huge lion, although very old – and it was snarling and trying to get at me. It was so close that I could see how all its teeth were broken.

"A lion is a most beautiful animal, ma'am, but when it is a few inches away and trying to eat you it is the most terrifying thing in the world. I later learned that this same lion was credited with the deaths of several children and as many women in the area."

I waited in suspense.

"The lion was huge, ma'am, and it had me pinned down and was staring into my face. In fact, some of the saliva from its open mouth had dripped onto my own face. I was terrified. To tell you the truth, I wet my pants. The lion was by now tearing at the canvas that lay between us. I was filled with fear and was struggling. I realized I could not move my left leg and was in great pain. I later discovered that the lion had broken my leg when he had sprung.

"Then I struggled to find calm. The beast was pressing down with all four paws. I was sweating and gritting my teeth and concentrating with all my might to keep my fear at bay, because I realized that my own fear was driving the beast on to eat me. I had been trying to scream and wrestle, but now I fought back my terror. Then, to my amazement, the lion just walked off and stood some distance away, watching.

"But that is not the end of the story," Mutwa continued. "Seeing the lion move off, I struggled under the canvas to free myself. And then, of course, the lion returned to finish me off. It was now using its front paws to tear at the canvas in an attempt to get at me under the tent. I could feel the terrible scratching of the claws at the canvas. Then once more I fought for calm. I remembered my grandfather's words, and now I tried to put them into practice. I said to the lion, 'You are my great brother. I respect you.' I was talking to the lion with my mind, you understand, ma'am, with all my will. 'I am not your food,' I told him. 'Please do not eat me. I bear you no ill will. I smile upon you. I do not have sharp teeth to injure you. Please leave me in peace.'

"And then, ma'am, I saw the lion simply walk away. I became unconscious and some time later I was found under the tent and taken to hospital.

"That lesson taught me, ma'am, that ferocious beasts, like ferocious humans, are driven on by the scent of fear. It also taught me that if you can conquer fear, you will not receive violence in return. If we humans can overcome this thing called fear, we can overcome the ills of this world and live in harmony. The trick, ma'am, is to face your fear and look into it as if it is the face of your lover.

"Our mistake," Mutwa was saying, "is that we forget that lions – all animals, in fact – are blessings from God.

"Our tradition tells us that the Great Earth Mother, Nomkhubhlwane, is capable of changing her shape into any animal at will. Most significantly, she can change into a lion or lioness. Her name means 'she who assumes the animal identity.' It is Zulu for 'shape-shifter.' You see, ma'am, our belief that the highest gods were part animal and part human being teaches us to treat animals with great reverence. Since our gods may take the head of a lion and the body of a human being, we treat all lions with love and respect."

"So why is it, then, that all the spiritual leaders seem to be associated with lions, Credo?" I asked, mulling over the patterns that had begun to emerge in my research.

"Ma'am, you are asking a very important question. Do you believe you are ready for the answer?"

The gravity of his response made me stop in my tracks. "Credo, I simply want to know," I said. "I need to understand. The more I investigate, the more questions keep coming up."

Mutwa smiled. "Even to this day there survive initiation schools in different parts of our continent, where the spiritual mysteries of Africa are taught. There we learn how it is that our gods and goddesses were capable of changing shape, and why they appear to be part animal and part human being. We learn, too, how we human beings might attempt the same feats. Our African forefathers gave us this wisdom because they understood what we ourselves should never forget: that is the oneness of the human being, in which the animal and the deity co-exist." He paused. "Why this should be the case, ma'am, is a very deep mystery indeed."

"So this would partly explain the belief that kings transmigrate into lions at death?"

"Yes, ma'am, yes. But that belief is itself only a sign of a deeper mystery."

I waited in silence.

"The lion is both the symbol and surrogate of the king. It is his totem. In Africa, the belief in reincarnation and transmigration of souls underlies the very basis of our thinking. When you die, it is believed that you are reincarnated into the totem animal of your tribe. For this reason, the Zulu people never willingly kill the lion; it is a sacred beast, symbolic of their king."

"But Credo, isn't it true," I asked, "that, throughout history, a young man – not only in the Zulu tradition but in most traditions – needs to kill a lion in order to become a man and in order to become lionhearted? And then he will wear the skin of the lion."

"Yes, ma'am, it is true. But not quite true. True lion combat is the exchange of souls. No lion is supposed to be killed unless it is a man-eater. Even our greatest kings did not kill a lion which was in the wild, not harming human beings. Only if in old age or sickness or injury, or for negative reasons, it became a man-eater. That is one of the oldest laws of Africa."

"As I understand it, Credo, there are two traditions running through Africa: the lion heroes and the lion priests. Is this correct? In the West, we would compare these with the very different stories of Hercules and Androcles: the one slays the lion while the other befriends it."

"In the Great African Tradition, ma'am, we do not separate the lion hero from the lion priest," he responded.

"I'm afraid I do not really understand, Credo."

Inhaling slowly, Mutwa continued. "Let me tell you a story, ma'am. In the history of the Zulus, there was a king called Mageba. He was a great lion warrior, but also he had the wisdom of high priesthood. He had studied the stars and knew what the gods intended of him.

"When he was still a prince, he was honored with the formal headdress and skin of a lion which had guarded over his territory for many years, and which had finally grown old. In this condition – at the stage when the mane of a lion gets blackened with age, ma'am – Mageba's warriors had dispatched the old lion. Mageba understood omens and knew that this symbolized his coronation as a lion king. For it is an old African belief that if you wear the skin of a particular animal, the qualities of that animal become part of you. Mageba understood this, but he also understood a lot more. Because, along with the lion skin, Mageba's warriors had brought a healthy young lion cub which had been captured during the hunt. The young king fell in love with the lion cub and cared for it as if it were his own son, for indeed it had become family. Wherever he went, the lion accompanied him. Whenever he sat on his chieftain's chair, the lion sat by his side.

"The young lion grew into a magnificent specimen," he continued, tilting his head in his characteristic manner. His eyes were obscured behind his lenses, but a slightly quizzical expression showed in his eyebrows. "Only one imperfection marred the lion's otherwise perfect physique, and that was an old injury to his paw as a result of the warriors' capturing him when he was small. But when he began to show the first signs of growing a mane, King Mageba decreed that he should be released into the wild to wander with the other lions of the bushveld.

"He told his warriors: 'I cannot keep another king as a slave in my village. He must return to his own kingdom as is the will of the Great Creator Spirit, uNkulunkulu.'

"Several years went by after the lion was set free, and then one day a terrible war broke out between the Zulu people and the Mangwani people – at the time when the Zulus were trading with the Portuguese. King Mageba was a powerful and fearless warrior, but there was one occasion when he was strategically separated from his men, and was trapped and wounded, almost fatally. His shield was in tatters as the Mangwani battle axes rained down on him, and his body was wet with the blood of the enemy, as well as his own."

Mutwa paused for effect, but I dared not interrupt.

"Then, at the point when he was about to expire, the point when he believed he was drawing his last breath, a pride of lions leapt out of the undergrowth and tore some of the enemy warriors to shreds, scattering the remaining Mangwani army in all directions. The lions were led by a proud young male which Mageba suddenly recognized, from the slight deformation in his front paw, as the very same lion he himself had hand-reared."

My heart leapt at this turning point in Mutwa's tale. Although the Zulu king was crowned with the lion headdress in the lion hero tradition, there was no mistaking the familiar shamanic theme: a lionhearted human whose love for a lion saved him from death. Mutwa's story helped explain to me how the twin themes – lion hero and lion priest – might be combined in one. Maria, the most heroic of women, would not have harmed a lion to prove her prowess.

"In victory," Mutwa concluded, "Mageba returned home with his army intact. His men watched how, all the way back to the village, his friendly lion and pride of lionesses followed to ensure the king's safety. It is said that the lion later accompanied him on many expeditions when King Mageba went to trade with the Portuguese."

The aging shaman looked up at me, in closing: "This is but one story that I know, ma'am, relating how the king of the wild may protect a human king. The Zulu nation to this day honor their king as a lion, and call him Ingonyama."[5]

"So," I concluded, "this story shows how certain men can be lion priests and lion warriors at one and the same time?"

"Yes, ma'am, yes. And, ultimately, a lion king, too. The lion priest is the true lion warrior of the spirit. It is such individuals, ma'am, whom it is said live on in the form of lions."

"I see, I see . . ." I was starting to make sense of some of Maria's cryptic explanations.

"You mean, when a human portrays the qualities of a lion, he can eventually become a lion?"

"It is a matter of spirit, ma'am. In spirit, they are one and the same."

He was watching me intently as I thought this over.

"You see, ma'am, when you are close to an animal in spirit, we believe it can read your mind. King Mageba cried out for help, and the lion heard him – although he may not have uttered a single word. In the same way, Maria spoke to the lions of Timbavati. You may call it telepathy, we call it mind-call."

"I'm beginning to understand, Credo."

"Do not forget what you have seen – there will be many who will not believe you."

"How can I forget?" I smiled at the memory. "I saw Maria pass through the Timbavati lions unharmed – and several other people saw it, too."

"Many people see things which they do not care to remember." A silence fell between us momentarily.

"You yourself have been to Timbavati, have you not, Credo?" I inquired.

"Yes, ma'am, yes. I went to Timbavati hoping to see a White Lion walking free in the bush. I never saw a single one. If, ma'am, I had seen a White Lion, it would have helped me to make a very important decision regarding my life. But I didn't. I didn't see a single White Lion and so I never made that very important decision which would have freed me from all nonsense. And I asked the people of Timbavati: 'Where are your lions? Where are the holy Children of the Sun God?' Because that is what they are called. I never received a straight answer.

"Instead, ma'am, I received strange news. A lion which was suspected of being the father of one of the white cubs was being threatened by trophy hunters. They wanted to shoot Ngwazi."

"Yes!" I interrupted. "Credo, I've seen Ngwazi."

"So he is still alive?" the shaman asked, with a whimsical smile.

"Very much so!" I said, recalling his dominant presence in the Timbavati territory.

"That is good, ma'am, that is good. You see, when I heard about the trophy-hunting expedition, I was so angry that I demanded to be taken to within a few meters of Ngwazi. There he sat, a majestic and beautiful creature. An ordinary South African lion, yes, but a beautiful creature. We believe that lions are more sacred, more special than any other animal, ma'am. Have you ever noticed how lions have the body of a carnivore but the tail of a herbivore – like a donkey's, ma'am?"

"I hadn't thought of it that way, Credo."

"That is part of a very great mystery. But to continue with my story. Upon seeing this great African lion, I stood up in the jeep and I blessed him. And then I said to everybody: 'Please spread the word that any man who shoots Ngwazi will be cursed unto the 16th generation, and he will be killed by his own bullet.'" He paused dramatically. "That, ma'am, is what saved Ngwazi."

Mutwa's powers of protection aside, this struck me as a brilliant tactical move.

"Do you know why human beings hunt animals for pleasure, ma'am?" the shaman asked me.

"I don't know, Credo. It seems to be a macho, egotistical thing. Men trying to prove their manhood, or something. They seem to think they are imbued with the power of a lion if they can kill a lion."

"They are wrong, ma'am." He paused. "You do not receive the power of something by killing it. You receive its power by touching it." Mutwa paused again. And I waited in suspense.

"You do not get the power of the bull by slaughtering it. You get the power of the bull by taking it by the horns – and somersaulting over it. In our Bushman tradition, ma'am, this is what our bravest warriors did with the sacred eland. Do you get the power of the king by murdering him?" he asked rhetorically. "No. You inquire of him respectfully whether you may exchange some of you for some of him." The words were regal and dramatic, yet heartfelt.

"You know, ma'am, the lion is the sacred totem of my family, on my grandfather's side. And not only am I sworn to protect women of any race or any tribe – even female baboons I must honor – but lions, being my family gods on my grandfather's side, I must protect."

He paused, looking deeply weary all of a sudden. "I have learned this the hard way, ma'am. The reason why my life is in such a mess, I believe, is that early in my life I was often present when lions were shot and sometimes I, too, unknowingly took part in the shooting of these sacred animals."

Mutwa had earlier mentioned his time in Kenya as a youth working in a safari camp, and I imagined that what he was referring to here was his involvement in the tracking and shooting of lions. I wondered how he had reconciled this with his grandfather's initiations into lion shamanism, and felt compelled to ask more; but the time did not seem appropriate.

Mutwa sat before me, his head downcast and his eyes obscured beneath thick lenses. I realized that I should not prolong the encounter.

"You are tired, Credo?"

"Yes, ma'am, I am tired."

"Should I keep my questions for another day, then?"

"Yes. If you please, ma'am."

But I needed to ask the golden question: "And the White Lions, how did they come to Timbavati in the first place?"

"That, ma'am, is another story. I see I have talked too much already, ma'am. That is the problem with my life. We Sanusis are taught to respect the Silence. But it is she who keeps telling me that now is the time to deliver the Great Knowledge to the world, before it is too late."

"Who is she, Credo?" I inquired.

"She is Amarava, ma'am, the woman to whom all my teachings are dedicated."

Naturally, my first thoughts were that she was a flesh-and-blood woman, a muse who had inspired the shaman to enlightenment. Then I recalled Maria telling me that Mutwa was always accompanied by the Great Mother of the First People, a primal goddess from the spirit world who had been his spirit guide throughout his life. Maria had explained that she had first appeared to him during his period of *twasa,* or sickness, before he was initiated, when he was tormented by recurring visions. Amarava had appeared to him and told him to be unafraid of the weird things happening to him. She had soothed him, telling him her name was Amarava and she had come to be his "bride."

There was so much more I needed to ask, and Mutwa was tired. But, before I left, I had to probe a little more about Amarava, the great inspiration of his life. Mutwa declined an answer. "I cannot – I may not – speak about Amarava!" He was shaking his head with a nervous laugh, as if he feared the repercussions. "It is she who has taught me all I know," he explained. "But she can also be vengeful!"

Despite his apprehension, he seemed animated by the mention of her name.

"You know, ma'am, Amarava is a bringer of enlightenment and wisdom to this earth. Do you know that she taught me how to make a telescope? It was at the time of man's first landings on the moon and our people wanted to see. Perhaps you know, ma'am, that the Bushman people of Africa have eyesight so keen they can see the mountains of the moon, and hearing so sharp they can detect the sound that heavenly bodies make in their movement around the sun. Did you know this, ma'am?"

"No, Credo, I'm afraid I didn't."

"Well, this is true, ma'am, but the Bushman shamans wanted to see more. They wanted to see the spacecraft's landing on the moon. It was Amarava who gave me the knowledge of how to construct a telescope so as to enlarge the moon many times over. And do you know what tools she told me to use? The base of ordinary glass bottles. Do you know, ma'am, I still have this telescope to this day."

Despite himself, Mutwa had begun to talk about Amarava. And he went on now to inform me that although she was a spirit, she was also quite real. So much so, she could manifest herself to others. He said Amarava was the reason his first marriage had dissolved. He said his first wife imagined he was having an affair – which was not the case at all. The same injustice might have destroyed his second marriage, to Cecilia, only now he knew how to explain things to her. Cecilia had come to him weeping with accusations that she had seen another woman in their bed, and he had calmed her, saying, "My darling, do real women have hair of green and skin of red? What you have seen is Amarava; perhaps one day you will come to understand . . ." And so Cecilia had learned to live with this apparition as an inevitable fact of their lives together. In describing the incident, Mutwa and I had simultaneously seen the humor in this ridiculous situation – his wife mistaking an apparition for a real-life lover – and we both laughed aloud.

"I now realize I cannot live without Amarava," he continued soberly, "but I respect and fear her completely."

"Why?" I asked.

"She has great powers of enlightenment and retaliation," he said. "All I wanted in my life, ma'am, was to be an ordinary greengrocer on the corner."

I let out an involuntary chuckle at his modesty.

'Yes, ma'am! Sometimes I still believe this is all I want, but it is not to be. When Amarava first came into my life, I feared her – like I feared that man-eating lion in Kenya. I struggled and I resisted, believing she was my opponent and not my guardian!"

He went on to explain how for years he had wrestled with the presence of Amarava in his life. He tried every conceivable means to rid himself of her. He prayed to be released from her. He willed her away with all his willpower, but she always returned. Finally, he resorted to making a trip to East Africa, where he tracked down a renowned exorcist in Dar es Salaam, and elicited his help in shedding the spirit of Amarava. He paid this famous man a substantial sum of money and the rituals were duly performed. After the exorcism, he was relieved to discover that Amarava had indeed gone away, and he returned to South Africa to get on with his life.

Mutwa gave me a rueful smile as he recounted this part of the story.

"About six months later, however, ma'am, a message came through a person I had never met – from another country altogether. This person reported to me that he had been instructed that a woman called Amarava had a message for the man Mutwa. The message was: 'Do not mess with me. I am back!'"

He sighed. "From that day on, she has been inseparable from my own existence, and I have finally learned, ma'am, to reconcile myself with the great joys and agonies she brings."

I was touched by this amazing tale, but, unschooled in the ways of shamanism and spiritual matters, I had no idea how to respond.

With that, we parted. I was ready to return the very next day, but unfortunately our next meeting would still be a long way off.

5

CREDO: THE WORD OF AFRICA

Our wise men hid their wisdom in what seem like children's stories – to protect it. . . . True, the black man of Africa had no mighty scrolls on which to write the history of this land. True, the black tribes of Africa had no pyramids on which to carve the history. . . . But this they did and still do!
– CREDO MUTWA ON THE GREAT ORAL TRADITION

Despite repeated efforts, I was unable to reach Credo Mutwa for the next six months. The day after I had first met him, he was said by attendants to be unwell. A few days later, the story had changed, and I was passed from one anonymous individual to another, all claiming to have no idea of his whereabouts. Soon I understood that in all probability he did not wish to be contacted, so I curtailed efforts to trace him.

What followed was a protracted period of mulling over what I'd been told, and contemplating what I was prepared to believe. Where there were gaps, I attempted to fill them by taking time to read Mutwa's published works. His temporary disappearance was fortunate, really: had I been given any further revelations, I doubt I would have been able to digest them. The fact that he had not even begun to address the question I had specifically come to have answered – the story behind the White Lions of Timbavati – was not of primary importance. The other disclosures, and the exciting questions they raised, were quite enough to ignite my curiosity about lion shamanism.

When I mentioned to colleagues that I had met Credo Mutwa in person, I was warned that I was opening myself up to the ramblings of an "old charlatan," although this cautionary advice generally came from people who had had no direct contact with the man himself. It seemed Mutwa's reputation was irreparably damaged in the eyes of the establishment. After this first meeting, I was left with only my own instinct and Maria's shamanic guidance for support. As far as I was concerned, Maria's inspired actions spoke louder than words. The high regard in which she held Credo Mutwa required no better recommendation.

Nevertheless, the shamanic material that Mutwa had been generous enough to impart was so dauntingly unfamiliar that its implications and consequences sometimes kept me awake at night.

Amarava – Enlightenment-Bearer

First of all, this notion of Amarava intrigued me. Was she a figment of Mutwa's imagination? It was easy to view her in Jungian terms as the shadowy female archetype, the *anima* figure contained within a man's psyche, to whom he is wedded more intimately than to his own matrimonial wife. But even Jung's powerful psychological explanation was inadequate. It could not explain, for instance, how this archetype could manifest in material reality, and be seen by others.

I noted that Amarava was not only able to assume physical form, but also take on different guises, sometimes part human and part animal: most significantly, part lion.

In one of Mutwa's books (a dictated work entitled *Song of the Stars*), the lion shaman describes a terrifying period of psychic disturbance, during which Amarava appeared repeatedly to him:

> Even now Amarava was transforming. Her color changed from red to gold, her breasts sprouted udders, her hands turned to terrible claws. A lion's tail curled from her backside, and it lashed angrily . . .[1]

In his writings, Mutwa records how his entry into shamanism was precipitated by a sudden illness. This important detail reminded me of how Africa's great medicine man fits into the immeasurably long-standing shamanic tradition. The scholarly study on this subject by Mircea Eliade, *Shamanism*, shows how shamans are initiated into profound knowledge after a period of pathological, often near-fatal, illness. Credo Mutwa was no exception.

One is tempted to dismiss this characteristic shamanic experience as a "mental breakdown," but even a clinical term fails to explain the heightened powers that ultimately arise out of this condition. Scholars of shamanic practices, such as Eliade and Giorgio de Santillana, help us to understand that such psychic turbulence, rather than being "mental illness," is a prerequisite for the initiate's access to enhanced states of awareness. I now understood that this was the experience referred to by Maria of Timbavati as *twasa*.

The problem appears to be that the role of shaman is not a choice the individual makes but, rather, a destiny which is bestowed upon him or her.[2] Because such individuals, like the rest of us, suffer from fear and doubt, they wrestle with the inevitable outcome and make the transitional process all the more difficult for themselves. This is why the election of a shaman so often appears to involve the sudden onset of this unexpected and unwanted ailment but then moves into gradual reconstruction, with the emerging shaman capable of feats that go beyond the merely human – an example of the evolutionary principle that what does not kill makes one stronger.

Once recovered from this psychic illness, newly endowed with "non-ordinary powers" – to use Carlos Castaneda's term – the shamanic student is then initiated by older traditional healers into their secret ways. Having survived his own ordeal, he assumes the mantle of the "wounded healer." In 1937, at the age of 16, following his shamanic "illness," Mutwa was reunited with his grandfather and set aside his Christian upbringing to take on the so-called ceremony of purification, the first step in the path toward shamanism. From this point on, the Earth Goddess, Amarava, was the spiritual inspiration behind all his actions.

Even as a youngster, before this illness, Mutwa was tormented by repeated psychic images of his leonine *anima* figure. He explains, "A very strange part of my life concerns Amarava."

> In my youth I had not known very much about her; but in my dreams and in my visions was a figure who kept appearing to me, with red skin and greenish hair. I did not know what to do. I wanted this woman to stop bothering me and go away. But I never told anyone about it. I was praying to be released from these disturbing visions . . .[3]

Upon reading this, I recalled the explanation he had given in my own meeting with him, as to how he had feared Amarava when she had first come into his life, just as he had feared that man-eating lion in Kenya. And how he had resisted her guiding presence, believing she was his opponent and not his guardian. It led me to reflect on my own recurring dream of a lion roaring into my face. It seems that, once the initiate stops combat with the leonine forces within him- or herself, and accepts his or her role as spiritual guide, the shamanic healing process begins.

Much of this material sounded bizarre and potentially dangerous, but if I were to define the overarching feeling I received from Mutwa, having met him in person, it was a radiant sense of power and light.

Vusamazulu, the Outcast

From Maria's words, and from what I went on to uncover in newspaper clippings and library archives, the picture I gained of Credo Mutwa was that of a man of great magnitude and deep pathos. His is an extraordinary and very moving life story.

Mutwa was born on 21 July in Umsinga in Zululand, just outside Durban, in the early 1920s. (Traditionally, the exact year of a Sanusi's birth may not be disclosed.) After growing up in the apartheid era in a household dominated by a Christian father, separated from his mother and her shamanic roots, he was abandoned on the streets of Sophiatown, and left to fend for himself for much of his early life.

To walk the shamanic path was the first agonizing decision of his life, a spiritual route that he had resisted on pain of death. After finally accepting his true calling, he was initiated and trained by the greatest of Africa's healers, awarded the highest of Africa's shamanic honors, and entrusted with the deepest secrets of the African continent.[4] He received his shamanic training in various parts of Africa: north, south, east, and west. The Great Knowledge is spoken about only in places of initiation, and preserved only in the memory of those who guard the Umlando. Having himself been honored with the title of Guardian of Umlando, he was also entrusted with the custodianship of some of the most sacred of Africa's secret treasures.

Then came the second most agonizing decision of his life: to break with the very shamanic tradition he had suffered such pains to enter.

Cast out and ostracized by the paternal line of his family for having followed the path of shamanism, he was now outcast by the shamanic priests, too, for having committed secret oral traditions to the written word. But having vowed to expose inherited tribal secrets for all to see, Mutwa continued on his new path. The more I read about the consequences of his brave action, and the numerous personal afflictions that followed, the more I marveled at what had compelled him do to this.

Not surprisingly, it turns out that his task of writing down the Great Knowledge is dedicated to the figure of Amarava.[5] He explains that behind this decision stands the goddess "who has been telling me to transmit these secret teachings, the legends and mythology of the Zulu people, to the rest of the world so that they may not wither away, and so that all of humanity may learn of them."[6] It is a monumental, unfinished *oeuvre,* the sole purpose of which is to deliver to the rest of humankind, against all odds, the shamanic memory over which he has guardianship.

His first controversial book, *Indaba, My Children* ("Communicate, My Children") was published nearly four decades ago. The impression one gets from Mutwa's African tome is that the history of Africa, like that of Europe and Asia, is one of bloody battles, pillage, and destruction, yet embedded in the mayhem are jewels of spiritual enlightenment.

My training in ancient symbolism and mythology assisted me in understanding the legendary quality of Mutwa's historical epics, where the boundaries between fable and fact appear to merge. Without this training, I might have been taken aback at the immovable sense of conviction with which Mutwa puts pen to paper:

> Many strange things have happened in Africa . . . Many will find it hard to
> believe much of what I have revealed . . . but I am not the least concerned,
> because whether I am believed or not, everything I write here is true.[7]

These might have been the words of an arrogant man, yet instead my firsthand impression of Mutwa was that of a humble individual, fired by the courage of conviction and the love of humanity, swearing to tell the world the truth as it had been entrusted to him, so that modern consciousness might eventually gain an understanding of old Africa's heritage. It seems he has lived his life in an unfailing effort to fulfill this oath: "an oath whose keeping has become the only purpose of my intolerable life."[8]

While still a youth in 1932, he was a witness to his stepbrother's death after being whipped senseless by a farmer. Some years later he himself suffered an accident (involving an unprotected petrol tank) on the farm where he was working as a laborer, which impaired his eyesight for life. Subsequently, as a middle-aged man in love, he lost the woman he had hoped to marry when she was killed by police gunfire in the notorious Sharpeville massacre of March 1960. Mutwa was branded a traitor during the 1976 Soweto uprising for revealing Africa's secrets to the white oppressor. His family house was razed to the ground by an angry crowd, who almost succeeded in beating and stabbing Mutwa to death. There were many times when Mutwa went into hiding, his life under threat. In South Africa's complex political maelstrom, the shaman's greater wisdom refused to allow him to take sides – making him "the enemy of all sides."

Of the many tragedies that have plagued Mutwa's life, most poignant is the appalling death of his son, Innocent Mutwa, whom he had intended to be his successor in the secret traditions. Mutwa's firstborn was the only natural inheritor of the Great Knowledge, and had already been inducted into the ways of lion shamanism. It is at the same time ironic and tragic that the young man who bore the name "Innocent" (thus named from birth) became the victim of cold-blooded political murder in 1986. He was in his twenties.

In the wake of Innocent Mutwa's killing, will the Great Tradition – which has been handed down through generations in Mutwa's direct line – die with Credo Mutwa?

Ancient Knowledge That Saved a Kingdom

On gathering information on Mutwa's history, I felt a deep compulsion to understand more about the "Great Knowledge," and why Mutwa considered this secret font of wisdom so important that he was prepared to dedicate a life of persecution to its delivery. In one of his published works I had come across a reference that gave me intimations of the nature of this knowledge. "In Africa," Mutwa writes, "we find many stories which seem at first glance rather childish and primitive but which on closer examination are revealed to hide mind-boggling facts about the depths of knowledge our forefathers possessed . . . these long-forgotten people reveal in stories the wisdom that they handed down to us over the missed centuries. The fact is that they were wiser than we are and possessed knowledge regarding things of which we are only now becoming aware."[9]

In my reading I came across an extract from the Great African Tradition, recounted by Mutwa in traditional story form, which cast light on his own life story. His method of documenting past events was quite unlike our history books. It sounded more like fable than fact – yet it rang with a deep authenticity, and its meaning resounded clear and true through simple, childlike words.

Mutwa begins the story by explaining that it carries a message "which will come to you when the story has ended." Although the Sanusi himself never spells out the parallels, I later realized how profoundly significant this ancient story was to the more recent autobiographical events of Mutwa's own life.

Entitled "The Ancient Knowledge That Saved a Kingdom," it tells the tale of Nalindele the medicine woman. Drawing on the inherited oral records, Mutwa explains, "There was a tribe somewhere in Southern Africa whose name we [the guardians] have forgotten. They had settled for so long that the storytellers could no longer tell exactly how long they had been [t]here."[10] It is known, however, that the event took place in the land of the Barotse people, during the reign of a king called Ndenge.

This particular tribe had been prosperous and peaceful, but Mutwa explains that, with time, and due to complacency and forgetfulness, the people disregarded "many important things which their long-forgotten ancestors had known about."[11]

Then, after a terrible comet is seen in the sky, conditions change on earth. A drought ensues, and famine follows. Household cats – symbols of guardianship – flee back to their natural habitat in the bush, while in the village of King Ndenge the children lie starving. In the midst of the "great darkness," an unknown woman arrives. She asks for safe passage through their land to another land where her brother is king. Clearly, she is a *sangoma*. She has a lovely daughter who is blind in both eyes, but "there was a beauty in her that was timeless, a wisdom that no amount of blindness could erase from her face."[12]

This woman carries a great knowledge, and seeing the suffering of these people, her first gesture is to offer them an understanding of nature and the edible "food in the bush"[13] of which they are completely ignorant. Through her ancient wisdom, derived from the Bushman people, she understands how to turn poison into cure. Instead of gratitude, however, Nalindele is met with suspicion and sarcasm, since the plant that she knows to have nutritious healing properties is believed to be poisonous.

The king promptly dismisses the *sangoma*'s ancient knowledge and, in desperation for a quick remedy for the troubles in his land, seizes upon the idea of sacrificing the beautiful blind girl to appease the gods. Alas, this atrocity does take place, and "she [is] done to death in a horrible way, then bound in a net and thrown onto a great pile of wood and burnt."[14]

One can only sympathize with the medicine woman's dreadful loss. After her beautiful child is murdered and ceremonially burned, Nalindele appeals to the Barotse people:

> "It is not the Gods which are angry with you," [cries] the grief-stricken Nalindele.
> "It is your own ignorance that is to blame!"[15]

Astoundingly, despite her appalling victimization, the medicine woman does not repay the dreadful deed with revenge. The cruel sacrifice to the gods has failed, and the drought has only worsened. But when the beleaguered people come begging for help, the medicine woman takes pity on them once more, and begins to introduce them to the very knowledge that their own forebears knew only too well. I found that detail deeply telling – how the "wounded healer"[16] heals the people who have wronged her by introducing them to wisdom that they themselves have forgotten. Mutwa concludes:

> The wise woman, Nalindele, became a helper of people who had forgotten about their past. She reminded the people of King Ndenge the one thing

that had brought about their suffering was that they had forgotten many things their ancestors had handed down to them.[17]

Mutwa concludes the story with the significant detail that even today, in the land of the Barotse, "when a person is in need and another person comes out of nowhere to help," rather like a guardian angel in our Western tradition, this person is known as a "Nalindele."

Voice of the Zulus

This extract from ancient oral history moved me, inviting as it did comparison with Mutwa's own tragic life story. I did not yet know Mutwa intimately, but my heart went out to him every time I identified a parallel between his own story and the tale of Nalindele.

I knew the facts of Mutwa's life, since they were public knowledge. Innocent was put to death by ritual burning by a gang of hysterical activists. In the African tradition this is the greatest of all tragedies, since death by fire is believed not only to destroy the human body but also the eternal soul.

Only once after I came to know Mutwa intimately did he allude to this heart-breakingly painful episode. The thought of it brought tears to his eyes. Yet, astoundingly, when speaking of the way he himself was savagely maltreated at the hands of a hysterical mass of activists, he was still able to show humor.

"When a gang of angry thugs wants to kill you," he explained, "excuse me, ma'am, but you shit yourself! However, when a whole ocean of people descends on you, it feels like it is happening to someone else." On both his left and his right arm, he showed me the brutal scars where he had been hacked by pangas and beaten with clubs. "When a Coca-Cola bottle smashes against your skull – let me tell you, ma'am, it is a most mind-opening experience!" he added. At one point, the crowd poured petrol over Mutwa, intent on setting him alight. How the horror finally resolved itself remains a mystery. It appears that only after the shaman finally summoned all his powers of prayer did the mass of incensed humans disperse.

As Mutwa recounted his life story to me, I felt the mythic dimensions of the man. Even the shaman's name itself – Credo Vusamazulu Mutwa, the name he had inherited at birth – had profound symbolic connotations. "Mutwa" means "Bushman" in Zulu and Xhosa (the -twa itself is also the root of the word twasa – the state of calling to shamanism).[18] Mutwa's own genetic lineage may be traced back to both Zulu and Bushman origins. Vusamazulu means "the Awakener" (or the "voice," or the "roar") of the Zulu people. Finally, his Christian name, Credo, refers to "the creed" or "the Word," meaning "I believe" in Latin. Some eight decades on, the great man himself more than amply lived up to these profoundly symbolic titles conferred upon him at birth. His birthplace and date of birth (I would later discover) were equally prophetic, providing critical clues to the mysteries surrounding the White Lions.

If his own story were handed down in oral history from this day forth, I realized that it would appear as yet another mythical tale in the Great Tradition. Yet, movingly, his story was true.

Wisdom from the World's First People

It is also deeply telling that, like Nalindele, the medicine woman of old, Mutwa's knowledge comes from the Bushman people. In Southern Africa, today's Bushmen represent the last surviving echo of First Man. With their origins traceable to the Stone and Ice Ages, the Bushman (or Khoisan) people are the direct descendants of Africa's original human inhabitants and the world's first true humans.[19] Unfortunately, the Bushman culture was all but destroyed by genocidal tactics up to and including the early 1900s, and has been under duress ever since.

Bushman history is a grim testimony to humanity's barbarity. Trophy-hunting sorties were organized by colonists to kill Bushmen, as if they were yet another species of wild animal to be eradicated in the Cape. Bushmen were hunted like lions – for sport. Appallingly, Bushmen heads on spikes and flayed Bushman skins are preserved in museums to this day.[20] The British, the Dutch, the Afrikaners, and certain African tribes were all responsible for the extermination of these gentle people, eliminating along with the people themselves a culture of more value than we can ever realize. In effect, we are all the Barotse of Mutwa's tale, brutally oblivious to ancient wisdom that may have life-saving significance in our contemporary situation. While colonists regarded Bushmen as wild prey to be eradicated, I felt all the more sickened when I remembered that, in a very special sense, the Bushman shamans were wild animals: their powers of interspecies communication were so acute that they were believed capable of assuming leonine form at will. This was one aspect of ancient Bushman knowledge that I myself had closely investigated in my quest to understand Maria's connection with the Timbavati lions. Today it would seem that not a single Bushman lion shaman survives. Regrettably, I have had to rely on secondhand reports in archives. This was one clan of lion shamanism – the original clan – to which I would never gain direct access. In this bleak context, Mutwa's knowledge of ancient Bushman culture was all the more important.

As the world's "First People," the Bushman ancestors developed an understanding of lion–human interactions that provided the founding bedrock beneath other shamanisms. In former times, tribes such as the Tsonga/Shangaan (Maria's tribe), the Zulu (Mutwa's tribe) and the Xhosa (Nelson Mandela's tribe) acquired their knowledge from a long history of cultural exchange and intermarriage with the Bushman people.

Rather than a quaint and poetic fireside tale, Mutwa's story of Nalindele is directly applicable to our present circumstances. This, after all, is what Mutwa himself has continued to do – hand over ancient knowledge – despite the persecution he has received at the brutal and ignorant hands of humanity. I could not help seeing humankind reflected in the Barotse tribe, which had lost its roots and its ancient knowledge. In their treatment of the wise woman who had attempted, to her detriment, to enlighten them, I saw Mutwa's own efforts laid bare. Nalindele's selfless action gave me insight into the motivation that lay behind Mutwa's monumental decision to break a sacred oath and hand over ancient secrets. It occurred to me that, like the victimized healer in the story, Mutwa might be prepared to suffer for humanity because he believed the lost knowledge of Africa that he was imparting could save the world.

When Maria talked of Mutwa symbolically through the bones, he was represented by a large distinctive relic, which turned out to be an antbear vertebra. After I inquired why this animal should symbolize Mutwa, she explained that it dug holes that many other animals used as houses, implying that the Sanusi's wisdom provided shelter for other people and cultures across the globe.[21]

According to Maria, Mutwa "carried the pain of Africa on his shoulders" and, given what I had learned of his history, it did seem as if this one individual bore the karma of an entire continent upon his large but humble shoulders. If today the Barotse people still use the word *Nalindele* to mean "guardian angel" or "patron saint," it occurred to me that perhaps one day we may use *Mutwa* in much the same way.

Guardian of Africa's Soul-History

In this African shaman, I now began to see a monumental but alienated figure, at the same time revered and disparaged, deified, and denounced: Credo Mutwa, the greatest lion priest in Africa, as well as Vusamazulu, the Outcast.

In his book *Indaba, My Children*, Mutwa alludes to the process of selecting the traditional bearers of Great Knowledge:[22] "There are men and women, preferably with black birthmarks on either palm of the hands, with good memories and a great capacity to remember words and repeat them exactly as they heard them spoken. These people are told the mystery of the tribes – under oath never to alter, add or subtract any word."[23]

On the one hand, *memory* means a process of learning, by rote, tribal history preserved through the centuries. On the other hand, together with this highly specialized memorizing art, there appears to be another form of "memory" entirely – a kind of shamanic "recall" of events that supersedes individual lifetimes and personal experiences. Primary to the role of the shaman is the notion of "memory" as something approximating cross-cultural or "archetypal" memory, and the ability to bring the past into the present, along with the future.

The Great Memory

The writer Laurens van der Post wrestled with this idea when he attempted to describe the difference between what he called "the Great Memory" and "the little memory," which he had witnessed in the Kalahari Bushmen. He talks about the Great Memory as:

A dimension of memory which has haunted me all my life . . . an over-arching memory which does not belong to man so much as to life itself, and no matter how much one may forget and ignore it, it never forgets or ignores whatever form of being is invested with life. It is a memory of all the life that has been; it is imparted to one through natural instinct and feeling, and yet it is also full of premonition of the future, and more. For my part, I can only say that to the extent to which I had become aware of it through the play of instinct and feeling in myself and intimation of dreams and images coming to me unsolicited and of their own accord – strong, real and often contrary to all that the world and time surrounding me demanded – it remained somewhere and somehow in supreme command of all that I possessed of meaning. I came to call it to myself the Great Memory.[24]

Similarly, the "memory" that a Sanusi carries represents more than oral history; and is synonymous with a heightened, or deepened, level of consciousness: something that goes beyond the individual in terms of both time and place, and approximates the condition of spiritual awareness and wisdom. When I thought of Mutwa's Great Knowledge, the word that came to mind was *enlightenment*. In this way, the secret tradition was both inherited knowledge passed on through generations of an initiated élite, and also ancestral knowledge inherited directly from what might be termed the "spirit world."

Mutwa was born of the Zulu and Bushman peoples. Yet if I understood him correctly, he was not only the guardian of the soul-history of these particular tribes, but the guardian of an entire continent. He carried a memory of events that took place in locations far afield from his own stomping ground, long before his own lifetime. He also carried the knowledge of realms of the sacred, inaccessible to most people. I now believed Mutwa to be the guardian of Africa – the continent that gave birth to the human species.

6

HUNTER OR HUNTED?

I have a vision of the Songlines stretching across the continents and ages; that wherever men have trodden they have left a trail of song; and that these trails must reach back, in time and space, to an isolated pocket in the African savanna, where the First Man shouted the opening stanza of the World Song, "I am."

– BRUCE CHATWIN, THE SONGLINES

African shamanism draws a vital connection between the king of the beasts and the evolution of man. What was the soul-history of man's affiliation with the big cats? When and how did the notions of lion hero and lion priest begin?

Birth of Man, the Hunter

As more and more research raised the same questions, I remembered a tantalizing piece of archeological speculation by acclaimed British adventurer and travel writer Bruce Chatwin. He poses the idea that early man and prehistoric felines might have co-existed in the same caves in Africa during a onetime Ice Age. Chatwin died before he could fully develop his ideas, though the picture he paints in *The Songlines* is so compelling that I have never forgotten it. Now, attempting to understand the intimate liaison between modern-day shamans and felines, I realized that this might provide a key to the origins of Africa's culture of lion shamanism.

My first step was to track down the primary material on which Chatwin's notes were based: the anthropological thesis of leading South African paleoanthropologist Dr C.K. Brain entitled *The Hunters or the Hunted?*

Chatwin had been so intrigued by Brain's archeological findings and the questions they provoked that he described the scientist's thesis as the "most compelling detective story" he had ever read. Brain's work more than satisfied my desire to find a scientific explanation for Africa's lion culture and the remarkable were-lion phenomenon I was tracking.

It involved the abundant and conclusive evidence of hominid remains that was discovered in the Sterkfontein Valley caves – a group of several caves (Sterkfontein, Swartkrans, Kromdraai, and others in the same valley) that provided early man with shelter from the cold climatic conditions, and housed Ice Age fossils that have preoccupied modern archeologists for the past three-quarters of a century. These are primarily classified as *Australopithecus africanus* (Southern African ape), small-brained creatures that exhibited both ape and human characteristics. They were herbivores who lived by uprooting bulbs and shoots and picking berries. They occasionally used basic tools. These "ape-men" lived from approximately 4 million to 2.5 million years ago.

The crux of the mystery is this: while the caves were the habitation of these ape-men, it seems they were also the lairs of big carnivores.

Hominids and Sabertooths

The biggest carnivores during this period of prehistory were saber-toothed felines of two distinct types – the *Machairodontinae* and the *Dinofelis barlowi*. Both of these extinct cats had rapier-like upper canines which would have served as lethal weapons. The *Machairodontinae* was a very heavily built predator with a long tail and hugely extended and curved upper canines that were flattened on both sides like two sabers. The *Dinofelis barlowi*, also known as the false sabertooth, had a short tail and enlarged upper canines that were not laterally flattened as in the true sabertooths.

The regular occurrence of *Dinofelis* fossils in the Sterkfontein Valley sites suggest that they were using the caves as lairs. What puzzled archeologists was why so many hominid and baboon skeletons existed alongside the feline remains in the same caves in the partial absence of prey species such as antelope. This evidence began to suggest an uncomfortable question: might our ape-men ancestors have been the main prey of the carnivores?

Brain's technique was to subject thousands upon thousands of bones to meticulous forensic examination in order to determine factors such as cause of death. He concluded that some of the primates were killed by the carnivores, their bones revealing unmistakable marks of violent death. A key exhibit is an australopithecine's cranium with two punctures around the base which correlate exactly with the fossilized lower canines of felines found in the same cave – evidence that hominids were hunted and eaten by prehistoric cats. Big cats generally dispatch their prey with a bite to the neck, thus silencing any distress calls that might attract other hungry predators. They might also drag their prey by the skull, which would account for the two perforations in the base of the ape-man's cranium.

All in all, careful analysis of evidence in the Swartkrans fossils led Brain to conclude that the felines (in particular *Dinofelis*) might be "a specialist killer of the primates."[1]

And it was this idea that seized Chatwin's macabre imagination:

> Could it be . . . that *Dinofelis* was a specialist predator on the primates?
> . . . Could it be . . . that *Dinofelis* was Our Beast? A Beast set aside from all
> the other Avatars of Hell? The Arch-Enemy who stalked us, stealthily and
> cunningly, wherever we went? But whom, in the end, we got the better of?[2]

The evidence led Brain to consider two options: either the early hominids were dragged into the caves by the prehistoric felines or, more curiously, they shared them with the big cats.

The period under consideration represents a major climatic upheaval of northern glaciation, when catastrophic plunges in global temperature resulted in the freezing of the north polar ice cap, approximately 2.5 million years ago. In Africa, bitter cold and droughts prevailed (although apparently not glaciation). This suggests that the *Australopithecus* may have been living together with sabertooths simply because they had nowhere else to shelter. As Chatwin puts it, these Ice Age circumstances would have resulted in the predators having "a living larder at their own front door."[3] He goes on to visualize their predicament:

> . . . without defences but their own brute strength; without fire; without warmth but their own huddled bodies; night-blind, yet forced to share their quarters with a glitter-eyed cat, who, now and then, would have prowled out to grab a straggler.[4]

Evolutionary Leap

The fact that climatic conditions forced early man to live closely with predators might not be worthy of decades of painstaking archeological research were it not for the extraordinary fact that two different forms of hominid remains were discovered in the same cave: the australopithecines already mentioned, and a more evolved hominid related to our direct ancestor, *Homo erectus.*[5]

Initially, Brain believed that the deposits under consideration were representative of a sustained evolutionary period, perhaps a million years of continuous prehistory. After years of careful analysis in Sterkfontein, Brain determined that there were two distinct layers, representing two entirely different glimpses of past ages, and that each represented a short-lived period: possibly less than 10,000 years.[6] The two separate prehistoric strata were termed Member 4 and Member 5 respectively, with Member 4 representing the older period of prehistory as the layer showed a close correspondence between hominid and sabertooth, and Member 5 representing the more recent period as the layer that contained significant stone implements and skeletal fossils related to our direct ancestors.[7]

This points to the fact that something extraordinary occurred between these two layers of prehistory. Brain analyzes it as follows:

> During Member 4 times the cats apparently controlled the Sterkfontein cave, dragging their australopithecine victims into the dark recesses. By Member 5 days, however, the new men not only had evicted the predators, but had taken up residence in the very chamber where their ancestors had been eaten.[8]

Reading the evidence, one cannot help but wonder what happened between the periods of humankind's prehistory known as Member 4 and Member 5. The answer is that the step up from one layer to the next may be understood as an abbreviated representation of the evolution from *Australopithecus* to *Homo erectus* (Southern African ape to early man), an evolutionary leap in the development of the human species.

In 1981, Brain came to the conclusion:

> At Sterkfontein, the interface between the top of Member 4 and the bottom of Member 5 represents a time interval crucial in the course of human evolution. During this time the gracile australopithecines disappeared from the Transvaal scene and the first men appeared. In this interval, too, the evolving men mastered a threat to their security that had been posed by the cave cats over countless generations.[9]

Almost two decades after the publication of these conclusions, the evidence is considerably more refined. Since then, Brain has concentrated his efforts almost exclusively on the neighboring Swartkrans caves, where the evidence, too, has convinced him of the importance of predation on the evolution of human intelligence.[10] The question raised by the particular circumstances in the cave is whether the proximity of hunter and hunted prompted the emergence from ape to human.

The discovery at the Sterkfontein Valley sites fascinated me, since it seemed to take me back to the origins of the tradition of lion heroism, in which initiates evolve into manhood through confrontation with lions.

Evolutionary Lion Heroism

C.K. Brain's hunted-to-hunter thesis sheds extraordinary light on man's evolutionary beginnings in relation to the big cats. Throughout Africa, countless generations later, this same evolutionary event is re-enacted in initiation rites in which man faces leonine combat in order to become a man.

Having apparently traced the African lion–human tradition back to its source, I yearned to talk through the implications with Credo Mutwa, lion priest of Africa.

As usual, Mutwa's whereabouts were virtually impossible to determine. The long journey I made to his hometown of Mafikeng was unsuccessful. I was told by neighbors that the shaman had moved on days before my arrival, without leaving a forwarding address. There was no further way of contacting him. I tried to telephone the sources who knew him, and who might by sheer luck be with him at the time, but none of them could be of any assistance.

I had to be content with delving deeper into his published books. I had managed to locate a recent publication, *Isilwane, the Animal,* which recorded, in no particular coherent sequence, some of the oral wisdom that Mutwa carried in memory. There was much of interest in the texts, but it was one account, in classic fireside-story form, that caught my imagination. The fable tells how fire was discovered by man – or rather how the tools for making fire were stolen from the gods and given to man. The parallels between Mutwa's symbolic tale and the archeological findings at the Sterkfontein Valley caves were uncanny.

The shaman's story is set many thousands of years ago, in an age when First Man and Woman walked upon the earth: Kintu and Mamaravi, the parents of the human race.

In his poetic turn of phrase, Mutwa describes the climatic conditions in which they found themselves, a prehistoric Ice Age:

> The earth herself began to stiffen with the intense cold. There was now frost in her hair and icicles dangled brightly from her eye lashes. She began to tremble as she fought with all means within her reach to bring the sun back to life again . . . The sun's condition grew even worse . . . The earth began to freeze . . . The sun no longer rose in the heavens . . . The forests were dark, brittle and frozen. The plains were covered under a thick blanket of rock-hard snow. The streams and the rivers no longer flowed, being held captive. Under great snarling boulders of merciless ice, the waves of the ocean were frozen and the sands of the coasts were hard, cold and cruel with ice . . .[11]
>
> The beasts were in hiding and those birds that still survived no longer flew through the air but cowered in caves and holes in the ground living a miserable and shivering existence. The animals no longer grazed upon the plains of the earth, but starved in caves and in caverns deep under the ground.[12]

Upon reading Mutwa's fable, my thoughts turned to those australopithecines huddled together for warmth in the Sterkfontein Valley caves. He describes the early humans "cowering in the rocky womb of a cave, fearful of the biting spirit of the cold."[13] But while Kintu and Mamaravi, like most of the animals around them, were on the point of expiring from hunger and cold, the situation was reversed for the feline hunters that were preying on the weakened herbivores.

The turning point of the story comes when a lion enters the cave that houses Kintu and Mamaravi. Kintu grabs a stone and hurls it at the lion, killing it.

This is the lion hero at full ferocity, emerging victorious over the feline predator. What follows in Mutwa's tale is symbolically sound in the African tradition of lion initiation:

> "Here is meat, my wife," said Kintu to Mamaravi. "The lions eat animals, and we, to prevent starvation, must eat this lion." . . . He butchered the lion, which he and his wife ate raw, wolfing the warm flesh like the wild animals that they themselves – though human – had now become.[14]

In the light of the Sterkfontein hypothesis, this moment in the cave illustrates the prey-to-predator metamorphosis: the transition of vulnerable humanity to courageous, lionhearted humanity. The shift of power from the hunted to the hunter is perfectly symbolized in the action of the hunted human eating the feline hunter. From this point on Kintu, caveman, becomes Kintu, lionman.

The Gift of Fire and Tool Invention

Significantly, anthropologists pinpoint meat consumption as the turning point in human evolution, a "hunting hypothesis" reinforced by its correspondence with the acquisition of fire, and tool invention.

Brain points out in the conclusion to his thesis that man could only have managed his critical evolutionary transition from prey to predator "through increasing intelligence reflected in developing technology."[15] He cites the mastery of fire and the development of crude weaponry as the prime advancements that "tipped the balance of power" in man's favor. These technological advancements distinguished early man from the australopithecines who, powerless to control the predators that preyed on them, were ultimately hunted to extinction.

Since the art of hunting is considered a critical barometer in human evolution, finding an accurate date for the advent of meat eating in our species enables us to interpret the very origins of human behavior. As Brain puts it:

> The taste for meat is one of the main characteristics distinguishing man from the apes, and this habit changes the whole way of life. Hunting involves co-operation within the group, division of labor, sharing food by adult males, wider interests, a great expansion of territory, and the use of tools.[16]

Just as Credo Mutwa's story of First Man confronting a lion parallels the scenario in the Sterkfontein Valley caves, so it struck me as no coincidence that the lion shaman's story deals with meat consumption simultaneously with the discovery of fire and tool production – the key indicators of hominid evolution.

> Most mythologies include the story of how fire was stolen and given to man, but Mutwa's story was particularly interesting because it was not so much fire, but the tools for making fire, that were acquired.[17]
>
> There, upon the mat, he [Kintu] saw fire sticks, and also there upon the mat he saw a stone, which, if you strike it with another stone, emitted sparks.[18]

And in the end,

> After many, many years, a sickly sun, now recovered from his pretended illness, showed his face over the mountains of the East, and the world was somewhat

warmed by the returning Lord of Day. But it was still cold, for a long time still and yet Kintu and his wife were happy in their cave, because they had kept the secret [of fire] ... a secret that was not only to benefit them, but their children's children's children down to the very days in which we live.[19]

This, then, was the fable of how early man and early woman became meat eaters through combat with lions, and how fire was stolen from the gods and given to humankind – a gift that was finally to separate humans from the animal kingdom.

Hunted to hunter: C.K. Brain's thesis was scientific; Mutwa's fable was symbolic; yet it seemed to me that the two contrary ways of approaching reality described the same event in humankind's evolutionary history.

7

GREAT HUNTERS AND MIGHTY PREDATORS

Weighed down by his quiver and his lion skin, he shouted,
"The huge lion of Nemea lies dead, throttled by these hands!"
– OVID, MYTH OF HERCULES

If Mutwa's mythological story was the shamanic retelling of the events that took place in the archeological sites at Sterkfontein, then it raised some important questions. First, how had Mutwa come by this information from prehistoric times? While C.K. Brain argued the case for the hunted-to-hunter evolution from *Australopithecus* to *Homo erectus*, based on the analysis of mountains of fossil evidence and the careful application of the scientific method, Mutwa drew his wisdom from another source entirely. Along with the stories locked into the oral tradition, the Sanusi appeared to carry with him ancient knowledge that extended beyond individual consciousness into humankind's collective memory.

If our species made a great evolutionary advance as a result of close proximity with felines, it is not unnatural to suppose that we would have trace memories of this pivotal developmental event embedded in our primal unconscious – that region of the mind to which shamanic individuals have access while in self-induced trances.

This possibility, however, raised a second question. Unlike the heroic tradition of lion combat, the culture of lion shamanism celebrates respect and kinship with lions, which is not reflected in the archeological Sterkfontein-Swartkrans evidence. For this reason, Brain's version of the hunting hypothesis could only partly account for the origins of the African culture of the lion. The scientist's theory provided me with a neat explanation for the initiation rituals of the lion, but it could not easily explain lion priesthood. Clearly, the story went deeper still.

When I finally managed to connect with Credo Mutwa again, the formalities of our greeting were immediately followed by pressing questions that had arisen out of the Sterkfontein Valley findings and Mutwa's mythological material. We settled ourselves down in two worn armchairs in the center of another Soweto house, accompanied today by a bevy of Ndebele women (minders or possibly trainee healers, I could not be sure), who were stitching traditional rag dolls up on an old Singer sewing machine and sitting on benches beading them. Among them was Mutwa's wife, Cecilia – although, in the absence of introductions, I would only discover this later.

Some time before, I had become intrigued by the fable entitled "How the Cat Came to Live with Human Beings,"[1] which contained the same notion of guardianship that Maria had introduced in respect of the feline species.

"You know that tale of how cats came to live with humankind, Credo?" I began. "Well, why is it exactly that you say cats are our keepers and not the other way around?"

The familiar mammoth figure sat before me in work clothing, with his head characteristically tilted to one side.

"In our tradition, ma'am, cats are much more than pets. They are magical creatures, and our protectors," he said. "They protect us from vermin that are harmful to us – as you know – but they also protect us from invisible enemies that we fear more than anything. The African people sing a praise song specially composed for this animal."

Mutwa paused and took a deep breath. "It goes like this . . ."

He broke into a song of praise in Zulu, and I found myself mesmerized by the spectacle of a great Sanusi singing a eulogy to a cat! It could have been ridiculous, but instead it was deeply moving.

After he had finished, he went on to translate for me:

> You are the cat, tamer of human beings, not tamed by them!
> You are the animal we all fear, favorite of sorcerers, darling of witches, treasured by *sangomas*.
> You are the cat, guardian of the village, protecting us from enemies we both can and cannot see!
> Sent by the sky gods to shield the world from invisible foes and visible vermin.
> Oh, cat, master of life!
> You guard me while I sleep,
> I honor you, dear cat,
> And feed and nourish you, for it is said that the gods and ancestors will bring eternal suffering upon any human who stoops to harm you.

After a moment's silence, Mutwa went on to explain that kings throughout Africa used to employ a special servant whose job it was to protect and care for the cats. This man was called "the Keeper of the Cats." And he was always a fearless individual, because he had to be prepared, if necessary, to die for the felines in his care.

"At one time, my grandfather toyed with the idea of training me as a Keeper of Cats," Mutwa explained. "You see, ma'am, because cats are considered magical animals, and have great powers, sorcerers or witch doctors unfortunately have been known to abuse these powers. It is not something we like to speak about, but there are those who will steal a cat from a village in order to gain powers from it through devious means. I do not like to talk of these things, ma'am, I prefer to tell how cats are used for good purposes, for purposes of divination, for instance, where *sangomas* may tell fortunes by simply gazing into the eyes of the feline."

"Is that because the *sangoma* is able to receive telepathic messages from the cat?"

"Yes, ma'am, and it is a very accurate form of divination indeed."

This reminded me of the black cat's association with magic and witches in children's fairy tales.[2] But rather than pursue this line with Mutwa, I went on to more immediate questions.

"The other story I want to know about is the one of how man came to be given the gift of fire."

"Yes, ma'am?"

"Well, my first question is about the archeological site of the Sterkfontein Valley caves in which, you may know, early man and saber-toothed cats possibly once co-existed. This is the site believed by prominent archeologists to represent the evolutionary leap of man from his ape ancestors to true man. In other words, Credo, is it the place where the 'hunted' evolved into the 'hunter'?"

"It may well be, ma'am," he commented. "What is your question?"

"You know Darwin's theory of evolution? What is your understanding of the Sterkfontein site which is thought to represent man's development out of apehood?"

Mutwa laughed. "I don't subscribe to the theory that man was once an ape," he said, his eyes twinkling behind his thick lenses. "It is a theory with so many loose things on it."

I had come to anticipate the unexpected from Mutwa, yet this response took me by surprise. "Don't you go along with the theory of hominid evolution?" I inquired.

"There are things which I know and have seen that demolish the theory of evolution – as the scientists present it," he replied.

"What things?" I asked. My first thought was that Mutwa's position was preposterous. If I hadn't nurtured such deepening respect for the shaman and his knowledge, I might have considered it laughable.

"There have been found, for instance, ma'am, in dense rock, spheres and spheroids which show all the signs of having been produced by a technology compared to which our own technology is like the Stone Age."

"Exactly where were these artifacts found?" I queried.

"In pyropheline rock in a hill quarry which I explored with Mr Boshier before the machines cut it up. These spheres were discovered inside this rock and must have been created by human beings who were already in a high stage of development millions of years ago – since that is how long it would have taken for that material to have hardened into the rock."[3]

"But couldn't these spheres have been natural and not man-made, Credo?"

"No, ma'am. These shiny spheres of reddish-silver material display special qualities. When positioned on a smooth surface, for instance, they rotate in sympathy with the earth, even when on a velvet base in a glass box."

"So you believe there was a technologically civilized culture millions of years ago?" I asked tentatively.

"Yes."

I contemplated this awhile. Raised as I was on Darwinian theory, such recalcitrance in the face of our "civilized" Western understanding was difficult to absorb. Yet, if it is indeed the case that there existed, many thousands or even millions of years ago, a civilization that had access to a technology "compared to which our own technology is like the Stone Age," then there were questions that remained unanswered.

Later, I would come across current material on the revised dating of the Sphinx, and the increasingly substantial case being made today for lost civilizations whose knowledge is manifest in every aspect of great monuments such as those of Giza and Stonehenge. When I did start reading archeoastronomers such as Graham Hancock, Robert Bauval, Adrian Gilbert, and John Anthony West – contemporary theorists who throw down the gauntlet to evolutionary historians – I had reason to think time and again of the lion shaman's words. In fact, Darwin's theory itself does not rule out the possibility of the rise and fall of civilizations. Darwin allowed for catastrophist principles, so the idea that species could evolve to a certain stage of advancement, then be destroyed by climatic conditions, and begin the process again, is not irreconcilable with his evolutionary theory. But at the time, I was surprised and disappointed by the High Shaman's response.

"We are not the first intelligent race to walk the planet," Mutwa concluded.[4]

"I see, Credo," I responded quietly, biting my tongue. "And Sterkfontein?" I asked, attempting to catch the thread of my unraveling grip on the past. "What do you think happened in the Sterkfontein caves?"

"You mean what happened between First Man and lions?"

"Yes, Credo. Did our human species evolve physically and technologically through interaction with prehistoric cats?"

"That is only a small part of the mystery, the little piece that makes sense to the scientists." He looked at me quizzically. "Why should it surprise scientists that early man may have lived together with prehistoric lions, ma'am? Have they moved so far from their roots that they cannot see the truth?"

"You mean there is more to the picture than they credit?"

"Yes, ma'am, there is very much more."

I contemplated a while, watching the attendants engrossed in their beading and listening to the hum of the sewing machine. In Mutwa's narrative version of this evolutionary turning point in humankind, there was something that bothered me. Now I made an attempt to clarify this uncomfortable detail.

"Credo, in your tale of Kintu and Mamaravi in the cave," I began, "your emphasis is really on how man came to be given the gift of fire, not so?"

"Yes, ma'am."

"Your story of fire is at the same time the story of how First Man came to eat meat."

"Yes, ma'am. It is."

"What worries me, Credo, is that in your story it is not any meat that Kintu eats – it is specifically lion meat!" I observed.

"That is so, ma'am."

"So is this fact or is it fable?"

"It was an exchange, ma'am, which is the case for all hunters and their prey, all the way down the food chain. Even the herbivore consuming from the plant kingdom is a story of the sacred exchange of souls."

This curious comment reminded me of Mutwa's shaman grandfather singing to his fig tree (which he called a "person") and how the tree in turn rewarded his gratitude with plentiful fruit.

"I still don't really understand, Credo. In respect of Sterkfontein, if you don't believe that we are descended from apes, what then happened between us and lions in this site?"

"The secret of those caves is an exchange of souls, ma'am. A sacred contract."

"You mean that is when we became lionhearted? When we, instead of the lions, became the king of the beasts?"

"That is the case, ma'am. No animal's soul can be taken against his will. It was a gift that lions gave to man at that time."

"But if it was a sacred contract," I responded, feeling unaccountably distressed at what was as yet incomprehensible to me, "then we've broken it. We haven't honored the gift that lions gave us!" I was thinking of the fine balance of nature, the delicate chain of being that we appear to have broken; the global ecosystem that we humans have systematically undermined and, it would appear, irreparably damaged.

"This is unfortunately the case, ma'am," came the shaman's somber response.

Bringing a soul dimension into the evolutionary picture refined the view of the relationship between carnivore and prey. It reminded me of the notion of hunting magic employed by Bushman shaman hunters, in which their pictorial representation of the hunt was believed to have an influence on the outcome of the actual hunt. Mutwa's words were beginning to help my understanding that, far from primitive superstition, shamanic "magic" was, in fact, attunement to the long-forgotten laws of nature. It now occurred to me that shamans worked with the real connection between different things, but at a more profound level than was apparent to the rest of us.

The thought of the desecration and havoc that modern man has wreaked upon his natural heritage gave me the first intimations that we ourselves, rather than the shaman with his primitive magic, have lost our reality principle.

The shaman believes that no prey is killed by chance, but rather (at a soul level) offers itself up for the taking, according to God's plan. By influencing the hunt, therefore, the shaman is identifying and honoring the soul connection that he or she believes exists between the hunter and the animal that becomes his prey.

Early this century, Sir James Frazer described this phenomenon in his famous study of magic and religion, *The Golden Bough*. He recounted how hunters from "primitive" tribes in different parts of the globe all valued their prey so highly that there was a sympathy, or a communication at a spirit level, between hunter and hunted.[5]

More recently, through close contact with the last surviving Bushman hunters of the Kalahari, South African field researcher Louis Liebenberg bore witness to some of these hunting beliefs in action. Liebenberg records the deep respect with which the hunters regard their quarry, venerating the animal both as man's equal and as precious livelihood, which amounts to an unspoken contract between two species. Significantly, for the sympathetic relationship between hunter and prey, it is one of the founding beliefs in Bushman cosmology that all animals were once people.

This mesmerizing connection between hunter and prey is well documented in the recent documentary feature film on the last of the Bushman hunters, *The Great Dance*, which was made by brothers Craig and Damon Foster. The film records how, after hours of endurance running in pursuit of herd of kudu in the heat of the day, a Bushman hunter finally outruns the antelope. One particular kudu doe turns to face the hunter and seemingly offers herself up to his spear.[6]

This profoundly moving moment captured on film reminded me of an observation in Liebenberg's study, when he pinpoints the "inevitable contradiction" in the Bushman tracker once he starts identifying himself with his prey:

> To track down an animal, the tracker must ask himself what he would do if he were that animal. In the process of projecting himself into the position of the animal, he actually feels like the animal. The tracker therefore develops a sympathetic relationship with the animal which he then kills.[7]

Liebenberg refers to the "sympathetic relationship" that exists between the Bushman hunter and his prey but, from Mutwa's own words, I had inferred that a similar level of interspecies communication might have operated between emerging man and the felines that he had to overpower as a means to survival.

Of Cats and Men

On this visit, I had brought with me something I imagined might be of interest to the lion shaman, and I decided to produce it now in an attempt to break the grim silence.

The night before seeing Mutwa, I had had what I considered to be an amazing piece of good fortune. With the White Lions in mind, I had been tracking down records of Bushman art in the vain hope of finding a depiction of a white feline in the ancient cave paintings. On the way home I had passed a bookstore, where a recent publication was displayed in the window. It was called *The Hunter's Vision*. My interest had been sparked by the title, and the fact that the work purported to be a collection of images from the "prehistoric art of Zimbabwe," and I had immediately walked in and bought it. I hadn't found a White Lion reference, but the book did reveal something equally exciting – a cave painting from Wedza (northeast of Great Zimbabwe National Monument) which illuminated the hunted-to-hunter theme perfectly.[8]

In his earliest writings (some four decades ago), Mutwa paid tribute to the Bushmen, at that time one of the most misunderstood and maltreated people on the globe. He insisted that Bushman cave paintings acted as a visual counterpart to the ancient memory carried by African initiates, corroborating closely guarded secrets contained in the oral traditions. "The Bushmen," he wrote, "though still living by force of circumstance in the ways of prehistoric man, were, and still are, the most intelligent and talented race in Africa. With their paintings in caves and shelters, they have made the most profound contribution to the 'documented' history of Africa, [recording] with their pictographic writing events that took place many thousands of years ago."[9]

Expert opinion has now caught up with Mutwa. Today's specialists on Bushman art, such as David Lewis-Williams, Thomas Dowson, and Peter Garlake, concur that cave paintings were largely executed by shamans transmitting wisdom received through shamanic trance.

If, as I was now beginning to understand, shamans are able to access an archetypal level of information within the residual memories of humankind, then it is understandable that traces of the lion–human evolutionary event might be revealed in atavistic dreams of shamanic initiates and stored in their meticulously preserved oral history, just as they are preserved in Bushman rock art. With this in mind, I was pleased to show Mutwa my discovery.

In a distinct three-part series, the Wedza work functions like a moving scene painted on rock, transporting the viewer right back to the very origins of bipedal man.[10] Working from left to right, the first part shows a saber-toothed feline with the body of a badly mutilated hominid lying beside him. The second part shows two tusked creatures not unlike the first, except that these are clearly neither hominid nor feline, but in fact a perfect combination of both species. Their hind legs resemble human legs – and in fact are closely replicated in the humans of the third part. Their feline forelegs could equally be human forearms, with the paws slightly distended, like fingers on a human hand. These dangle beneath them, as if no longer carrying weight, and are raised a little off the ground, suggesting that these creatures are poised to rise on to their hindquarters and stand on two legs. But their heads with pointed ears and long snouts are pure cat: to be precise, pure saber-toothed cat, the tusks being the primary feature.

The powerful cinematic quality of this shamanic painting allows one to virtually witness the evolutionary process taking place – even right down to a detail such as the feline's tail, which is lengthy in the first section, but progressively shortened through the sequence until it is nonexistent in the humans of the third section. In this third and final section the transformation is complete. Two perfect representations of bipedal man are proudly shown. There could be no better depiction of "mighty hunters," broad-shouldered, well-endowed and, of course, heavily armed – with magnificent oversized bows and arrows. And to emphasize the point that these are meat-eating humans, their full attention is directed at two immaculately painted antelope. The evolution from prey to predator is accomplished.

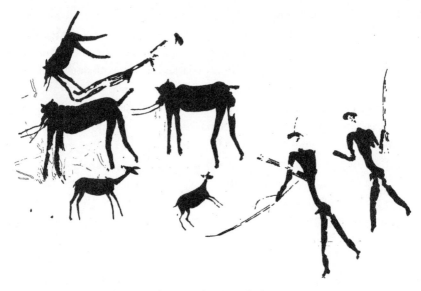

The Wedza painting depicts the stages of transition from hunted to hunter.

"Wow!" Mutwa said. I had never heard him use this expression before. "That's wonderful!" he added.

I briefly outlined for Mutwa the hominid–*Dinofelis* hypothesis. "Because there were so many bones of this second type of saber-toothed feline – with shorter tusks – in the same cave as the hominids, the scientists are beginning to suspect that *Dinofelis* might have been the main predators of early man."

"Forgive me, ma'am," the shaman responded. "But that is poppycock, hogwash. How can they add two plus two and make 35?" Mutwa had not so much as lifted an eyebrow in delivering this colorful retort.

"Are you saying they are mistaken in this hypothesis, Credo?"

"What I am saying is that it is rubbish, ma'am."

"How do you explain the apparent co-existence of hominid bones with *Dinofelis* bones, then?"

Mutwa paused for a long time. Then he sighed. "Much is locked up in secrets that we may not reveal."

I hesitated. "Are we suggesting that there was some kind of cooperation between early man and prehistoric lions, Credo?" I ventured. He had removed his eyes from the reproduction, and he was focusing straight ahead once more through his frosted spectacles.

"We live in a strange world of separatism, ma'am, a world in which things that really belong together and which ought to be seen as part of a great whole are cruelly separated."

"Why do you say that, Credo?" I probed, trying to get beneath the words to the heart of what the shaman was saying.

"Because, ma'am, Western man has come to believe that he is the master of all living things, and that nature is there to be tamed at best; despised, broken, and destroyed at worst. It has led to a very dangerous situation, ma'am: the belief that human beings can build a shining technological future without animals, and trees, and other life-forms." He shook his head. "Until this attitude is combated and erased from the human mind, Westernized human beings will be a danger to all earthly life, including themselves."

"But how do we combat this, Credo?" I questioned, noting the sadness rather than anger in his voice.

"Ma'am, I say we must take a great spiritual step backward. We must embrace the original view of creation: that everything around us is part of one great and interconnected whole. We must change this habit of regarding ourselves as superior or special creatures. This misconception has led us to the very brink of destruction."

He paused solemnly, his pupils dilated behind the thick lenses.

"We have become denatured. In old Africa, ma'am, we believed that human beings could not exist without animals, birds, and fishes or trees. We believed that the universe was not only all around us – but also within us. For this reason, many African gods were depicted as part animal and part human." He looked at me gravely. "If your God had the body of a man and the head of a lion, I ask you, ma'am, would you shoot lions for sport, or commercial reasons?"

"I should hope not, Credo," I said, trying to see the connections he was making. "But how would you say this relates to Sterkfontein?"

"Ma'am, it is all part of the same mystery."

He paused, then reconsidered. "It is mysterious, ma'am, but it is no riddle. Take the Sphinx, for example. It is a giant carving of a man-lion, is it not? There is no Sphinx riddle. A secret, yes, and it is there for everyone to see."

This had never struck me before. Of course: the Sphinx, both human and leonine, was the ultimate symbol of lion shamanism and the unity between man and nature.

While various scholars have argued that the Sphinx was originally a lion, the fact that the Egyptians carved their pharaoh's head into its leonine body is testament to a belief system that identified the deified pharaoh with the power of the king of the beasts. While I was still trying to come to grips with this ancient yet remarkable revelation, Mutwa himself had apparently moved on.

"Man must make two connections," he said. "He must reconnect with the earth and he must reconnect with the stars. We may not talk about such things as power, ma'am. But in Egypt in those days, the high priests possessed an art which we call the 'star thing.' We may not speak about this thing, ma'am, for it is a very powerful force. Through it, they were able to enter the minds of animals, such as lions, and harness their power so that these animals would build their sacred monuments. I may not say more."

He was losing me. "Are we talking about mind power here, Credo?" I suggested.

"You might call it that, ma'am."

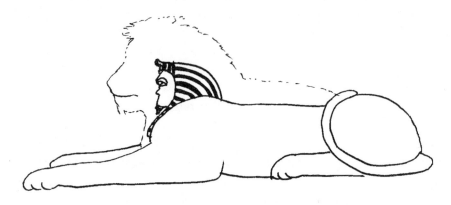

Proportions of the Sphinx indicate that the head was probably recarved. The question as to why the monument is represented as part lion and part human goes back to our earliest evolutionary origins.

"Well, in my Egyptian research," I observed, attempting to return the conversation to concrete examples from Egypt, "it's true that I've come across a lot of carved reliefs relating pharaohs to lions."

I was thinking of the murals depicting the twin theme of lion priesthood and lion heroism. Pharaohs were regularly shown either in combat with lions, or enthroned with friendly lions at their side.[11] There are scenes of rampant lions pacing beneath the pharaoh's chariot as he heads into battle.[12] Rameses II was known to be accompanied wherever he went in peace and in war by his own lioness, Anta-m-Nekht, whose name meant "Goddess Anta loves me." Lions, like the pharaohs themselves, were considered no less than royalty.[13]

"Ma'am," Mutwa responded, with a wry smile, "that may be so, but the Sphinx is older than the days of the pharaohs – by many, many, many thousands of years, ma'am."

"So does the Sphinx somehow relate to hominid events at Sterkfontein?" I proposed, attempting to make sense of this revelation.

"Ma'am, it is part of the same mystery."

The women's sewing machines were singing in my head. "I see. So this is what we call the Great Knowledge, Credo?" I queried.

"It is part of the Great Knowledge, yes, ma'am." He paused again, perhaps detecting the puzzlement in my eyes.

"If you continue to follow the footprints of the White Lions," he said slowly, as if taking me through the steps in his own mind, "you yourself will eventually come to know the secrets of the Great Sphinx."

"Is that so, Credo?" I asked, attempting not to sound incredulous at the thought of unlocking humankind's oldest riddle.

"You do not know it yet, ma'am, but you yourself are on the path of the shaman," Mutwa observed.

My head was reeling. At the same time, I was aware of a dull pain in my stomach: a combination of fear and excitement. Myself a shaman? I recalled Maria's intimations to this effect. On being questioned as to why strategic bones continued to roll off the mat in my direction, she had finally revealed that this meant I was destined to be a *sangoma* – "Not one who digs roots and heals people," she had said, "but one who carries the flame of light, like Mu-twah."

"Forgive me, Credo," I said now. "Thank you for all this information, but you must excuse me. I can no longer think straight."

I retraced my route until I reached the concrete highway, feeling buoyed up and strangely dissociated from the Johannesburg traffic, which was virtually stationary. As usual, once I had allowed the unfamiliar ideas to settle, I would regret not having asked numerous other questions that demanded urgent answers.

8

THE WHITE LIONS ACCORDING TO THE GREAT KNOWLEDGE

Science without religion is lame. Religion without science is blind.
– ALBERT EINSTEIN

Prior to this point in evolution, our species was a natural part of the ecosystem. After imitating the hunting and meat-eating functions of the feline predators, we found ourselves at the very top of the food chain: the kings of beasts and rulers of the earth. In this position, there was an overriding incentive to view ourselves as different and better. Yet shamanic wisdom teaches that both these perceptions are deeply mistaken: we are not different from the natural kingdom, nor superior, but remain a critically integral part. It is precisely our tendency toward egotism and virtual reality that has created the most dangerous of all illusions in our minds – that of omnipotence.

King of the Food Chain

In Timbavati's teeming bushveld, I blended scientific theory with shamanic knowledge. Both made good sense.

On game drives, and occasionally on foot, I was lucky enough to observe prides of lions lounging, fast asleep under mopane trees, with their paws curled up luxuriantly or, if rudely disturbed, crouched on all fours and staring back at me with the tufts of their tails flicking angrily. Mutwa's humorous observation that these great cats have the fluffy-tipped tail of a donkey pinned to their rears suggests the symbolic fusion of carnivore and herbivore.

Occupying the top of the food chain, lions effectively include the herbivores within their biological makeup, as well as the plants upon which the herbivores feed, and so on, right down to the nutrients from the soil upon which the plants feed. This begins to make sense of the persistent connection that shamanism draws between lions and the earth itself.

In the introduction to *Isilwane, the Animal*,[1] Mutwa records the principles of nature conservation that were strictly adhered to in the Great African Tradition. In the old African way, every clan has a totem animal, after which the clan was originally named.

This totem must be protected by the tribe within the tribe's territorial boundaries, under all circumstances. It must never be harmed in any manner – or devastation will ensue. This decree effectively means that it is also essential to protect the animals that co-exist with the totem animal, for the totem animal cannot survive without its fellow creatures. Ancient tribal law protects not only the food upon which the sacred animal grazes and the animals that graze alongside the sacred animal, but also the animals that prey upon the sacred animal. As an example, Mutwa recounts how some of the Bushman clans had the eland (antelope) as their totem. But they knew that protecting the eland was not enough. The plants that fed the eland, as well as the lion that fed upon it, needed to be protected. This was essential to ensure the survival and nourishment of the fittest antelope, since, if the harmonious balance was not maintained, the eland might overbreed and destroy the very grasslands upon which it fed.[2] The preying lion co-exists with all of the animals in the animal kingdom, therefore it is ultimately the duty of every single clan to ensure the lion's protection and preservation.

In describing this decree, which was sacrosanct to tribes throughout the African continent, Mutwa could only lament the loss of the Great Tradition, and the subsequent extinction of the vast herds that once graced the African plains:

> What many people do not realise is that these huge, wild herds existed because the native people of Africa regarded them as a blessing from the Gods – as something unbelievably sacred and vital for the continued existence of human beings . . . No-one ever interfered with these great migrations because they really believed that wildlife was the soul, the very life-blood, of Mother Earth. When white people came to Africa, they had been conditioned to separate themselves spiritually and physically from wildlife . . . Many hundreds of years ago, a wise old man called Pinda Moleli prophesied that one of the first indications that the end of the world had come would be the disappearance of herds from the African plains. The herds have almost disappeared and Pinda Moleli's prophecy appears to be coming true.[3]

Mutwa's somber conclusion reminded me of how humankind's attempt at royalty, at the top of the food chain, has been miserably ineffectual at upholding and maintaining the sacred laws of nature.

The shaman's words also reminded me that the end of the world is not a sudden, unexpected event. Rather, it is the consequence of humans systematically eroding their own natural habitat – actively working toward their own extinction. We are killing the lions that we should be befriending.

When I questioned Maria on the widespread shamanic notion of lions as civilization-bearers, she restated the idea of the lion-as-teacher, not without betraying a flash of exasperation. "They bring us wisdom," the interpreter explained. "The White Lions guard the land. Without them, Maria says the earth will die . . ."

In the Great African Tradition, the lion is said to be the wise judge, since he takes down sick or weak prey, and so maintains nature's laws. In the kingdom of lions, the king of the beasts once achieved a perfect balance of law and order at the top of the food chain. In the kingdom of man, can we humans truly say we have achieved the same harmony and balance? When it comes to preserving our earth, which of the two species, man or lion, is the more responsible custodian of our natural resources?

I had not thought of it this way before.

Conservation Value

The notion of a human being who can pacify lions is identifiable with "power." Although it remained a mystery to me what powers shamans possessed that could turn lions from foe to friend, I no longer doubted the authenticity of this shamanic process. Maria was a powerful woman. What made the figure of Timbavati's Lion Queen all the more compelling was that the creature with whom she co-existed and communicated was not only the king of beasts, but also the rarest lion on earth: the White Lion of Timbavati.

All lions are a majestic sight in their natural environment. But my sightings of Timbavati's great lions were enlivened by an additional magic, since these tawny lions might well be carriers of the unique white gene – just like those lions from which Maria had once rescued us. Sadly, 1991, year of the rescue, was the last time a White Lion was spotted in the wild in Timbavati.

Whenever I thought about the White Lions, I felt an aching loss, remembering that those legendary beasts that once stalked these plains were now all but extinct. After their brief appearance for the first time in living memory, they had died out in the wild – or worse, been actively hunted down by poachers and trophy hunters.[4]

For some reason, many landowners in the Timbavati region do not view the extinction of the White Lions as a great loss, nor do they see their arrival in the first place as representing anything remarkable. Astoundingly, White Lions are considered to have no "conservation value." Since the White Lion is classified as *Panthera leo,* along with the ordinary lion species, the extinction of the White Lion is not considered a loss since it represents no threat to the lion species in general.

Over my many years of visiting Timbavati, whenever I asked landowners, rangers, and conservationists why they believed the White Lions had cropped up specifically in this particular place on our globe, I received the same answer: chance.

At first I had no immediate grounds for assuming otherwise, but Credo Mutwa and my instinct kept telling me that "chance" was simply not a good enough explanation for the sudden appearance of this unique animal.

First reported by a conservationist in Timbavati in the 1970s, the White Lions soon became lauded as a curiosity and genetic freak in nature magazines across the globe.

Chris McBride believed he might have been the first human to spot them; in fact, legends of their existence lie deep in the ancestral memories of African shamans.

In contrast to the conventional view of conservationists and game rangers, which maintains that the aberrant white gene is a random mutation of no consequence or "conservation value," shamanic wisdom views the White Lions as the highest form of enlightenment bearer or teacher. Maria's perspective led me to view the White Lions not only as a unique strain in and of themselves, but as symbolic custodians of a message specifically intended for humankind at this particular time.

It was this version of the truth that I began to consider as I again sought access to Credo Mutwa, from whom I was to learn the extraordinary tale of Timbavati's White Lions according to the Great Knowledge.

Blue Blood, White Genes

Much to my frustration, it was impossible for many months to contact Sanusi Mutwa. His intermediaries stonewalled all efforts to get through to him. It continued to perplex me that such a commanding figure should surround himself with characters who did not appear to have his best interests at heart.

The set of advisors who had attached themselves to Mutwa at this stage of his life were the latest in a long line of patron figures who apparently set out with the positive intention of protecting the great man and his words, but ended up controlling and exploiting him. Mutwa's history showed a repeating pattern in this respect, and in the years that I've known him this pattern has replicated itself several times over. It has occurred to me that these exploitative people may in part be responsible for discrediting Mutwa, after discovering that their attachment to him failed to bring the material returns on which they had bargained.

For the moment, however, there was no way of reaching him except through a particular advertising agency, which (quite amazingly) believed that it owned him and had, in fact, made the shaman sign a contract giving them rights to every word uttered. I set up an appointment and a sum was negotiated with them for my hour's session. This time, we met in the heart of the leafy suburbs of Johannesburg, at an appointed place and at an agreed time.

In contrast to the bleakness of the Soweto box house, the Johannesburg apartment had the plush anonymity of an international hotel. A Scandinavian-style table in beech-wood veneer stood in the center of the room, and a suede-covered lounge suite was positioned impersonally around a glass coffee table on thick wall-to-wall carpeting. The advertising executive stood ready to monitor every detail of my encounter with Mutwa. As we waited, I reminded myself how deeply wounded the great shaman was by the brutal tragedies of his life, and I began to imagine how vulnerable he must be. I came to the conclusion that he no longer trusted his deeper instincts in respect of individuals who attached themselves to him, and he no longer expected fair treatment, since he had been cursed with ill treatment most of his life. It was a desperately sad condition to witness. Despite his courageous act in defying the High Oath of Secrecy, Mutwa was after all, at one level, merely a simple man who lived in dire fear of the consequences of his actions. He believed in the curse that had befallen him and, alas, in believing it, he perpetuated it. Having endured great sacrifices in bringing enlightenment to the world, Mutwa's love for humanity was clear to the point of trusting and believing indiscriminately in humankind's good intentions. Unfortunately, our species did not always live up to his high expectations.

Waiting in the Johannesburg apartment, it seemed as if I had seen the same scene many times before in home-and-leisure catalogs. But once Credo Mutwa entered, his singular presence filled the room.

His mood seemed low, and there were no immediate signs of recognition.

"Good evening, Credo," I greeted him informally.

"Good evening, ma'am."

The executive explained to Mutwa that I had come with a request to hear the story of the White Lions, and the medicine man nodded slowly. Although appearing even more sizeable than I remembered him, Mutwa carried himself with grace. We moved over to the central table, where I sat down beside him, with the advertising executive diagonally across from us.

My overwhelming impression was once again that of a man who suffered from a privileged knowledge with dignity and humility.

We began with some background information about what he had recently been up to, and he mentioned the small piece of land that he still hoped to acquire one day. At this point, some ten minutes into our interview, the advertising executive moved out of the room to answer a call on his cellular phone, and Mutwa and I exchanged some quiet words.

First, I informed Mutwa of the latest isotope findings in respect of the fossilized bones at Swartkrans, and the evidence indicated that, while living in the same caves as our early ancestors, *Dinofelis* was not preying on them.

"Of course he didn't," responded the shaman emphatically. "This is known from African legends. In places of initiation, they tell us there were two kinds, ma'am. There was the big predator with a long tail and very long teeth, like swords – the great Ngewula. He was ferocious. Then there was the big predator with a shorter tail and shorter teeth, like knives – the lesser Ngewula. He was different. Not all predators murdered human beings. And even those who did, even the fiercest, could be tamed – and were tamed. This is known all over Africa. Even if the scientists find, through their experiments, that there are human remains in the bones of these lesser Ngewula, it is not correct that humans were being murdered, ma'am. This is nonsense. These beasts might have come across a human being that was already dead, or dying. That is possible."

"How do you account for the fact that *Dinofelis*, the lesser Ngewula, appears to have been living with the ape-men in the same caves?" I inquired. "Is it possible that these predators were not our arch-enemies, but actually our guardians?"

"Look into your heart, ma'am. I believe you know the answer."

My heart was pounding. I pictured the *Dinofelis* with his savage canines. "The most fearsome of all beasts . . . our protector?" I asked.

"Even the fiercest of predators can be tamed." By way of example, my great orator friend recounted another story from the Great Knowledge, much like the rescue of King Mageba from death at the hands of his enemies by his own friendly lion. This story involved lion priestesses, the matriarchs of the Magaliesberg mountains, and how they were rescued by a great saber-toothed Ngewula which appeared out of the mountain mists and devoured their enemies.

"But I thought sabertooths were extinct a very long time ago – many, many thousands of years before the time of the Magaliesberg matriarchs," I observed, not wishing to spoil Mutwa's story.

The lion shaman smiled enigmatically. Alluding to the sabertooth's disappearance, he recounted a delightful short tale of how the sabertooth was banished from the earth, "after he accidentally bit the bottom of the Great Earth Mother, thinking she was a hippopotamus."

In a more serious vein, Mutwa then informed me that this prehistoric predator was, in truth, not altogether dead. Intriguingly, he instructed me that there had been several sightings in the Magaliesberg mountains (which encircle the Sterkfontein Valley) – particularly, it seemed, under unusual weather conditions. In firsthand accounts, this extraordinary beast has been described as substantially larger than a lion, with very few spots on its pelt.

Unlikely as it may have been, it was tantalizing to visualize the existence of a prehistoric predator believed to be long gone, particularly in view of the colony of prehistoric coelacanth fish discovered near Sodwana on South Africa's Natal coast. The coelacanth is found in the fossil record of 60 million years ago, and has remained virtually unchanged to this day.[5]

"So what was going on between our prehistoric ancestors and these sabertoothed cats at the Sterkfontein Valley caves?" I persisted.

A flicker lit up Mutwa's face before it was quenched in solemnity. "Much is held secret, and much must remain so." Appreciating the taboos that Mutwa had broken in delivering ancient knowledge to a wider audience, I had learned to curb my frustration at not always receiving immediate answers. Despite Mutwa's having broken the Oath of Silence, there were many occasions when the shaman made it clear that certain information was withheld from me on the grounds of my own lack of shamanic initiation. With the subject closed, a protracted silence followed, which was finally broken by Mutwa.

"You have come for the story of the White Lions. Let me begin by asking you a question, ma'am." Once again, I wondered whether this was an indication of his doubts as to my readiness, or fitness, to receive the secret story behind the White Lions.

"What do you think those stones are for that stand on their own in Timbavati?"

"You mean those strange bladelike stones embedded in the ground? I don't know," I replied. "But I have wondered whether they have some symbolic meaning. They've always appeared incongruous to me, in the middle of the African bushveld."

"They are astrological stones," he explained. "They are there for a purpose."

"I see, Credo." This immediately captured my interest, but I hoped the story of the astrological stones was not a decoy to distract my attention from the subject of the White Lions, which, after all, was the reason I had tracked Mutwa down yet another time. Only later would I realize that each one of his pointed questions was a concise clue in the White Lion mystery.

"And ma'am, what do you feel when you go to the land of Timbavati?" Mutwa continued.

"I feel an intense sense of peace, Credo – and also excitement!" I admitted, my memory sweeping over the many magical moments I had spent in Timbavati since childhood.

Mutwa smiled. "You know, ma'am, when a *sangoma* is sick of spirit he needs to reconnect with the Great Earth Spirit. There are very sacred places of great energy. There are places of earth energy. There are places of water energy. And then, finally, there are places of star energy. Timbavati is a place of star energy." I recalled then how Mutwa had described his own visit to Timbavati in our first meeting, a pilgrimage that was precipitated by an illness or depression from which he suffered.

"Credo, you told me when we last met that you had gone to Timbavati hoping to see a White Lion walking freely in the bushveld. And, of course, you never saw a single one – because they are extinct in the wild. You told me that if you had seen a White Lion, it would have helped you to make a very important decision in your life."

"Yes, ma'am. A very important one," he responded.

"As it was, you didn't see a White Lion and so you never made that very important decision."

"Yes, ma'am."

"May I ask, Credo, what is so important about your seeing the White Lions? What was the decision you needed to make?"

Mutwa sighed, raising his eyebrows so that they appeared like two question marks above the frames of his glasses.

"Would you rather not tell me about this decision?" I asked, hesitantly. "Is it too personal?"

"Yes, ma'am," he retracted. "It is a very important thing – a very personal thing . . ."

The advertising executive had returned, looking efficient and slightly harassed, and the three of us sat in silence for a moment. "I will tell you the story of the White Lions of Timbavati, ma'am," Mutwa began. "It has never before been recorded. It must not be changed by a single word."[6]

"You have my word on this, Credo," I said.

I prepared myself for a fabulous tale in the great tradition of epic storytelling.

The advertising executive shifted in his seat, watching us impassively. His thoughts seemed to be elsewhere.

Mutwa settled himself with his hands placed one above the other on the table, and I could tell from the expression on his face that he was preparing for a long slow delivery of an important story. Never before set down in writing, yet unchanged by time, the tale of the White Lions of Timbavati was about to be presented by one of Africa's pre-eminent guardians of tribal history.

"I am ready," I told Credo as I switched on my tape recorder.

"First of all," Mutwa began, "if you want to know the mystery of the place called Timbavati, you must please find the real meaning of the name Timbavati. Many people don't know what this name really means. The name Timbavati really is 'Timba-vaati': *Timba*: 'to come down (like a bird)'; *vaati*: 'to the ground.' So Timbavati really means 'the place of coming down.' The place where something came down – in the ancient Tsonga language."

Mutwa paused, perhaps re-evaluating whether I was a fit recipient for this revelation.

"So what came down at Timbavati, you may ask," he continued, with a rhetorical question. "What is the story of this place?"

I waited in silence.

"Many years ago, long before the white people came to South Africa, there was an empire which had succeeded an even greater empire before it. Ruling the people at that time, in the area in which today we find the Kruger National Park, was a female chief, a queen, called Numbi, 'the Ugly.' Numbi, though lacking in beauty, was a very wise woman indeed. She was a woman of great spiritual power. She was a Rain Mother of her people. In fact, the Rain Queens of the Eastern Transvaal are really a continuation of an ancient matriarchal system which goes back many hundreds of years in Southern Africa.

"It is said that a terrible illness attacked Queen Numbi. Her legs swelled and her stomach swelled. She was very close to death when her people prayed to the ancestral spirits for a sign which would help to save the queen's life. For many months the people prayed. For many months nothing happened. One day when Numbi was very close to death, night fell, the stars appeared in the sky; there was no moon, only the stars, and animals were sounding off in the bush: lions roaring, hyenas laughing, and owls hooting. It was then that loud shouts were heard from many villages in the vicinity of Numbi's great royal village. People were shouting, 'Aaayeeeh! Yeeehhhh!' There was great excitement.

"'What is going on?' asked the queen Numbi, propping herself up on one elbow on her sick bed. An elder crawled into Numbi's hut and told her that a strange light was coming out of the skies. A star was falling to the earth. A very great star.

"'Oh, Great One! That star shines like the sun at midday. It has lighted up the whole land as if it was daylight!'

"'Take me out! Take me out immediately!' cried Queen Numbi. 'This sight I must see!'

"Servants arrived to obey the queen's command. They supported the weakened woman out of her hut and out into the open. She was covered by a jackal-skin blanket, and her hair was as white as snow in stark contrast to the polished ebony of her face and shoulders.

"It was true! It was true. Something was happening out there.

"The old woman looked up and saw a great ball of light, bigger than a meeting hut, coming slowly down into the bush. It was as if in a dream. The thing came down with incredible slowness. Slowly it came down, illuminating the whole landscape, bathing it in its eerie bluish-white light. It circled down in the bush somewhere, and there was a great halo of bluish light where the thing had come down.

"'*Timbi-lé! Timbi-lé!*' cried the people. 'It has come down! *Timbi-Lé Vaa-ti!* It has come down to the ground!'

"People wanted to rush forward to go and see what that thing was. But fear held them back. But Queen Numbi was a woman beyond fear. She was not afraid of anything. She called to her two oldest and most reliable servants, Namasele and Ngwandi, and she ordered these women to support her on either side and to lead her toward that thing down there in the valley.

"The women walked for a long time, they were old, their bones were creaking and their joints stiff, but at last they came to the place where this strange spherical light was sitting like a newborn sun upon the ground. The women heard a strange humming noise coming from the sphere of light. For a long time they stood there, squinting into the glare of the strange star lying on the ground. It was huge, it was big, but it radiated very little heat. The women were amazed.

"'Great One, Mother of the People,' said Ngwandi, 'we must go from here!'

"'I agree,' said Numbi. 'Let us go, my faithful ones. We might accidentally anger the gods.'

"The women turned away to go, moving slowly, and all of a sudden Ngwandi saw something move behind her. She said, '*Maaai!* Look!'

"And the queen turned and there stood a god who had emerged from the glare of bluish light. The god was a being of pure light, yellowish light; he had no features to his face. They could make out shoulders, the head, the body, the limbs. And the being was walking toward them. They stood, and the being lifted its right hand, a hand of fire, a hand of light, without any fingers.

"And Numbi said to her servants, 'Look, my servants, the god raises its hand in salutation to me, Numbi. The god wants me to approach it . . .'

"'Do not do so, Great Mother!'

"'I will do so. I am the queen.'

"Numbi walked slowly toward the god. She moved with shambling gait on weakened knees. And she came close to the god and lifted her hand. And the god came close to Numbi and placed its hand upon hers. And then the god disappeared. One moment it was there, the next it was gone. Only its footprints in the soft sand testified to the fact that it had been there.

"Numbi was there, standing a dark silhouette against the glare of the star. And then she turned, and as she turned to face her servants, the servants noticed that Numbi's eyes were glowing.

"She walked toward them, and she said, 'Ngwandi, listen, my two little sisters. You must go now, return home.'

"'Where will you go, Great One? Why do you want us to leave you here . . .?'

"Numbi said, 'The gods want me. That is why the god came.'

"The two old women gripped each other like things gone mad as they watched their queen walking slowly toward the glare of the unknown thing. She walked and walked and walked, and then, in the bluish glare, the women made out human forms, yellow ghosts against the blue. And the glare swallowed up Numbi and she was seen no more.

"The two old women could not run away from that sight. For a long time, they stood there transfixed and then they left, moving as fast as their old limbs could allow them. And then, just as they reached Numbi's village, the star that had come from the sky rose slowly toward the dark heavens, once again bathing the entire landscape in its eerie light. It moved faster this time. Like a thunderbolt, it sought the distant skies and disappeared.

"Then it was observed, many years after Numbi's disappearance, many years after the strange star that had come to ground, all animals that stayed within that area where the mysterious object had settled on the ground were giving birth to snow-white offspring. It is said that at one time people saw many white leopards at Timbavati. The people saw herds of antelope, impala, and eland which were snow white with blue eyes. Some of these elands grew up and only had one horn instead of two. And some of the impalas and elands had strange malformations involving their hooves or their horns.[7]

"And a pride of lions had also moved into the area where the strange star had come down from the sky and it was observed that they too started giving birth to white offspring with blue eyes.

"Many kings who ruled after Numbi declared Timbavati a sacred place, especially after two elephants – a bull elephant and a cow – were seen which were unbelievably white in the color of their skin. These elephants avoided the light of the sun and used to graze when the sun . . . was either setting or before it rose. It is said that these elephants mysteriously disappeared after that – but the sacred White Lions were born again and again in that place. It is for this reason that a great King, Npepo I – the original Npepo – declared this place to be a sacred place where no hunting was allowed. It was not Paul Kruger who declared that this should be a place only for the animals, it was King Npepo, not only because of the repeated birth of White Lions but also because of white leopards and white baboons as well.

"At one time, we are told, the great King Shaka made a sacred pilgrimage to Timbavati. King Shaka was not only a great warrior but also an amazing prophet who made many predictions, some of which have already come true.

"This, ma'am, is the story of Timbavati."

Mutwa paused, holding his hands gently in his lap, and waited.

"Was that the end of Queen Numbi?" I asked.

"No, ma'am, it was not. Our guardians tell that she returned to rule her people. She was now believed to have special powers, and there are accounts of extraordinary deeds which were performed by her."

"I will preserve this story in the exact words it was told to me, Credo," I assured him.

"Thank you, ma'am, thank you," he said. "Understand this, ma'am, just as these stories reconstruct Africa's long past, so our present story is added to the long scroll of memory and handed down to future generations. The stories of the Guardians of Umlando do not have an ending, ma'am. The story of the White Lions continues today, and is added to during our own lifetime by today's Guardian of Umlando."

For a protracted moment I mulled over Mutwa's story, imagining how the original episode would have been related firsthand to the tribe's most highly respected shaman, who would have gone on to relate it word for word to the next initiate, and so on through the generations. In this way, the story would retain much of its original flavor, as if the orator himself were present at the time of the occurrence.

"Do you have any questions?" the advertiser prompted me.

"Well, yes, as a matter of fact I do," I replied.

My immediate question had to do with the date of the White Lions' first occurrence. I asked Mutwa if he knew of the precise date for the "fallen star" which, according to his account, preceded the birth of the first White Lions.

"Ma'am, we cannot say exactly," he responded. "It was before the establishment of the Zulu nation, in the time of Numbi. That we know."

"And Numbi was a real person, not a mythological figure?" I asked, reminded all of a sudden that one of the gates to the Kruger National Park was named after Numbi.

"Yes, ma'am, a real person. She has direct descendants who are alive today."

"And the Zulu nation, when was that established?"

"Over 400 years ago."

"But if they have been around for over four centuries, surely one would expect a white pelt to have shown up somewhere?" I asked Credo, thinking of McBride's query as to evidence of their prior existence.

"Yes, ma'am," he said gravely, "one would. It is known by the Guardians of Umlando that a skin – a *kaross* – of a White Lion which had died of old age was given as a gift to King Dinizulu, son of King Malandela. After this time, the king began to receive very important dreams about the future of the earth and the Zulu people."

"May I ask the nature of the dreams, Credo?"

"No, ma'am," he replied. "We may not speak about them."

The detail of the white *kaross* indicated the existence of the White Lions long before the current sightings. It occurred to me that precise dates were lacking because an oral tradition, which predated our own calendar, would have recorded significant events as having occurred during the reign of so-and-so, or after the happening of such-and-such.

From the chronological sequence of African royal dynasties, one could then calculate "generational" time in line with our calendar, and so arrive at approximate dates for the oral records.[8]

"So the White Lions haven't suddenly cropped up in this day and age as people imagine?"

"We live in prophetic times, ma'am – the White Lions have returned recently as prophets of this new age."

"But 400 years is not recent, Credo."

"Ma'am" – he smiled – "400 years is a very short time in the lifetime of our planet."

"I see," I said again, trying to accommodate this idea of the lions as "newcomers."

"The White Lions are very old beings, ma'am, as old as life itself. Their appearance in the reign of Queen Numbi is their most recent arrival on this planet."

"I see, Credo," I found myself falling back into my usual comment, unable to articulate any immediate response.

"But why are they white?" I proceeded to ask what appeared an elementary question.

"We believe, ma'am, that camouflage comes from the soul of the animal. The White Lions appear white." He paused. "They can also appear invisible."

"Appear invisible" – it was an interesting concept.

This, then, was the Tale of Timbavati according to the Great Knowledge. I was only too aware of Mutwa's reputation for telling tall tales. With this in mind, I had come to suspect that many of the misunderstandings might, in fact, have arisen from the listeners' inability to translate symbolic and mythical language into reality. Having specialized in symbolism in dream psychology and medieval literary texts during my university studies, I felt fairly well equipped not to repeat this mistake.

Nevertheless, for all my training, I found myself wondering what, if any, sense I could make of this truly weird and wonderful new perspective on Timbavati's White Lions. A small incident had occurred that gave me intimations of the integrity of Mutwa's story. Several minutes into the tale, I was embarrassed to discover that my tape recorder was not recording, and had to interrupt Mutwa midsentence. After I had readjusted the machine, he had to take another deep breath, and began his story again – in precisely the same words as the first time.

"Credo," I said after some consideration. "You said earlier that Timbavati was 'a place of star energy' and that the strange stones were 'astrological stones' with special purpose . . ."

"Yes, ma'am."

"May I ask: what is their purpose? Is it related to the White Lions in some way?"

"Ma'am, when I saw the strange bladelike stone in Timbavati which had been planted in the ground in a slanting position many, many, many years ago, I recalled the story that had been told me many times."

He paused, and I waited.

"Tell me, ma'am, have you ever struck the stone in Timbavati?"

"I can't say that I have, Credo."

"Well, ma'am, if you strike this strange knifelike stone, you will find that it gives a sharp ringing sound – for it is a rock gong of unbelievable antiquity. It has, in fact, been brought to Timbavati and is not native to that part of the Transvaal. It is identical to those one finds in the Zimbabwe ruins: strips of ringing stone which in ancient times were used to summon warriors during times of trouble or, more particularly, in rituals to do with the worship of the moon or the sun."

"But how did the stones get there?" I asked, intrigued that there should be a connection between Timbavati and Great Zimbabwe, a mysterious ruined citadel regarded as the most significant archeological site in Africa after Giza.

"It is said that one great king whose name was Ndnebete made a pilgrimage to Timbavati, and in salutation to the spirits of Timbavati he brought with him one or two strips of radio stone, and two of them still remain where he planted them, although one is standing at a weird angle."[9]

"Do they have magnetic energy?" I asked on impulse.

"I do not know, ma'am. All I know is that with that stone, if you stand against it, you get healed. And if you lean against a stone of that kind after a thunderstorm, you get nauseous."

"Does the stone point east?" I tried again. "Is it a marker of that kind?"

"No. The stone probably used to stand upright and somebody pushed it over a long time ago. Maybe something collided with it."

"So it is connected with the Great Zimbabwe ruins in some way?" I reiterated.

"Yes, ma'am. These rock gongs, these strips of – I do not know what stone – were used at Zimbabwe to greet certain stars in the sky. For instance, if the stars of spring, the Pleiades, rose in the east, there was a wild tintinnabulation when the king's attendants played these rock gongs in order to salute the stars and to mark the plowing season. Then, also, ma'am, if a comet was seen in the sky, three of these long strips of stone were rung. And their notes were like no other note in that place, so that everybody knew when these stones were sounded there was a great and terrible star in the sky."

"So Zimbabwe was a site for communicating with the stars?" I asked, thinking of Africa's long-standing archeological enigma and how it still inspired controversy today.

"This custom was not only confined to Zimbabwe," Mutwa continued, "but in Zululand there was a stone called Mcemcemce. Now, that stone my grandfather used to sound. It was a rock gong which was high on the mountain. My grandfather used to travel to that mountain to sound that gong whenever the stars of spring appeared, and also whenever a star such as the one we call 'the eye of the wolf'[10] – which is the planet Mars – moved to a certain position in the heavens.

"Another thing, ma'am. You should know that Timbavati was originally a place of much metal smelting. You can still see in some places the ancient furnaces which were used. In one place I counted a whole line of 16 ancient metal-smelting furnaces, and these were of a very sophisticated kind."

"I see, Credo," I said, suspecting that this was yet another critical clue, but not yet knowing how to pursue it.

"What you have said, Credo, makes me wonder if the White Lions are a symbol of how we might save our planet, which is in serious trouble . . ."

"They are, ma'am," he said simply. "They are a symbol."

"Do you think that we have something very serious to learn from them?"

"Yes, ma'am," he replied. "Yes, yes, yes."

"What, Credo? What is it that we must learn from them?"

"Ma'am, that is a very serious question indeed."

"I see that, Credo. I see that," I prompted him, thinking over all I had learned so far. "What exactly is this enlightenment and wisdom that they are offering us, Credo?"

"Ma'am, we will talk more," said Mutwa with understanding, as if the time or the place was not right.

"Thank you for telling me about Timbavati," I said, realizing that I should conclude things. "I am beginning to see how important it is. From my own experience there, I felt that it was important."

"It is, ma'am."

"I knew that the White Lions had special meaning, but I could not fully understand."

"Our people believe that the lion is a beast like no other. It is something more important, more sacred. All catlike animals, from domestic cats to lions, were brought to this earth, we believe, to protect human beings and other life-forms."

"They are our protectors," I said, repeating this idea, which was now becoming a refrain in my quest to understand Africa's lion culture.

"Yes."

"And so the White Lions, particularly, would be our protectors?"

"Yes, ma'am."

Standing up to leave, I said, "You must be very tired, but I have one last question, if I may – an important one."

"Yes, ma'am," he said patiently.

"Do you think it a good idea that people know Timbavati is a sacred place? Do you think it will do good or bad?"

"Ma'am, if people know about Jerusalem, is it a good thing or a bad thing? If people know about other sacred places, is it a good or bad thing? It is bad if a sacred place is desecrated, destroyed, or obliterated. But if the story is known, then that sacred place will be preserved."

"And the White Lions? If their story is known – will they be preserved?"

"We must have hope and faith that this will be the case, ma'am. We must trust that it will do good if people know how important lions are, and how gravely important the White Lions are, and how gravely important it is to preserve our earth, if we can."

"That is what I was hoping," I told him. "That the knowledge you are helping me to uncover will do good."

"All knowledge is good, ma'am. It is how it is used that may be harmful."

"I see, Credo. Thank you," I responded.

"Our great kings many hundreds of years ago protected areas as sacred and free from hunting, except by royal decree," he explained by way of conclusion. "Only the king was allowed to hunt, and on sacred occasions only. There were ancient laws in Africa that governed human beings' behavior toward the earth and the animals which lived on it – these, if broken, were punishable by death. In the great history of Africa, Timbavati has long been known as a sacred site. For many centuries, ma'am, long before the white president Paul Kruger, the Shangaan kings forbade hunting in the Timbavati area, for they knew that this game reserve was not only a sanctuary for animals but also a sacred place of the gods."

9

WHITE LION GENETICS

The White Lions of Timbavati, the lions of the star that fell to the earth,
must not be allowed to vanish from the pages of our country's history.
– CREDO MUTWA

After my visit to Mutwa I came away feeling elated. What an amazing story! The inherent meaningfulness of the symbolic language infused my spirits, requiring no explanation or analysis. The mythological magnitude of Mutwa's storytelling spoke for itself, and the conservationist message was as radiantly relevant today as it must have been in the bygone days of the African elders. Mutwa's imperatives resounded in my head: "How important lions are, and how gravely important the White Lions are, and how gravely important it is to preserve our earth, if we can." Far from being of no conservation value, the White Lions, I saw now, embodied critical principles of conservation of our earth, and key symbols for our day and age.

Then, after settling down for a late-night cup of coffee after the interview, I began to think.

Although at a personal level I tend to give people the benefit of the doubt, my academic training simply would not allow Mutwa's account to stand at face value. If his oral knowledge contained primal truths, how could I verify them? Was it fair to a sacred tradition to attempt to do so? Knowing by now that secret wisdom was encoded in these seemingly childlike tales, I appreciated that the extract of oral history was a symbolic rendition of the events rather than a blow-by-blow factual account. I realized that what made Mutwa's White Lion story hard to credit was its presentation: it was not a familiar Western-style historical record, but rather a fireside tale. We are accustomed to history recounted in bare factual point form, not vivid story form. Unlike historical archives, Mutwa's tale of Timbavati had an atmospheric quality, a vivid immediacy, as if told by a firsthand witness rather than a fastidious scribe with attention only to hard facts.

Nevertheless, factual details had emerged, such as the dating of the White Lions' appearance. What should I make of these? King Dinizulu's White Lion *kaross* might well be in the secret possession of the guardians of tribal history, but I would be unable to verify its existence without gaining direct access to these forbidden realms. Yet Mutwa's account made it perfectly plain that White Lions existed in Timbavati long before Chris McBride's "discovery" of them in the 1970s. But how could I substantiate this?

In respect of the White Lions' arrival, there are key two questions I needed to ask: first, when exactly did the White Lions first appear at Timbavati; and, second, why did this unique lion strain suddenly materialize in Timbavati and nowhere else on the globe?

McBride puzzled over their origins, too, as does anyone who stumbles across a unique animal type: "If a strain of White Lions does exist in this part of South Africa, why has it never shown up before?" McBride wrote. "If there had been White Lions here at some point, you would at least expect to find a White Lion skin somewhere."[1]

In respect to their first appearance in Timbavati, McBride records his chance discovery early in October 1975. He had been studying a lion pride in the Machaton territory of Timbavati and, having witnessed a mating ritual, was expecting one of the females – a lioness he had nicknamed Tabby after his daughter, Tabitha – to produce cubs. On the day in question, McBride himself was sick in bed, and his sister, Lan, who was visiting briefly, went out on a game drive with the rest of the family. Hoping that Tabby had already given birth and that they might catch her in a rare moment with her newborn cubs, they headed straight for her favorite resting place.[2] McBride recounts the unforgettable moment:

> As [Lan] approached the spot . . . she suddenly braked and switched off the motor.
>
> "Look, James, a lioness," she whispered.
>
> "Where?" he asked, searching the terrain without any success. Lions are notoriously difficult to spot, even when you are right on top of them.
>
> Then he saw her. It was Tabby, only about 25 yards from the track, under a shangani [tree]. She lay there, quite unconcerned, looking back at the jeep. Beside her was the remains of a wildebeest kill on which she'd been feeding.
>
> In absolute silence, Lan, James and Johnson sat and waited.
>
> Within a minute, a little head popped up behind the lioness. To Lan's amazement, it was snow white.
>
> Then another little head appeared – tawny.
>
> And yet a third – snow white again.
>
> Lan was staggered. She'd heard of very rare albino cubs, but these [Timbavati lions] had yellow eyes – normal lions' eyes. It was quite clear that they weren't albinos [as albinos would have pink eyes]. They were ordinary, seemingly healthy lions. Except that they were pure white.
>
> She drove back to me – "like a maniac," as she put it. She found me in bed, reading and unable, because of the flu, to get as excited as I should have about the news.
>
> "Are you sure they're not just pale?" I asked her.
>
> She was furious. "No. They're white. Pure white," she insisted.[3]

Everyone's first reaction was disbelief. The idea of pure White Lions was unprecedented. Only on reflection did the full impact of this unique discovery finally dawn on McBride.

As he had been studying the Machaton pride for months prior to this chance discovery, McBride was able to be quite specific about the birth dates of the first White Lions. "I tried to reconstruct the timing," he writes. "The cubs were roughly two weeks old when we saw them, and knowing that the gestation period of lions is between 106 and 110 days, there wasn't much doubt that what we had seen and photographed on 6 June had resulted in the birth of these white cubs."[4]

What he had seen and photographed was the mating of one of the pride males, Agamemnon, with the lioness he had named Tabby. Working forward from this date of 6 June, he could safely calculate that the white cubs had been born in the second-last week of September 1975. He could also be sure that both parent lions were carriers of the white gene, since if only one were carrying the recessive white gene it would not have shown up – just as two brown-eyed humans both need to be bearers of a recessive blue-eye gene for it to appear in their children.

Birth of the Lion Kings

While the birth date of the first White Lions ever recorded by Western man could be precisely calculated, there is nothing to suggest that these were the first White Lions ever born. McBride himself makes this point. "It is quite possible that White Lion cubs have been born here in the past and simply disappeared before anyone has caught a glimpse of them. As it happened, we were unusually lucky to spot them when they were only a few weeks old . . ."[5] He admits that "[the] high mortality rate among cubs and the fact that lionesses keep their young well hidden in the riverine bush makes the chances of young White Lion cubs being seen in this area very slight." And he cites subsequent examples of Timbavati wardens who, in full knowledge of the existence of the white cubs, were unable to find them. Until very recently, he points out, the Timbavati region was almost completely uninhabited, so even if White Lions had existed, they would have remained undetected.[6]

Speculation that these newly discovered white cubs were by no means the first of their kind was further fueled once McBride came across another white cub, in the same region but of a different age and belonging to a different mother. Believing that these young White Lions would be "severely handicapped" by their coloring, and surmising that "over the millennia, evolution must have produced mutants of this type before, and the fact that none of them appears ever to have survived could very well attest to their inability to fend for themselves,"[7] McBride held fast to his opinion that they were probably not an overnight occurrence.

The question, then, remained: when did the White Lions first appear?

White Lion Antecedents

I spent the next few months researching this question, attempting to trace any record of the White Lions – written, spoken, or pictorial – predating McBride's photographic records. I determined that the first sighting of a White Lion by a European witness was in 1938. After I gave a radio interview on the subject of the White Lions, I was contacted by an elderly woman named Joyce Mostert, who recounted a firsthand experience at the age of ten, in which she and her family had spotted, at night, an entire pride of tawny lions – and one snow-white one.

To my knowledge, no living eyewitness accounts predate this sighting. Were there other means of tracing the origins of the White Lions, besides relying on Mutwa's oral testimony?

Many sources now corroborate Credo Mutwa's early declaration that the rock paintings of the Bushmen of Southern Africa depict profound knowledge that corresponds to secret information preserved by the guardians of tribal history. The one tradition is visual, the other oral; but the knowledge recorded in both is one and the same. It occurred to me that this offers one route for tracking White Lion antecedents. There are, however, inherent difficulties in relying on rock art as reliable evidence for dating species.

Other dating methods are equally inconclusive. At a genetic level, the origins of the White Lions of Timbavati's mutation remains an unanswered question. Either they were genetic remnants from a past epoch – possibly a previous Ice Age – or, alternatively, they were the result of an aberrant gene that cropped up recently. If they were Ice Age relics, the question is: how did they survive in this bushveld landscape throughout the millennia? If, on the other hand, they were recent genetic mutations, I ask: why here and why now? What circumstances prompted this freak genetic occurrence?

Credo Mutwa's story of the origins of the White Lions suggests the more recent option. They appeared just over 400 years ago, after an unusual event (which we'll call the fall of a meteorite of sorts) took place in the Timbavati region. Some years after this, "it was observed that all animals that stayed within that area where the mysterious object had settled on the ground were giving birth to snow-white offspring" – most importantly a pride of lions that "started giving birth to white offspring with blue eyes."

On the question of a fallen star, radioactivity in the distinctive Timbavati geology suggests possible factual grounds for the birth of unique White Lions. Something certainly prompted genetic mutations in this specific vicinity, and the radioactivity from a fallen meteorite is as legitimate a contender as any.[8]

The obvious question is: what were these snowy White Lions doing in a tawny landscape? How and when did they first appear?

Somewhat astoundingly – to my way of thinking – the game rangers in Timbavati have tended to adopt the attitude that there is nothing special about the White Lions. They cropped up here by chance, they suggest, and the white pigmentation was the result of a random mutation that might equally have occurred elsewhere. The fact that it hasn't occurred anywhere else in the world does not seem worthy of consideration. One might be satisfied with such a pragmatic attitude were it not for the number of unexplained circumstances that surround this genetic rarity.

Recent Mutation

Finding that there is virtually no background material on the White Lions or their genetics, I decided to contact Ted Sohn, an old Cambridge colleague of mine. Sohn has a doctorate in genetic engineering and molecular biology, and his dissertation addresses genetic mutation and hair color. The numerous e-mails exchanged between us gave me a deepening perspective on the genetic questions surrounding the unique Timbavati lions.

The genetic code that produces White Lions is unique. Genetically speaking, the color white is in fact a total lack of color. This indicates that the gene determining whether there is color or not is inoperative; but if that were the case, there should be no color in the eyes as well as the coat, in other words, the eyes should be pale pink. In this way, it seems the White Lions defy the normal rules of genetics.

"If a White Lion has gold pigmentation, then we may be talking of a different set of genes altogether," Sohn wrote to me. "The gene I was thinking about would give white skin and pink eyes."

"What about white skin with blue eyes?" I asked, remembering how Mutwa's reference from the Great Knowledge was corroborated by several recorded sightings of White Lions.

"Now that would be really unusual," Sohn responded. "For a lion or any other mammal to have white hair but colored eyes would mean a very rare and novel set of mutations. Something really weird is going on. Are you sure that the lions are really white and not just very pale brown?"

"Snow white, Ted. Snow white," I wrote back, thinking of McBride's photographic records. Moreover, Maria had given me the remains of a tuft of White Lion hair she had held in her possession after discovering it impaled on a thorn tree – which I decided to send on to Sohn as verification. I explained to the geneticist that some photographs showed them as slightly tawny, but that was only because their coats were covered with dust.

My discussions with Sohn, as with my probing into the origins of Africa's extraordinary lion culture, had left me with the distinct impression that there was far more to the legendary White Lions than met the eye. While the White Lions were no longer in the wilds of Timbavati, hope of their continuance lay in the tawny lions of the region. I took heart in Sohn's assertion that if just one gene-bearing lion still survived, the strain was not yet dead.

According to Mutwa's story, the White Lions are symbols for our time. For whatever reason, this unique lion strain declared itself some 400 years ago in this precise spot on the globe as a precursor of a new epoch. While there are suggestions of a mutation prompted by unusual circumstances in the Timbavati region, the origins of the White Lions appear to go back to the very beginning of time. I was intrigued by Mutwa's description of the White Lions as "very old beings . . . as old as life itself," and the new perspective he provided on their mutation in Timbavati, as representing "their most recent arrival on this planet." In his terms, their appearance in our day and age was, in fact, a reappearance.

Rather than satisfying my questions as to the mysterious antecedents of the White Lions, instead the shamanic lore that Mutwa passed down to me simply fired my curiosity. I knew that I needed to return to the great shaman to help focus the intensity of my investigations, and I sought another opportunity to do so.

10

GREAT ZIMBABWE:
RESTING PLACE OF THE LION

If the heart is the image of the sun in man, in the earth it is gold.
– JUAN EDUARDO CIRLOT, *DICTIONARY OF SYMBOLS*

At the first opportunity, early in 1997, I revisited Credo Mutwa, but the timing was inappropriate.

It was a brief encounter of less than half an hour – and was interrupted by foreign guests for the purposes of a documentary. Brief as it was, the contact with the lion shaman was worth every moment. I had driven 1,500 kilometers (about 930 miles) from Cape Town to Johannesburg to see Mutwa; his visitors had traveled from the other end of the earth. So I took the gracious option, and left.

In the short time we spent together, however, Mutwa dropped a couple of critical hints that would determine the next step in my journey.

Having spent the intervening period unsuccessfully attempting to trace Bushmen paintings with reference to white felines, I recounted my difficulties to Mutwa. He listened patiently, then alluded to the fact that there were important depictions in and around Great Zimbabwe. Zimbabwe's great ruins, therefore, formed the centerpiece to our short meeting. Intrigued by the connections Mutwa had earlier drawn between Timbavati and Great Zimbabwe, I had long since been mulling over his assertion that the strange bladelike stone I had seen in Timbavati was "a rock gong of unbelievable antiquity" used to communicate with certain stars, along with the "radio stones" of Great Zimbabwe. I wondered, then, what Mutwa meant by a pilgrimage of "Sun People" being led from Great Zimbabwe south to Timbavati. I also wondered about the ritual connections that the ancients identified between the heavenly sky and Timbavati's sacred land.

Now, in our short time together, I had a chance to put some of my questions to him. Like the new archeoastronomical theories about the Mayan and Egyptian civilizations having inherited a lost wisdom from a highly advanced civilization, Great Zimbabwe has long been attributed to a lost civilization – although which civilization exactly continues to attract a great deal of speculation. The problem, at first, was that colonials simply could not credit Africans with the sophistication and artistry demonstrated in the architectural marvel known as Great Zimbabwe.

Southern African colonials maintained it had to be a European achievement.[1] But now the official, categorical political line is that Great Zimbabwe was built by tribal Africans and cannot be evidence of an advanced civilization.[2] According to Credo Mutwa, this is not the case. He claims that relics from this lost advanced civilization are in the secret possession of shamans throughout the African continent. Amid continuing controversy over the site, Sanusi Mutwa maintains the origins of Great Zimbabwe are well preserved within the Great Tradition.

Since my allusion to ancient Bushman painting had raised the question of Great Zimbabwe, Mutwa began disclosing information about the enigmatic site, and I listened with interest, despite believing this was not the specific subject I had set out to discuss. If I had only known then how significant Zimbabwe was to the White Lion mysteries, I would have paid closer attention.

Mutwa summarized the historical sequence of events, saying that many thousands of years ago a sophisticated seafaring civilization built Great Zimbabwe on its present site. It is not clear where these colonizers originated, although he maintains they were the product of a true multiracial global civilization.[3] As usual, precise dating proved difficult, but Mutwa explained that Great Zimbabwe was constructed in a time when bronze weaponry was used, with the very masonry taken from a Ma-iti city, which itself had been destroyed. One of these bronze weapons was in his possession and, to my utter delight, Mutwa instructed one of his attendants to produce the relic for my scrutiny: a tapered sword of a magnificence I could never have imagined, let alone carried. This was known as the Sword of Shelumi and said to have been in the possession of King Solomon himself.[4]

Mutwa went on to explain that Great Zimbabwe was the most stable empire in Africa, lasting thousands of years, and was ruled by a succession of Monomotapa kings. *Monomotapa*, Mutwa told me, meant "Lord of the World"[5] and indeed, on their arrival, the Portuguese discovered a dynasty that was the most powerful in Africa. Mutwa disclosed a gruesome story, however: in their greed for gold, the Portuguese skinned alive the last of the Monomotapa kings to force him to reveal his hidden treasure. Mutwa said that Great Zimbabwe was destroyed by Nguni invaders (who came down from central Africa) at the end of the dynastic line, in the 15th century, and was never inhabited again.

This, in summary, is the story of Great Zimbabwe – *Zima-Mbje* – according to the Great Knowledge.[6]

It soon became clear to me that Mutwa's story did not square with the position of historians and archeologists today, who believe they have proved beyond speculation who built Great Zimbabwe, and when. Current orthodoxy dates the ruins to between AD 900 and AD 1500, maintaining that the structure was built by the Mashona and Karanga people. Although it is accepted that the Hill Complex is older than the inner wall of the elliptical "temple," the National Monuments Commission settled upon the medieval dating after testing two wood fragments that were discovered beneath the inner wall of this elliptical temple.[7] While the findings of earlier scholars, such as Hall

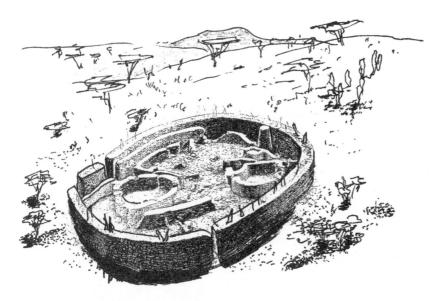

The elliptical temple of Great Zimbabwe, seen from the Hill Complex.

and Neal, are not impossible to reconcile with Mutwa's claims of an ancient seafaring nation influenced by the biblical King Solomon, an enormous rift appears to separate Mutwa's seemingly mythological inherited knowledge from today's orthodox opinion on Great Zimbabwe. I wondered which version would survive the test of time.

The famous relics from Great Zimbabwe are a collection of monoliths crowned by sculpted soapstone birds. Yet, according to Mutwa, these birds (now the national emblem of the country of Zimbabwe) were not the only animal relics found on the site. Most important were totem lions, some in ivory and one, amazingly, carved in wood and clothed in a sheet of pure beaten gold. These may have been ritual vessels used to "hold" the soul of the king. Mutwa was insistent on the critical importance of these lion artifacts – despite the fact that it is the soapstone birds that are associated with the Zimbabwe ruins.

The idea of a sacred golden lion excited me, and I will never forget my impression of Mutwa when he first told me of its existence. He was sitting incongruously in the sophisticated *faux*-leather easy chair, bedecked in ceremonial dress, waiting patiently for the foreign documentary makers to arrive. On his chest was a monumental breastplate from which hung massive crystals and jade artifacts set in beaten bronze. I later learned that this weighed a mighty 25 kilograms (about 55 pounds). Only someone of Mutwa's stature could bear the weight of half a human around his shoulders. In his hand, he held his eagle-crested staff. In that moment, I saw him suddenly as one of those enlightened beings – "the Shining Ones" – that world mythology records in vivid symbolic form. It was not his exterior appearance that called forth this sense in me, although admittedly the ceremonial artifacts were hugely impressive. The unusual sense of heightened consciousness I experienced was of an intuitive nature rather than anything I could have articulated logically. For a privileged moment, it was almost as if I was witnessing the very soul of this lion priest of Africa.

What precipitated this moment was my reminding Mutwa that Zimbabwe was identified with the Zimbabwe bird. "That is only half the story," he responded with a wry snort. "*Zimba* means lion, ma'am, as I think you should know."

"You mean Zimbabwe is, in fact, a lion shrine?"

"Yes, ma'am, yes! That is the clue to its mystery. Not only that, ma'am, but in our secret language the root word of Zimbabwe – *zim* – not only has to do with a lion but also has to do with gold. I may not say more."

As always, I had to hold myself back from being too obtrusive. But after considering a moment, Mutwa gave me a further clue about this sacred lion relic. He recalled that he had seen reference to the Zimbabwe lion totems in a South African newspaper – *The Sunday Times,* he thought – in the late 1940s or early 1950s, under the headline "Empire That Worshipped the Sun."

"But you have come to see me again about the White Lions?" Mutwa continued, changing tack.

"Yes, Credo," I said. "As always, there are so many questions that I'd love to ask you."

Alas, I could hear the voices of the agents and their clients ascending the staircase ahead of them. "Do not forget the White Lions, ma'am," were the lion shaman's closing words to me. "They are more important than you could ever realize."

Empire of Gold

After reluctantly parting from Mutwa, I took the opportunity to scour the university libraries of Pretoria and Johannesburg in an attempt to trace the article he had recalled.

Having grown up in South Africa, I had always been aware of Great Zimbabwe as a site of legend and mystery. As a child, I had read Rider Haggard's adventure story, an early Indiana Jones–type quest into the riddle of Zimbabwe, based on associated legends of the Queen of Sheba and King Solomon's mines. Since then, the archeological community has set about debunking the mystique of the great ruins.[8]

One glittering thread continued to run through the labyrinthine passages of inquiry into Zimbabwe: *gold.*

In following the clues at the Sterkfontein Valley sites, I had shared Bruce Chatwin's sense of adventure in uncovering an archeological detective story. Now the quest for discovery was intensified. In the archives of the state library, dusting off old volumes of Africana, I felt as if I were taking real-life steps into an archeological treasure map. It was apparent that Zimbabwe had been established as the chief gold-yielding center of the ancient world by Western chroniclers as early as the 16th century, during the Portuguese colonization – a fact that was subsequently forgotten by Europeans after the Portuguese plundered the lands and erased the memory of native African gold wealth.[9] Only in the late 19th century was the importance of Great Zimbabwe re-evaluated by European researchers such as Thomas Bains.

By the turn of the 20th century, hundreds of ancient gold-working sites had been traced and mapped.[10] The prodigious wealth and scale of this gold-bearing land of Zimbabwe (then called Rhodesia) prompted researchers to question whether the Rhodesian goldfields were not, in fact, the fabled source of the precious metals of King Solomon's Temple, described in some detail in the Old Testament of the Bible.[11] Among the treasures discovered in and around the Zimbabwe ruins were engraved stone artifacts and fine earthenware that showed inscriptions thought to date back to the time of Solomon and the ages of Egyptian and Babylonian ascendancy.[12]

The Egyptian Queen Hatshepsut's famous expedition to the so-called Land of Punt emerged as a crucial clue in a long tradition that suggested Egyptian influence in Southern Africa.[13] The fabled Land of Punt, and where it might be geographically located, became a question of intense speculation.[14] The 19th-century researcher A.H. Keane, for instance, investigated whether or not the Egyptian deities arose from Rhodesia's gold lands. Might the ancient Egyptians have sourced "their Ra and their Hathor, and their other deities, as well as their gold, from this Rhodesia," he asks, "which . . . was at that time still inhabited by Bushman-Hottentots?"[15] Scholars such as Martin Bernal (in *Black Athena*) have argued for ancient Egypt's rootedness in Africa. My mind was filled with images of the famous golden mummy cases, pharaonic breastplates, gold scarabs, and ankhs. There are no significant goldfields in Egypt; could the precious metal for these treasures have come from the golden lands of Zimbabwe? But if Solomon and Hatshepsut's people were mining gold in the south, these activities would have long predated the current AD 900–1500 dating.

In respect to Mutwa's tantalizing mention of a golden lion discovered in the late 1940s or 1950s, try as I might, I could find no mention of the sacred artifact. A host of gold ornaments is recorded, and housed in national museums at Bulawayo, Harare, and Mutare; at the site museum at Great Zimbabwe; and in the South African Museum in Cape Town, a collection generally taken to be "a very comprehensive display of the artifacts."[16] The quantities of gold produced are described in awe-inspiring terms. Solid gold bracelets, lengthy strings of gold beads, golden head- and armbands, 22-carat gold plating, gold chain, gold wire of different gauges, bags of gold dust, even gold nails and tacks – but no lion.[17] There are several references to gold rosettes with embossed sun images – which reminded me of the lion's affiliation with the sun symbol – yet no reference to anything of a vaguely leonine nature. Remembering the controversy surrounding the Gold Rhino of Mapungubwe, which was kept hidden from the public in the University of Pretoria, apparently for reasons of racial politics,[18] I wondered whether a similar fate had befallen the missing golden lion.

At the time Mutwa published his work on the oral knowledge behind Great Zimbabwe, there was a great deal of dissension in the archeological establishment as to the status of the dynasty that ruled here, with prominent figures such as the editor of

The Times of London even maintaining Zimbabwe had a "vacant throne."[19] Mutwa's claim in respect of the Monomotapa dynasty is, in fact, corroborated by a Portuguese historian, De Barros (1496–1570), who at the time of the Portuguese penetration into Africa in the early 16th century recorded the goldfields and how these were centered in the land of a powerful king or emperor named Benamatápa (i.e., Monomotapa). He

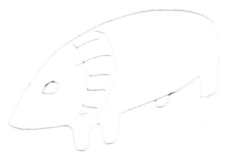

Credo Mutwa's sketch of the missing gold lion artifact of Zimbabwe.

describes the potentate, his gold mines, and his now-ruined residences of Zimbabwe.[20] He also describes where the Monomotapa empire was geographically located (the significance of which I would only come to understand later). He says that the gold-yielding empire was centered on the hidden source of the Nile (Lake Victoria/Tanganyika in Central Africa), as well as catchment areas to which the south-flowing rivers bore much gold, arriving at the land of the Mashona people (around Great Zimbabwe).[21] The location of the gold sites proved critical to the White Lion mysteries once the whole picture began to fall into place.

Africa's "Great Mystery"

After the intimations Mutwa had given about Great Zimbabwe, I was determined to make the trip to see the site for myself.

Approaching Great Zimbabwe, I felt a sense of awe. The rock formations cradling the great ruins are regarded as some of the oldest in the world. Having heaved themselves through the earth's crust in the earliest rock-forming epochs, they evoke the era to which Mutwa refers as *Kewebamatse*. This is the setting for certain of Mutwa's tales, including those describing First Man (Kintu) in caves with felines at a time "when the rocks had not solidified." Rather than a sense of scientific time, Mutwa's tales reveal a notion of ancient shamanic time, which Mutwa calls *Ndelo Ntulo*, "the time of the First."[22]

Like the natural rock fortifications, the ruins themselves are incongruously laid out in the midst of the bushveld. Walking around the circumference of the Great Enclosure, with its 6-meter-thick (about 20-feet) walls built from tons of hewn stone, rising starkly impressive out of the African wilderness, I followed the elliptical sweep of masonry, with the wilderness on one side and the enclosure on the other. On the great wall above me, balanced at odd angles along the ramparts like patrolling sentinels, were the distinctive monolithic flints that Mutwa had said had astrological significance.

The site was surprisingly peaceful. All around, the African veld shimmered with its own unique vibrant silence. And once we were inside the walls of the Great Enclosure, we were shrouded in a different quality of silent solemnity, occasionally disturbed by the droning of bees and laughter from wardens chewing sugar cane. Amazingly, there was not a single tourist.

From the ruins on the open plain, it is about half a kilometer's (about a third of a mile) walk northward to the Hill Fortress, which stands on a volcanic outcrop overlooking the walls of the Great Enclosure. The Hill Fortress of Zimbabwe encompasses the eastern enclosure with its circular platforms, which once held monoliths, some crowned by the famous soapstone birds.

After making the blistering ascent to the fortified ruins on the hill, I gained the full sweep of the ground plan of the famous site. Eagles were circling slowly in the sky above the elliptical enclosure with its curious stone tower, and I thought again of Africa's lion priest with his eagle-crested staff. It was as if his spirit hovered with me over this sacred lion site, guiding me toward hidden knowledge.

From the bird's-eye perspective of the granite outcrop overlooking the site, I was struck by the distinct impression that these great ruins were not an isolated mystery in the middle of a dark continent, but were somehow integral to unlocking other African mysteries. I could not, as yet, explain why the place gave me this impression. It had partly to do with the gravity Mutwa's words had imparted to the sacred site, and partly to do with the sense of symbolic consequence that the ancient stones themselves drew from me. Below me, the elliptical ground plan invoked womblike and fetal images – as if to suggest the birthplace of a continent.

It was only after returning to my hotel room that evening, when mulling over a map of the region, that the critical piece of the mystery dropped into place.

Mutwa had more than once implied a direct connection between Great Zimbabwe and Timbavati. He testified that the distinctive stone gongs in Timbavati were astrological artifacts carried to this region over long distances from the great ruins. In my own long journey from Timbavati to Great Zimbabwe, I had imagined the immensity of this mission. Humans on foot, bearing back-breaking stones over vast distances through wild bushveld, across rivers, mountains, and predator-infested valleys, so as to mark the sanctity of the Timbavati site. Tracing the route on a map, I wondered: why? To what purpose should such a thread have been drawn through the African continent? Like all the best teachers, Mutwa had left me to fathom the answers for myself.

Now I saw that the Timbavati–Zimbabwe connection was obvious. It took more than a bird's-eye perspective to make the connection; it entailed an aerial view of greater magnitude. In fact, it required a cartographer's knowledge of our globe. Both sacred sites were laid out in perfect alignment on the map of Africa – with the precision of a draftsman – on precisely the same longitudinal line, 31°14′ E. This was my first real indication that something other than chance was at work in the White Lions' arrival on our planet.

11

ZIMBA: GOLDEN LION SHRINE

The great healers were my husband, and two other men, both of whom gave me n/um
(supernatural potency). All are now dead. None were killed by God.
All were killed by people.

– WA NA GOSHE (WIFE OF BUSHMAN LION SHAMAN)

Eager to return to Mutwa with my exciting discovery, I was again frustrated to have to wait several weeks before we were able to make contact. I wanted to show him the geodetic alignment of Great Zimbabwe and Timbavati. I wanted to question him more closely about the leonine connection between the site of the ruins and the site of the White Lions. I needed more details on the lion relics of Zimbabwe. Had they been bought by a private collection? Were they gathering dust in a museum somewhere? Or had they disappeared into the secret possession of the Guardians of Umlando?

Golden Thread

In the meantime, all I could do was sift through research material in an attempt to find some reference to the missing relics. There was no doubt that a concentration of lion interest existed in and around the great ruins. To begin with, there was the name itself: Zimbabwe. The textbooks inform us that the word *Zimbabwe* means "stone hut."[1] It originates from the Mashona word for "home," and is short for *Zimaremabwe* in the Mashona (Karanga) language. *Imba* means "hut," and the prefix *z* as in *(z)imba,* means "large"; therefore the whole word means "large stone hut."

According to Mutwa, however, this is a superficial reading. The hidden meaning of the word, he says, revolves around the core word: *zim* meaning "gold" and *zimba* meaning "lion." Even today, *zimba* means "lion" in African languages such as that of the Matabele.[2] But why were the leonine associations of Zimbabwe not commonly known, and why was the bird of prey its primary association instead?

Still searching for any mention of the golden lion relic, I contacted the then Zimbabwean Minister of Culture, who assured me that to his knowledge no such artifact had ever existed. I approached various archeological departments in South African universities, none of whom were helpful in providing any mention, let alone record, of a golden lion.

Then I traced the Great Zimbabwe expert Roger Summers, the man who had excavated the site in the 1940s and 1950s, now in his 90s and rumored still to have all his wits about him. I gave him a call.

After introducing myself, and explaining briefly what my research was about, I asked him about the possibility of lion relics at the Zimbabwe ruins. I told him the discovery was supposedly made a long time ago, and that it was believed to have been documented in a newspaper in the 1940s or 1950s.

"Nineteen-forty is not very long ago, my dear," he responded. "For you, no doubt, but not for me."

It made me smile to see how the old gent's wit was still button-bright.

"You do know that I am over 90?" he said, without a hint of a quaver.

"I would never have believed it!" I replied, in all honesty.

He told me that at the time of his excavations, he had gone through every archive in Harare. If there had been any lion artifacts, he concluded, he would surely have found some reference. It was tempting to agree. Any discovery of lion artifacts should have been well documented – most notably if they had been made of gold. Yet the golden rhinoceros discovered in the 1930s in Mapungubwe, at the Limpopo, south of Zimbabwe, was withheld from public knowledge for decades.[3] During the time in question Summers himself was director of the Monuments Commission. He of all people should have known.[4] But in all his excavations and research into the ruins, he never came across any reference to any lion relics. This did not make sense.

"Hmm, it is possible that there was something in Johannesburg which did not get into the archives in Harare?" he mused. Then, in response to my pointed silence, he said, "My dear girl, I've been working on Great Zimbabwe long enough not to be surprised at anything – however seemingly peculiar."

In short, there was no record anywhere of a discovery of lion relics in Zimbabwe. Yet the more I researched the customs and beliefs of the people in the vicinity of the ruins, the more apparent it was that the lion played a central role in their culture.

Resting Place of the Lion

Meanwhile, the image of a golden lion had now begun to invade my dreams. I saw it emerging out of smelting works, and then – disturbingly – being melted down again. This, coupled with the roaring lion who continued to visit me at night, made my sleep increasingly fitful, and spilled over into my daily preoccupations.

I was desperately keen to see Mutwa again. The quest for the elusive golden lion was becoming something of a holy grail. I needed further direction from the lion shaman. Although I was loath to entertain the thought, the possibility remained that Mutwa's memory might be rusty with age, and the lion relics about which he spoke had never existed at all.

When we did finally meet again, my first question had to do with the golden lion, although, sensing that I was venturing into closely guarded territories, I tried not to be overly bold in my questioning. Having found nothing fitting his description of *The Sunday Times* article, I told Mutwa of my frustration.

"It concerns me that I've been unable to trace any record of a golden lion whatsoever," I confessed.

"You need to take another look, ma'am," he said simply.

His memory of the article relating to the lion relics was so clear that he not only remembered the title – "Empire That Worshipped the Sun" – but he recalled the closing sentence almost verbatim. He also said that the article was accompanied by a diagram of one of the lion relics, which he went on to reproduce for me – a young lion in outline with a pointed snout.

"But where might these relics be, Credo?" I wondered.

"I do not know, ma'am. That I do not know."

Also, I admitted to Mutwa that I had been unable to locate White Lion paintings in the vicinity of Great Zimbabwe – or anywhere else for that matter. Having failed to find any mention in library reference books on South African studies, I did not know how to proceed.

"Have endurance, ma'am. Remember: the lioness never gives up until she has tracked down her prey."

He then proceeded to give me further clues, which fueled my determination to keep on track. He told me that the Sword of Shelumi (which we will come across again later) was created by the Lemba people, an African tribe said to be of Jewish origin. When Mutwa had written about this tribe many years ago,[5] his claims had been dismissed as nonsense. Genetic testing, however, has now determined the Lembas' Jewish ancestry.[6] Many tribes claim responsibility for the building of Great Zimbabwe, but, given these clues, I was encouraged to favor the Lemba people's claim to have been among the original builders.

"It was the Lemba who were responsible for crafting this sword for Shelumi," Mutwa explained, now running his hand along the flat side of its blade, which, he maintained, had once been very much longer than its present length of less than a meter (about a yard, or three feet).

Imagining scenes of bloody battle and carnage of the kind described in this early work, *Indaba, My Children*, I asked Mutwa what the sword had been used for.

"It was a sword used to fight, and win, many a spiritual battle," he instructed me, and an entirely new picture began to form in my imagination.

He also informed me that, like certain other tribes in Africa, the Lemba hold sacred a great mountain that, under certain conditions, may roar like a lion.

"I am beginning to feel exactly what you told me, Credo," I explained, "that, in following the footsteps of the White Lions, I will be led all the way up Africa to the Nile Delta, with the Sphinx and its riddle."

Mutwa smiled as if approving the connections I was making; but, at the same time, a grave expression darkened his face.

"The White Lions guard a secret, ma'am," he said somberly. "A secret which can save humankind."

"Are we in need of saving, Credo?" I inquired, feeling a clawing pain of trepidation in the pit of my stomach.

"Desperately, ma'am," Mutwa replied. "And time is short."

The pain I felt was one I could not fully identify. Sometimes my responses to Mutwa were as yet half-formed impressions that seemed to arise from deep within me, rather than my own rational thoughts. Being in the presence of a great *sangoma* was an otherworldly, transfiguring experience, and the safe structures that had once held fast in my mind often dissolved and shifted uncomfortably. As Mutwa spoke these words, I visualized a clear picture of a golden lion – resembling very closely the beautiful Gold Rhino of Mapungubwe – but then the vision disappeared again, as if melting into nothing. For some reason, this figment distressed me, too, and I tried to get a grip on my logical thought processes again.

"You said that the secret meaning of the word *Zimbabwe* had to do with lions and gold, Credo?"

Mutwa smiled. "That is so, ma'am. Just as Timbavati was also originally a place of much metal smelting – which is guarded over by the White Lions."

Since my discovery that Timbavati and Zimbabwe were on the same longitude, I had considered possible implications for this curious alignment. That there might be metal-smelting sites in common was a connection on which I had not bargained. Unclear of what significance this might hold, except as a possible link in the trading of precious metals, I asked Mutwa directly.

His response alerted me that I was venturing close to the mark. But rather than withhold all information, he offered an important detail. "You should know, ma'am, that at the helm of Africa's highest shamans are the Sacred Blacksmiths, who are initiated in the secret art of investing knowledge in sacred metal-smelting practices. I cannot say more."

"Are you one of these Sacred Blacksmiths, Credo?" I asked on impulse, realizing I was now overstepping the mark.

"I am, ma'am," he replied, as if the matter was now closed.

I had to hold myself back from probing further. "May I tell you something that might interest you, Credo?" I inquired instead.

"Yes, ma'am, please tell me."

"If you look on a map and you draw a straight line from [Great] Zimbabwe to Timbavati – a longitudinal line – it goes exactly from the great ruins to the birthplace of the White Lions."

"And beyond."

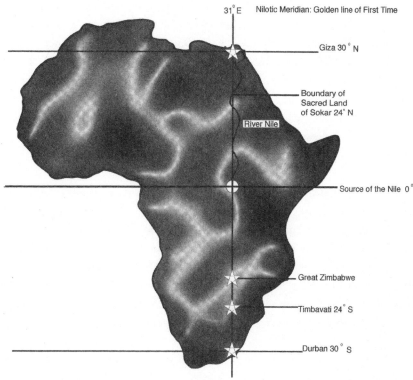

Key sacred sites along the prime meridian.

"And beyond?" I queried.

"The mystery that links Zimbabwe to Timbavati is the same thread that runs beneath the African continent."

"I see, Credo," I said, stopping in my tracks. "And does that thread have something to do with the lion symbol?"

"Yes, ma'am. It does."

But how? I was not following. Mutwa considered a moment. As if reaching for another scroll from his oral knowledge, he now proceeded to unroll it.

The Great Underground River

"African legend tells us, ma'am, that there is a great river flowing beneath the continent together with many tributaries. It is said that this great river flows all the way from North Africa down into what was called the Transvaal, down under the Free State and beyond."

While this obscure reference seemed unrelated to our present discussion, I knew Mutwa well enough to suspect a critical connection somewhere. One day, I would see how the different fragments that had come to me piecemeal would add up to one cohesive and astoundingly clear picture.

"Now, this river was regarded by scientists simply as a figment of the black imagination," the Sanusi explained, continuing on his obscure train of thought. "A superstition at best, and a total falsehood at worst. But, one day, scientists experimenting in the Chinhoyi [or Chinoia] caves in the land once known as Rhodesia – now Zimbabwe – put a special dye into a pool inside the great caves, and that dye was detected in the waters of the Mulopo Oog [Mulopo Eye] in the Western Transvaal, known as Wondergat. This showed conclusively that there was a huge underground river with many tributaries which flowed under the African continent . . ." He looked up at me through his dense glasses. "What does this prove to us?"

I hesitated.

He posed another question. "Where does this mysterious river flow to eventually?"

"Do you know where it might end?" I inquired.

"No, I do not. But I do know that our people – storytellers from as far away as Kenya, Zaire, and Zululand – speak a lot about this underground river in our places of initiation: the river that is said to hold the continent of Africa together."

Some of Maria's words were coming back to me as he spoke. She had explained that the White Lions had their origins in the Milky Way and in a river that never ran dry.

"And is this great subterranean river somehow connected to the Milky Way?" I asked Mutwa.

"The Milky Way is the known as 'the river of stars' – yes, ma'am. That I can tell you."

"Maria told me that the White Lions originated in the stars, in the heavenly river that never runs dry. Are we also saying, Credo, that there may be a sacred underground river running beneath Timbavati's dry riverbeds?"

Mutwa listened, nodding, with his hands demurely in his lap. "Perhaps, ma'am, perhaps. We take it further, ma'am. We even take it that for every river that flows to the sea, there is a deep river underground directly under that river which flows in the opposite direction. Rivers would not flow if they did not have counter-rivers."

I paused expectantly. But he ventured nothing further, for the moment. "And what is the name of this sacred subterranean river in the African continent?" I asked.

"It is called *Lulungwa Mangakatsi*. It is the old African term for 'river underneath,' the 'river below.'" Then he added, "Do you know that the Nile is a man-made river, ma'am, not nature-made?"

Now he had entirely lost me. "The Nile, Credo?" I asked, trying not to sound too incredulous. "The longest river in the world?"

"That is what we are told, ma'am."

I was having trouble understanding the connections, particularly as they were not what we were taught in geography classes.

I parted from Mutwa once more, little knowing how Africa's lion priest had planted more seeds of knowledge that would blossom into a new awareness in due course. In fact, that very afternoon, the stirrings of new knowledge began to grow. I was due to meet up again with archetypal lion man Gareth Patterson, the fierce campaigner who had written seven books on his experiences with lions. From our first meeting, we had struck up a rapport. I had long admired his tireless efforts at saving lions destined for trophy hunting,[7] and he, in turn, was fascinated by the White Lion mysteries that I began to disclose to him. Patterson's many books recount his firsthand contact with the lions he had taken care of after George Adamson's death in Kenya. He describes in real physical terms the joy and tragedy that he suffered in his intimate lion experiences. Yet in private he and I discussed the psychic and spiritual dimensions that seemed to lie behind his real experiences with lions.

As we talked over lunch, I informed Patterson about the geodetic lineup of Timbavati and Great Zimbabwe. When I got onto the legend of Shelumi and the golden lion, I suddenly saw his eyes grow leonine and intense, and he reached for a book he had been reading.

"Take a look at this," he said.

In it, the author, Tudor Parfitt, described his search for the "lost tribe of Israel," the black Jews believed to inhabit the continent of Africa. Patterson pointed me to a passage, no more than a couple of lines long, in which there was mention of the legend of a sacred White Lion rumored to guard the precincts of Great Zimbabwe.

The author's quest to find the lost tribe of Israel had led him directly to the Lemba people in the vicinity of Great Zimbabwe, a tribe whose traditions echo ancient Jewish customs, and whose genetics show direct traces of the Judaic bloodline. Like other African tribes, the Lemba believe their ancestors become lions after death and might prowl around sacred sites in lion form.[8] The Lemba people also venerate a great lion mountain, which they believe is able to roar and even set itself alight. There is a specific lion connection, however, that made the Lemba people of particular interest to my White Lion quest, and it was this that Patterson wanted to point out to me.

Having insinuated himself into a Lemba *kraal*, the author was led by the wise man Sevias to a site considered to be the Lemba "holy of holies." In the valley, in front of a sacred mountain known as Dumghe, it was said that "strange and mysterious things took place," most notably that "a White Lion . . . was sometimes seen." Also, wailing sounds could be heard throughout the night, which the people attributed to the ancestral spirits weeping for the land.[9]

The author goes on to describe an evocative journey to this mountain, as he follows the guide Klopas along a path:

> On all sides rocky outcrops pierced the turf topped with gigantic bal-
> ancing boulders created over the millennia by the erosion of wind . . . [It
> was believed that] the fierce weather might bring out the animals sacred to
> the mountain.
> "What animals?" [the author] asked.
> "The lion," hissed Klopas.

"Is there a lion?"

"Yes, there is a White Lion," he said.

"No one would harm this sacred lion," murmured Sevias piously.[10]

That was all. But it was enough to reveal another mysterious connection between the White Lions of Timbavati and the sacred lion site of Great Zimbabwe, situated due north.

Although enigmatically, Mutwa had indicated that the White Lion mystery was directly associated with the riddle of the Sphinx. On mulling over the connections, my immediate conclusion was that the culture of lion shamanism might well have been carried by initiates from Egypt to sites in the south, such as Zimbabwe and Timbavati. However, Mutwa subtly insinuated something more than simply a cultural, or philosophical, link between the lion mysteries.

His hint that the sites might somehow be linked by an underground river, and his related assertion that the Nile itself had been redirected by man along a specific course, had sounded too far-fetched for my immediate comprehension. Yet, barely a few days after my latest meeting with him, I found myself catapulted out of sleep – with the answer to the riddle he had given me. I was staying with my sister and her family at the time, who are fortunately sound sleepers. Had they discovered me wandering around in the middle of the night, dragging book after book from the shelf in the hope of finding the right atlas, they might have considered me deranged. Not for the first time in my dealings with Mutwa, the material was so extraordinary that it could not immediately translate into everyday reality.

Deep into this particular night, I finally located a world atlas detailed enough to show the information I was looking for. And there it was: the connection at which Mutwa had so tantalizingly hinted. The connection between Great Zimbabwe, Timbavati, and beyond: the connection between the White Lions and the Great Sphinx of Giza. All three sacred sites were on precisely the same longitudinal line, 31°14′!

As yet, I had no way of fathoming the reasons for the seemingly strategic alignment on this meridian, but scrutinizing these clues on the map of Africa, I saw the three sites as shining beacons in the treasure map of the White Lion mystery.

12

LION PRIESTS AND EAGLE SHAMANS

The sun is in all hunting mythologies a great hunter. He is the lion . . . whose pounce at the neck of the antelope slays it; the great eagle whose plunge traps the lamb. . . .
– JOSEPH CAMPBELL

My immediate sense of the miraculous in identifying three sacred sites in perfect geodetic alignment was compounded as I continued to gather further information. This connection delivered the striking suggestion that the Great Sphinx of Egypt and the White Lions of Timbavati were somehow linked, and that Great Zimbabwe was part of the mystery.

Why should the reappearance of today's White Lions in the flesh align cartographically with the two greatest archeological monuments on the African continent: Giza and Great Zimbabwe?

My first thought was that lion spirituality must provide a critical clue. Giza is the site of humankind's oldest leonine monument, the Sphinx. Its surrounding territory of Memphis is the principal site of the worship of the lion-headed goddess Sekhmet. Great Zimbabwe is "the sacred site of the lion." Finally, Timbavati is a sanctuary for White Lions and a sacred site of the gods. All three sacred sites on the African continent – Giza, Zimbabwe, and Timbavati – are consecrated to the lion.

I sat in the sparse Johannesburg townhouse that Credo Mutwa was now temporarily occupying, presided over by an expansive half-finished painting of his own, depicting our earth and its moon from outer space. I informed him about my discovery that the three sacred sites shared a meridian on our globe.

"The sites' alignment on this longitudinal line, Credo," I commented, "seems to imply some connection between the White Lions and the Sphinx."

"There may well be, ma'am. That is a big question. I may not say more. But this I can tell you: what started off the White Lions' story in this day was the coming down to earth of the strange object from which a group of glowing creatures emerged."

"But why should that be so, Credo?" I remained reluctant to accept this aspect of the oral knowledge.

"That I do not know, ma'am. But as Mr Shakespeare said, there are more things in heaven and on earth than in the affairs of humans."[1]

Today, Mutwa was draped in a wealth of material, clasped around his shoulders with a giant safety pin. I looked from the mountainous form of the lion shaman to his great painting behind. In one corner was a powerful rendition of a saber-toothed cat, a Ngewula. In the other, hovering above the sphere of the earth, was a magnificent eagle in flight. Strangely, the eagle was bearing a dove on its back. Beside the great raptor was a scaled-down man-made rocket ship suspended above the earth. This image of the great winged bird of prey reminded me of the Timbavati story. By association, I concluded that whatever came down to this sacred site "like a bird," must have been larger in spirit than any man-made flying object.

"Do you think Timbavati is the place where something will go back to the stars?" I asked on impulse.

"Yes."

His one-syllable answer was pronounced as if to close rather than open the subject. Nevertheless I attempted to pinpoint what exactly might ascend to the stars at this precise spot.

"That we may not say, ma'am," he said in response. As with many of his tantalizing clues, I was left in the hope that I might know the answer someday.

Lion-Eagle Priest

Meanwhile, I sat in respectful silence, perplexed and unsure of my next step. It was only much later, once I had encountered archeoastronomers investigating the ancient Egyptian mysteries (in particular, the belief that the pharaohs' souls ascended to the stars upon death) that I would have cause to remember Mutwa's hint about returning to the stars.

After a moment, the lion shaman seemed to reconsider and relaxed a little. Referring to his painting, he told me that the eagle, king of the birds, was venerated alongside the lion, king of the beasts. The Zulu people never wantonly slaughtered eagles, just as they never willingly killed lions, for they were sacred birds and beasts, symbolic of their king.

Elaborating on the theme as the day unfolded, Mutwa described how his grandfather had taught him the secret art of capturing an eagle and removing two of its tail or wing feathers – without in any way impairing the bird's flight or well-being. A trench was dug, in which the young boy Mutwa would hide himself. This was covered with green branches and young trees to resemble live foliage. Bait was then tied on top in the form of a rock rabbit. The success of his exercise brought great status in the tribal community, as it was both a delicate and a dangerous task. It trained the initiate to be bold and swift, since there were few precious moments, once the eagle had soared down to snatch the bait and had wrestled it free from its rope, in which the initiate could reach out and pluck the feathers. He would suffer severe lacerations if he hesitated or lost his nerve. Since Mutwa's story was recounted without the least bravado, I might easily have overlooked the heroism in it. Yet, having studied eagles close up in a wildlife rehabilitation center near Timbavati, having seen the size of their talons and been informed of their awesome ability to kill and lift sizeable animals from the ground, this story gave me new insight into Mutwa's courage.

"What was the objective of this exercise?" I inquired.

"The prize was two plumes from a live eagle, which would then return to the heavens, bearing its prey as reward for its pains,"[2] he responded.

This story of courage and affinity with nature reminded me of the vital difference between lion heroism and lion priesthood. Rather than slaying the king of the birds, the initiate's spiritual evolution came through working in accordance with the bird's living powers of flight.

As if reading my thoughts, Mutwa commented, "African warriors wore headdresses made from eagle feathers. However, no warrior in his right mind wore feathers of a bird he had killed – since this is believed to be very unlucky. The bird had to be alive when the feathers were taken, and then released."

We had lunch in this small room, which smelled strongly of turpentine from his oil painting. Although the circumstances were not particularly congenial, the warmth and radiance that emanated from Mutwa's person amply made up for them.

Our communication seemed to open up, and Mutwa followed his description of his initiation rite in respect of the great birds of prey with a parallel initiation rite in the face of the great beasts of prey.

"When you are initiated into the mysteries of the people of Okavango, ma'am, it is the case that you have to sleep at night buried up to your neck in the ground. It is a high form of initiation, since you are forced to face your fear – and get over it. The predators come over to you in the night and sniff your face. Four times I was made to perform this ritual, ma'am, in two separate places. It is a supreme trial. The predators come right up and smell you. You are trained to control your breathing and keep it constant. They can smell that you are alive and leave you in peace. You may not reveal fear, however, for fear smells very bad, and you may then be taken."

Having experienced the proximity of dangerous predators, I found it impossible to imagine enduring this ordeal without extreme terror.

"The Bushmen, ma'am, did this by habit," Mutwa continued. "They buried themselves up to their necks in their caves each night, and slept peacefully, knowing they were safe in this way. They only had a slight problem if they had to pass water in the night." His face lit up with amusement. "The next morning one of them – the only one who had his hands free – would dig the next one out and so on, until they were all dug out of their beds in the earth."

There was little I could say. I was still marveling at how the courage of the eagle priests was matched, even superseded, by the bravery of the lion priests.

"May I show you something, ma'am?" Mutwa inquired as soon as lunch was finished. "Have you seen the eagle on my staff?"

"When you were waiting for the documentary makers, I caught a brief glimpse of it," I commented.

It reminded me now: the great lion shaman had said, with reference to Great Zimbabwe, that this totem was only half the mystery. "I would love to look more closely," I added.

"Come with me, then, ma'am," he said, leading me to the adjoining room. He opened the door for me and I walked in – then stopped dead, stunned, as if suddenly walking from a dark space into a radiant light.

Leaning casually against the wall was Mutwa's eagle-headed ceremonial staff, symbol of his high title. But as I looked around the room I saw, piled up in the center, a mountain of dazzling artifacts. This was the first time Mutwa had allowed me a private view of the sacred relics over which he had custodianship, and a surge of excitement rushed through me. The experience had nothing of the sterility of viewing museum treasures through glass boxes. Although jumbled together in a heap on the bare floor, these precious artifacts resonated with gravity. I was drawn to them magnetically, but dared not lay a finger upon them. These were objects not of art, but of power.

Observing my state of awe, Mutwa said, "Oh, that rubbish!" referring to the priceless relics that had dominated his onerous and inspired existence. His dismissive remark might have sounded peevish; instead, I caught the spirit of his tone – and we both laughed out loud.

There were times when Mutwa disclosed secrets that he compelled me not to put into writing, the confidentiality of which I have, naturally, honored. There were other times he confessed to me that he would answer my question "no matter the consequences," ever mindful of the risks of releasing long-protected secrets into the public domain. Then again, there were many occasions when I had to be satisfied with Mutwa's response that "we may not speak of these things," or that he "may not say more."

Unlike Maria, Mutwa determinedly avoided the use of the term *power*. While Timbavati's Mother of Lions made no apologies for her own powers, the man she regarded as the greatest lion shaman in Africa was a person of astounding humility. In his persistent avoidance of all reference to his personal magnetism, I sensed his restraint, as well as due awe for something indescribably momentous that could both create and destroy.

As our rapport grew ever deeper, Mutwa spoke guardedly about the origins of the select priesthood from which he descended. He explained that the very highest ranks of the Sanusis originated from beings of semi-divine origin: a lion priest (*WaNdau*) and an eagle or hawk priest (*Ntswana*). These enlightened individuals, he said, were ascendant beings, imbued with stellar powers.

This reminded me of Mutwa's mysterious allusion to the fact that the high priests of ancient Egypt possessed an art that enabled them to enter the minds of lions, so as to harness leonine energy in building sacred monuments. He had mentioned that the Guardians of Umlando called this ancient art the "star thing." While he remained reticent in alluding to it, there were occasions when he described personal shamanic experiences and showed me examples that left me in little doubt that he himself possessed a quality along these lines. The few glimpses I caught of these processes made it clear to me that I was not spiritually equipped to understand their full implications. What I am sure of is that the fabled lion–human exchanges that I had been studying in libraries (that refer to Bushman shamans, in particular, taking on lion identity) are not simply academic in Mutwa's case. Furthermore, it appears that whatever Mutwa was alluding to in respect of the mind-power that helped build ancient monuments may be allied to the concentration of power that exchanges energy with sacred beasts such as lions. Mutwa's supremacy over the man-eating lion, using mind-call or mental telepathy, gave me intimations of this process – but clearly it went further still. He entrusted me with further information, held secret for centuries within an initiated priesthood, which had to do with the exalted notion of the exchange of souls, and the assumption of what might be termed *star identity* or *astral travel*. Taking account of my novice status in respect of lion–human spirituality, he gave me limited examples. These explained in concrete terms how, under duress, one might draw on this stellar source to effect changes on physical reality, both of an animate and inanimate nature. I understood that the root and nature of these powers were directly related to one's spiritual evolution. Always, Mutwa insisted that the exercise of power went hand in hand with reverence and a strong sense of responsibility.

The lion and the eagle are kings but are also sun symbols. In this way, they are symbols of light as opposed to darkness.

In closing, Mutwa identified the four successive steps of induction in the lion shaman's spiritualizing process:

> The first stage is the courage to face up to the lion.
>
> The second stage is the assumption of the lion-man identity.
>
> The third stage is the assumption of the lion-man-hawk identity.
>
> The fourth stage is the evolution into the lion-man-hawk-serpent identity, the highest leonine state: Guardian of Sacred Knowledge, known in ancient heraldry as the gryphon.

The African name for this sacred hybrid creature is Npenvu – the Beast of Truth. Mutwa told me that truth was as mighty as a lion, and as brave as an eagle. (The eagle and the hawk are used interchangeably.) When I inquired why this entity should have a serpent's tail, he told me that truth also bit – like a mamba.

Before I had paused to consider the magnitude of what I was proposing, I asked Mutwa whether one day he would introduce me to the ways of the lion shaman. Looking back on my request, I quaked at the memory of Mutwa's description of the eagle and lion initiation rites. In both, a single rash or fearful move would have endangered the initiate's life. In response to my spontaneous and ill-considered request, Mutwa gave me a long, hard look. He then informed me that only if I had a dream "sent by the spirits" would I be considered fit for induction into the rites of lion shamanism. He also told me that should I have this dream, he would recognize it immediately.

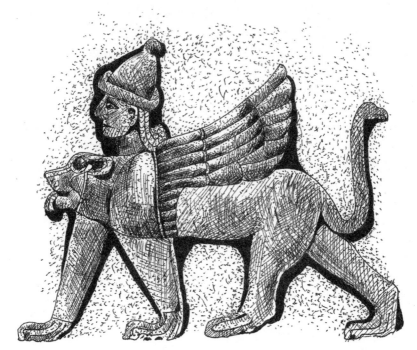

Gryphon, guardian of sacred knowledge. The assumption of the lion-man-hawk-serpent identity is the highest condition of shamanic lion priesthood. Late Hittite, dated 10th century BC (Ankara Museum).

I remonstrated myself for my audacity in demanding further knowledge, and thought of how much information the lion shaman had offered me already, and how little I truly understood.

Bow of Burning Gold

At Mutwa's suggestion, I returned the following day. Despite my brashness, it seemed that our intimacy had deepened. Not once in his presence was I made to feel inferior as a woman, and his gentle manner toward me reminded me of his touching admission that, in line with his family totem of lion protection, he was "sworn to protect women of any race or any tribe – even female baboons." He told me that in the Great Tradition, men were not superior in status to women. I was reminded how my investigations of world mythology had revealed lion goddesses of equal stature to lion-hero gods.

Today he was attended by one of his *sangoma* assistants, Virginia, the striking woman with long beaded braids and a fine-featured face of amber complexion whom I had seen there before. Mutwa's great bronze breastplate had been laid on the table, and she was attempting to make an impression on it with a rag and a tin of Brasso.

Among the ornaments attached to this massive breastplate, I noticed, hung two large pendants on either side of the chest.

"Those," Mutwa explained, catching my eye, "symbolize the breasts of the great Earth Mother, Amarava."

It was the first time since our initial encounter that Mutwa had mentioned this formidable deity's name, and in that moment it felt as if a tangible presence had suddenly entered the room. I began to wonder again just how closely his female spirit guide was identified with Mutwa's own character. He went on to tell me that, at the highest ranks of the Sanusis, the perfect human condition is neither female nor male, but a union of the two.

"When Africans honor you as a man of great wisdom, ma'am," he told me, "they give you a feminine name."

"So what is your feminine name?" I asked.

This would have seemed a natural enough question, but Mutwa gave a sudden chuckle, clearly taken by surprise, "Oh, no! That I will never tell."

Rather than deliberately withholding information, I realized once again that there was greater meaning attached to shamanic concepts than I could fully appreciate. Since names carry immense power, I suspected that Mutwa's feminine name might have direct bearing on the female spirit guide who was in constant attendance over him.

As I grew to know Mutwa better, I began to suspect that the reason for the repeating pattern of victimization in his life lay in his refusal to draw on the full extent of his own power. If Amarava was indeed his female counterpart, she was certainly not humble and vulnerable like Mutwa himself. As a fearsome deity of undisguised supremacy and enlightenment, she was identified with all those goddesses across the globe who dominate wild beasts, among them Sekhmet, the lion-headed goddess of Egypt, whose very name, I would come to learn, is synonymous with raw power.[3] While Mutwa, in all humility, might truly wish to be a simple grocer on the street corner, Amarava was unapologetically the supreme Earth Mother, the Great Mother of humanity itself.[4]

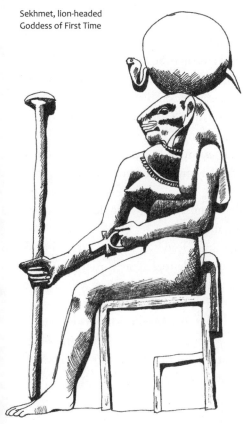

Sekhmet, lion-headed Goddess of First Time

In speaking of this deity with caution and manifest respect, Mutwa informed me that "Amarava was the mother of the First People on earth, and she will be the mother of the last."

He removed his thick glasses and wiped them thoughtfully before explaining further. "In dominating the beast of prey, she turns it into a beast of light. She is the great enlightenment-bearer, and I fear her and honor her absolutely – but I cannot always obey her," he added.

I came to see how it was his personal struggle, his all-too-human consciousness wrestling with his inner divinity, that left him vulnerable to outside attack. One can only wonder how different life would have been had he obeyed her every word and commanded his full powers through her.

I was reminded of this fatal vulnerability when we spoke about his political affiliations. Many times during the decades of apartheid rule, Mutwa was put under pressure to join the liberation struggle against oppression.

"I would not, ma'am. I would not," he explained to me. "I could not take up arms!"

Refusing to become a political figure on the side of the armed struggle, Mutwa was labeled a "sellout," an enemy of the people, and became a prime target for attack.

"What is it exactly that she asks you to do, and that you refuse?" I asked respectfully.

Mutwa shook his head gravely.

I waited in silence.

Looking pained, he said, "She has always commanded me to be the leader of this country – but I cannot!"

He shook his head slowly from side to side, and a silence fell between us once more.

Much as I respected Credo, it was hard for me to imagine this alienated figure as the leader of our country.

Virginia, the trainee *sangoma,* had entered, and Mutwa turned and gave an instruction to her in Xhosa. She disappeared and returned, bearing a massive metal bow. This, Mutwa informed me, was constructed from the axle of a motor car and I saw that, from end to end, it stood higher than a man and was thicker than his wrist.

"Amarava showed me how to craft this," he told me. "She has taught me everything I know. This would have been the weaponry of my warriors."

He paused, his eyes downcast. As was characteristic of Mutwa, the introduction of the giant bow had provided his story with a strangely mythic dimension in an age when battles were fought with atomic warheads.

"Amarava has instructed me all my life that I must lead my people out of mental servitude – but I cannot take up arms. I cannot, ma'am."

"Is she telling you that you should be the political leader of this country?" I asked, still finding the picture of Mutwa as some sort of presidential figure hard to credit.

"Ma'am, in the highest laws of the Sanusis, political and spiritual are one," the lion shaman replied.

Reminding myself again that Mutwa was, in my experience, a man entirely without ego, it now began to dawn on me why the fiery Amarava expected some kind of epic battle plan from a humble shaman. I realized that the great Earth Mother figure was not proposing that Mutwa should seize political control, with the attendant abuse of power and corruption often associated with such a leadership position, but that he should take spiritual command. When Mutwa used the term *my people,* my first thought was that he was referring to his Bushman or Zulu origins. Yet people from all nations made pilgrimages to see him and he was not being culturally specific. In accordance with his Great Knowledge, Mutwa the lion shaman was ready to lead all people from spiritual enslavement. What held Mutwa the man back was his lack of self-confidence in heeding his inner female counterpart: the leonine *magna mater,* Amarava.

In front of him now, he held the monumental welded-steel instrument in both hands, shaking his head slowly from side to side. I couldn't help noticing how the last rays of the highveld sun, slanting through the metal window frames, seemed to home in on Mutwa's sacred weapon. Remembering the symbolism behind the Sword of Shelumi helped me to understand his predicament.

"This instrument of death, ma'am," he said, drawing a painful breath, "has been used instead as a weapon of the spirit. It is a sacred bow. There are only three arrows that may be launched from it. These symbolize the three powers of God."

Resting the great bow against the wall now, Mutwa drew a sketch for me of an all-seeing eye, with three lines beneath the iris, resembling the paths of tears. The image was familiar, but it was only later that I identified a parallel motif in Egyptian iconography – where one of the three lines curls back expressively, like a twirled mustache.

Mutwa continued: "When the sacred hunter dreams of his lion – take note, ma'am – he must take three spears to kill it, or three arrows of God the Trinity. This is a symbolic and spiritual battle, ma'am, for no lion should be killed in reality. We perform this ritual with surrogates such as a wooden lion, or even a large watermelon, called *ingonyama.* The green arrow symbolizes earth, the red arrow symbolizes fire, and the transparent arrow symbolizes water."

Although Mutwa had drawn only three lines, he explained that there was an invisible fourth arrow, which symbolized air.

"And both male and female initiates perform this ritual?" I asked, picturing the strangely evocative sequence in my mind's eye.

"Yes, ma'am, yes. As I told you, there is no gender discrimination in Africa's ancient healing arts."

Now that my perspective had shifted from the immediate political picture to the more mythic dimension of Mutwa's words, I began to visualize the scroll of the future rolling out before me just as Mutwa's stories in *Indaba, My Children* recounted the past. If the warlike fierceness of an angry Amarava was anything to go by, the picture that was being conjured up in my imagination suggested that the titanic battles of history and legend might be child's play compared with what lay ahead. While the battles on those pages were fought by nation upon nation, kingdom upon kingdom and tribe upon tribe, the epic battle of the future, it seemed to me, might be pitched by the forces of light against those of darkness.

Falcon-Headed Lion God

Mutwa's revelations about the origins of the African high priesthood being traced back to the lion and hawk priests reinforced the connections I had made between the mysteries of Timbavati and Zimbabwe in the south and Giza in the north.

African shamans underwent secret initiation practices in much the same way, modern archeoastronomers believe, that pharaohs underwent awesome ordeals in order to "spiritualize" themselves – the assumption of the lion incarnation being understood as an evolutionary theory of the soul toward its highest essence. Although the ancients' notion of the pharaoh's soul returning to the stars was a much-discussed idea in Egyptological circles, I had always had difficulty comprehending it. Through the principles of lion shamanism and the battle for enlightenment, the ancient belief now began to make sense. There are two meanings of the word *light*. The one is the opposite of darkness, and the other is the opposite of heaviness. Both meanings seem to be applicable when it comes to the evolution of the soul. When we humans do dark, base, harmful, or degrading things, our spirit becomes heavy. We can feel this physically. We become burdened with guilt and shame, and lose our sense of connectedness with the shining stars. The more refined, enlightened, and connected we strive to be, the lighter our spirit. Perhaps this is what is meant by the path of ascension.

As always, the first step is to conquer fear. Fear is heavy; love and courage are light.

It now became clear to me that the four stages of lion shamanism were the very same principles by which the living pharaohs were believed to have attained spiritual evolution and finally ascended to the stars – to immortality.

There is a lot to suggest that the pharaohs, as living embodiment of the sun god Horus,[5] followed the same four-fold stages of initiation in the evolution of the human soul. Horus, the original falcon-headed god who assumed lion identity as the Sphinx, also came to incorporate the serpent identity (depicted as a cobra coiled around the sun disc). In direct parallel, the pharaohs wore breastplates symbolic of the outstretched wings of the hawk, as well as a lion *kaross* over their shoulders and the cobra on their headdresses. It would seem that the pharaohs themselves were attempting to achieve initiation into the highest consciousness, symbolized by the four-fold Beast of Truth, the gryphon.

While alive, the pharaohs were Horus on earth, but after death, they in were believed to became the god Osiris, the major figure in the Egyptian cult of immortality. In Egyptian astrology, Osiris is closely identified with the constellation of Orion – after death, the pharaohs became star gods. Just as the pharaohs returned to the stars after death, so, in the African tradition, Mutwa informed me that "the souls of kings return to the stars, awaiting reincarnation." In this way, African initiation practices echo the funerary rites of the ancient Egyptians.

That pharaohs and African kings, at a soul level, had an important leonine aspect, and later ascended to the stars, remained a profoundly interesting concept for me. I had no way of knowing at this time that this concept of a lion king's soul returning to the stars would become critically relevant in relation to the Timbavati–Giza meridian, and would take on real manifest meaning in respect of the living lions of Timbavati.

What struck me in these most recent lessons with Mutwa was how closely the ancient lion-bird knowledge surrounding the mystery of Zimbabwe followed the lion-hawk tradition of Egypt – a connection implicit in Great Zimbabwe's geographic alignment with the monuments of Giza.

The connection between Egypt and the southern sites emerged again once Mutwa began to tell me of "a very, very ancient tribe belonging to the land we call Lesotho: the Bakwama."

"This is one of the oldest and wisest of Africa's star tribes," he explained. "In their memory, they recall a mysterious land of huge square mountains which come to a point, a land which is ruled by a god with the head of a human being and the body of the lion."

"Like the Sphinx in Egypt?" I pointed out the obvious.

"Yes, ma'am. Exactly. Only, the Bakwama call this country Ntswana-tsasi – which means 'the Land of the Sun-Hawk or Sun-Eagle.' It is from this mysterious land of the gods that they say their ancestors came."

Knowing that the ancient Egyptians worshipped a solar falcon god, Horus, it was interesting to detect Egyptian influence extending to this southernmost part of Africa. More curious still, however, were occasions when Mutwa's Great Knowledge suggested the reversal of this position: rather than Africa's traditions originating in Egypt, it was Egypt's spiritual tradition that appeared to be rooted in the Great African Tradition.

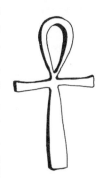

The Egyptian ankh.

I recognized the great bronze symbol hanging as a centerpiece from Mutwa's breastplate as the very same as that which the pharaohs are routinely depicted as holding in one hand. I was interested to hear from Mutwa that this symbol, the ankh, was not of Egyptian origin, but was lifted from sub-Saharan Africa, where it was known over the entire continent as the "Knot of Life" – the symbol of the one-legged Sun God Mvelinqangi, whose return was so long-awaited. I knew Mutwa better than to believe it was arrogance that had prompted these assertions of the African tradition nurturing symbols before they were immortalized in ancient Egyptian mythology. Instead, the ankh suggested an enlightened understanding that traced knowledge around the globe to one original source.[6]

The Talking Rosetta Stone

Of all the secret relics, the most extraordinary had to be the "Talking Stone" – a monumental block of masonry engraved with astronomical symbols and sacred writing in more than one script, which Mutwa explained was by many centuries the oldest of all the antiquities in his possession. On his instruction, it had taken two strong men to carry the artifact, housed in its metal box and sealed with steel cable, into the room to show me. Mutwa unlocked the seal with a key he carried around his neck, and expectantly I watched his attendant, Virginia, open the box.

Although dull with dust, the luster of the stone shone through. Without doubt, it was a Rosetta stone of sorts. Although its several texts (separated into columns) were entirely indecipherable,[7] there were several gracefully carved symbols that were immediately recognizable to me. Most conspicuous was a star symbol, representing Sirius, as well as a lion in a guarding position, and a leaping dolphin.[8] While the original Rosetta stone was found near the mouth of the river Nile, Mutwa informed me that this tablet was taken from the lintel of a ruined temple at the entrance of the House of Prayer in the South African territory of Venda, due north of Timbavati. Mutwa said the temple belonged to a lion king many centuries ago, who was known to Africans as Shelumi. Naturally, I had not forgotten the impressive Zimbabwean sword that was also said to belong to this king. Mutwa informed me that Shelumi was not black, but white-skinned. He was a friend, and guest, of the very first of the Monomotapa kings, Mutota. He was also the man who once acquired a wealth of gold. These details began to rekindle the biblical associations of Great Zimbabwe that, according to legend, was the source of Solomon's Old Testament treasure. As Mutwa spoke, the picture started to fall into place.

Mutwa confirmed what I now suspected – that Shelumi was, in fact, the biblical King Solomon, son of David (of the tribe of Judah). This piece of masonry itself appeared to be a much more ancient relic which had been incorporated into a temple of Solomon in the Southern Hemisphere.[9] Exciting as the prospect was, I wondered whether this could be true, remembering the legions of scholars who had dismissed Zimbabwe's association with King Solomon's gold mines.[10] If Mutwa's artifacts could be authenticated, it would shed an entirely new light on the question. Apart from Professor Barry Fell (of the International Epigraphic Society of California), few have given serious

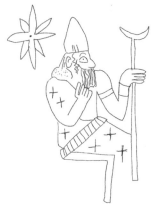

Engraving on the arm plate of Shelumi. This relic is in the custodianship of Credo Mutwa, Guardian of Umlando.

consideration to these artifacts. Fell is known for his work in deciphering the Easter Island inscriptions. After the professor of epigraphy[11] was shown the Talking Stone, he wrote a paper relating its inscriptions to the Ten Commandments.[12]

Even today, *shelumi,* in the Tswana language, means "lion," and, according to Mutwa, is also a term for the bones of divination. Mutwa also informed me that in Zimbabwe there existed a tribe who still revered King Shelumi.[13] As confirmation of Solomon's presence in the southern regions, the Guardian of Umlando went on to produce another artifact from his collection, a bronze arm plate with an engraved star and a fine engraving of a bearded king of distinctly Semitic appearance, which he said was worn by the lion king Shelumi.

Intrigued as I was at the time, I would have all the more reason to remember Mutwa's words, and the *Leswika la kuruma* – the so-called Talking Stone – once I ventured onto Egyptian soil and learned important details about King Solomon's association with the lion symbol.[14] It was only some time after this encounter with Mutwa that I would discover that the Venda area, which Mutwa claimed to be the location of Solomon's (Shelumi's) temple in the south, also carried powerful legends of White Lions.[15] This identified the site with the White Lion legends of Zimbabwe to the north and the living appearance of White Lions of Timbavati to the south. Venda itself is on precisely the same longitudinal line. The White Lion legends in the two different locations also associate the Venda people with the Lemba people, whom Mutwa had identified as two different strains of the same Jewish ancestry. The Lion of Judah was the symbolic totem of the royal Jewish line, as founded by King David, the ancestor of Jesus (for Christians, the ultimate monarch of that line). The lion is closely associated with kingship all over the ancient Middle East.

This and other evidence, including clues Mutwa had dropped about the presence of King Solomon in the south, led me to identify a poignant pattern in my interaction with the lion shaman. Despite feeling a sense of honor at Mutwa's entrusting me with such gems of knowledge, my opinion remained tinged with skepticism. The ever-deepening layers of significance only began to reveal themselves to me over time, after painstaking further investigation – when Mutwa, alas, was no longer by my side to share my sense of revelation.

13

UNDERGROUND RIVER OF GOLD

A great river flows under the African continent,
a river that is said to lead both into the future as well as the past.

– CREDO MUTWA

Following my discovery of a geodetic link between the White Lions' physical birthplace and the ancient position of the Sphinx in Giza, I had also become aware of curious resonances between the folklore of the Timbavati region and ancient Egyptian cosmology. This applied in particular to the notion of the Milky Way as a great river of stars.

In this bushveld region, the name Timbavati is commonly taken to mean both "river of stars" and "the river that never runs dry," much as the ancient Egyptians used the concept of the Duat to mean both "river in the sky" and "subterranean river." Why should a myth analogous to the Duat crop up in a remote part of Southern Africa?

It was understandable that the Egyptians might have compared their great river to the Milky Way, an apparent shower or overarching stream that existed in the heavens in perfect alignment to the Nile on earth.[1] As Adrian Gilbert and Robert Bauval remark in *The Orion Mystery*, "It is not hard to see why a Nilotic people with a sky religion should see a correlation between their river and the Milky Way. Just as the Nile divides Egypt into two regions, so the Milky Way divides the sky."[2]

But the same can't be said for Timbavati. The curious fact is that, in contrast with the Nile in Egypt, the Timbavati rivers virtually never flow. While the Nile was easily conceptualized as an eternal river, since it flowed constantly and flooded every year, bringing the rich silt on which the agricultural civilization depended, Timbavati is a land of dry dongas and empty watercourses in which water flows for only one or two days a year after occasional thunderstorms. Yet the word *Timbavati* refers to an eternal river, or starry river, or more specifically, a subterranean river. Why, in this arid bushveld region without visible rivers, should the myth of the celestial river be eternalized?

The River That Never Runs Dry

On one occasion, I raised this question with Mutwa. "You explained to me that the name Timba-vaati has to do with the descent of this star thing to this precise spot on the globe," I began. "But in the mythology of Timbavati, Maria has explained to me that the name Timbavati also has to do with a river that never runs dry – a starry river or an underground river ..."

"This is also true. Yes, yes," he said emphatically.

"Do you know, Credo, that the ancient Egyptians believed that the river Nile was an earthly copy of the Milky Way?"

"It does not surprise me, ma'am."

"But I need to understand this, Credo: why should Timbavati's knowledge be the same as that of the Egyptians?"

"Ma'am, all knowledge in the world is connected. It is all from one great source. There is nothing that the ancient Egyptians knew that we do not know. We believe that the Milky Way is the spinal fluid of the universe. There is a lot of water carried between the stars, and it may be distributed across space in this way. Amarava has told me water is not native to our planet, but came to us through the star which you call Sirius."

Although this notion delighted my senses, it eluded my rational comprehension, so I resisted pursuing it further at this stage. Instead, I followed a golden thread that Mutwa had dropped in an earlier meeting.

After his allusions to an underground river that "holds the continent of Africa together," I had spent time examining maps of our earth, and discovered an interesting fact. The 31°14′ longitudinal line is defined by the Nile Delta at the top of Africa. Since the Nile's course follows this line from its source at the equator, up the continent of Africa to the Delta, this exact parallel on our globe is known by Egyptologists, unsurprisingly, as the Nilotic Meridian. One of the interesting factors about the Nilotic Meridian is that it defines the center of the earth's landmasses. This is well illustrated by spinning a globe of the earth, on which it can be seen that one side of the earth is virtually all ocean, while the other supports a concentration of landmasses, at the geographical epicenter of which is the Nilotic Meridian.

"Help me to understand this mystery, Credo," I asked politely. "You told me that the present course of the Nile was man-made, not nature-made?"

"That is what is said, ma'am."

"And you told me that according to the Great Knowledge there are underground rivers running beneath rivers flowing on the surface."

"Yes, ma'am. Yes."

"Therefore," I concluded, "underneath the present position of the Nile, we are saying there may flow a deep subterranean river, which might in fact be associated with the Lulungwa Mangakatsi – Africa's legendary underground river?"

"It is possible, ma'am," Mutwa said with a slight smile.

This encouraged me to contemplate a moment. "So now I know that there is a sacred subterranean river under the continent of Africa and that this river has special qualities. Are we saying that it has qualities of energy?"

"Yes, ma'am, at the very least we are saying that."

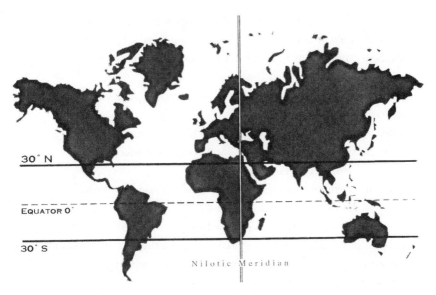

30° N

EQUATOR 0°

30° S

Nilotic Meridian

The Nilotic Meridian at the center of the earth's landmasses.

Although I sensed I was reaching a revelation of great import, I remained unsure where it was leading. Was Africa's great subterranean river best understood as a symbolic river of some kind, or was it a physical reality? On deeper reflection, was it not perhaps – as Mutwa himself had intimated – both? That is, a river in the physical as well as the metaphysical sense, a real flowing river – with special qualities. In my mind's eye, I began to visualize the notion of a "river" in terms of waves, streams, frequencies – in short, a subterranean current. I began to suspect that what was meant was an energy line of sorts beneath the surface of the earth, whether one understood it in terms of a faultline of Western seismology, or the more ancient notion of ley lines, such as songlines (Aboriginal), dragonlines (Feng Shui), or chakras (Indian).

"The next time you go to a flowing river in the veld, ma'am," Mutwa instructed me, "go at night – not with rubber-soled shoes but with leather soles. The nearer you draw to the river, the more you will feel this . . ." – he paused – "this thing, what you might call a vibration. Freshwater rivers are living, ma'am. And what is more, they contain memory – like a photograph. We Sanusis are trained to see the photographic images that rivers carry. This is even more the case when a river runs beneath the surface, where it forms invisible pipes of great power."

I paused, attempting as ever to accommodate Mutwa's unfamiliar information. "Are we saying there is some kind of 'power line' linking Timbavati to Giza, Credo?"

"Yes, ma'am, yes."

From my personal experience in nature, I knew that animals such as whales, elephants, and lions followed ancestral paths generation after generation. Why should this be? And why is water regularly discovered at the intersection of these paths? I had often wondered how shamans such as Maria divined water. For some reason, animals – like shamans around the globe – can tap subterranean energy currents. Similarly, the world's ancient tribes believe that walking these sacred paths is an act of creation. With these connections in mind, I was reminded that the Sphinx was said to be built upon just such a subterranean "power point." Why?

"If there is some kind of energy line linking Timbavati to Giza, Credo," I ventured, "what has it to do with lion worship?"

Mutwa smiled and tilted his head to one side in his characteristic fashion.

"Close your eyes, if you please, ma'am. What picture do you see?"

For some reason, I visualized a radiant golden lion.

"I see a gold lion – perhaps that missing relic, Credo," I said hesitantly.

"Yes, ma'am, yes!" he said, then paused dramatically.

Was this the clue he was giving me? I knew from world mythology that gold was equated with lions – just as lions were identified with gold, the so-called lion of metals.[3]

"Are we suggesting that the Lulungwa Mangakatsi has something to do with gold?" I asked cautiously, my heart pounding.

"This may be so, ma'am," Mutwa responded solemnly.

"A river of gold?"

He sat in solemn silence.

"Just as the white ant digs deep underground and returns through earth with gold dust, so we Sanusis work with the sacred metals of knowledge. I cannot say more, ma'am."

I knew only too well now that Mutwa's simple answers belied deeper truths, just as the childlike simplicity of his beast fables hid profound knowledge.

"So what does this have to do with Zimbabwe," I proceeded to ask cautiously, "where the word *Zimbabwe – zim* – not only had to do with a lion but also with gold?"

While the leonine associations of Great Zimbabwe are as yet unacknowledged, its affiliation with gold is commonly known.[4] It has long been known that Great Zimbabwe was a place of gold production and a thriving mercantile trading center in Africa – unlike Timbavati, where the ancient furnaces identified by Mutwa remain unknown to archeologists.[5] Mutwa told me that "what brought the Portuguese to this part of the world were long-standing legends about Prester John and Monomotapa – the empire of gold."

Although I tread warily here, to ensure I reveal no more than my Sanusi friend intended, Mutwa was prepared to go on record in respect of the secret societies led by Sacred Blacksmiths, whose knowledge of herbs and molten matter enables them to "recreate objects which God gave us many centuries ago," which have to do with "the soul of the earth but also the universe beyond."

In approaching the subject of precious metal smelting practices used by Sacred Blacksmiths (which entail combining earth matter with stellar energies), I realized I was approaching something of an alchemical nature that joined the physical with the metaphysical – the ultimate nature of which I had only the faintest inklings. There was no shadow of doubt that the High Priest was alluding not to the mercantile value of sacred metal smelting practices, but to something of a profoundly spiritual nature.

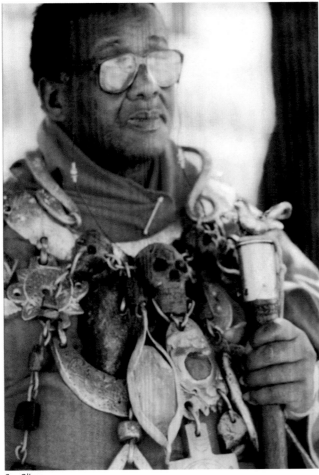

Credo Vusamazulu Mutwa. Africa's great lion priest; prophet without honor in his own country

Guy Oliver

Richard Wicksteed

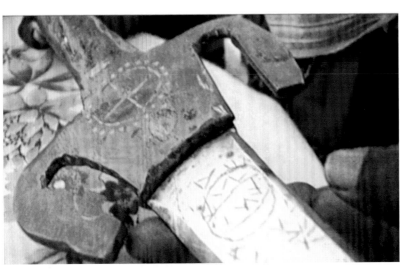

The Sword of Shelumi, with astronomical engravings on the hilt and blade

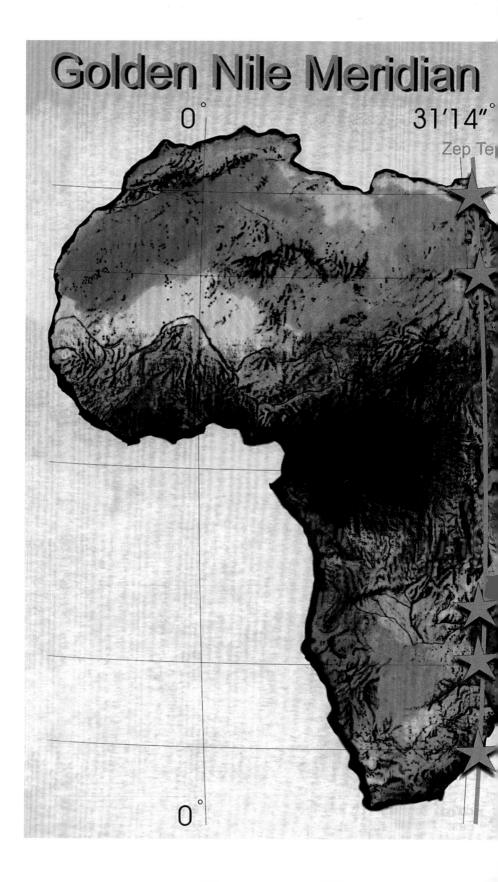

# of First Time

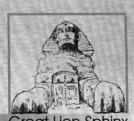

Great Lion Sphinx

30° N Giza
Heliopolis

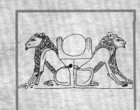

Akeru

24° N Philae

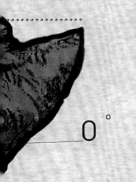

Melozo
Ethiopia / Sudan

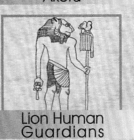

Lion Human
Guardians

0° Equator

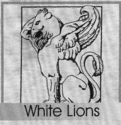

Zimbabwe Bird

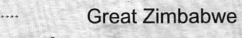

Great Zimbabwe

24° S Timbavati

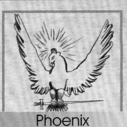

White Lions

30° S Durban (Phoenix)

Phoenix

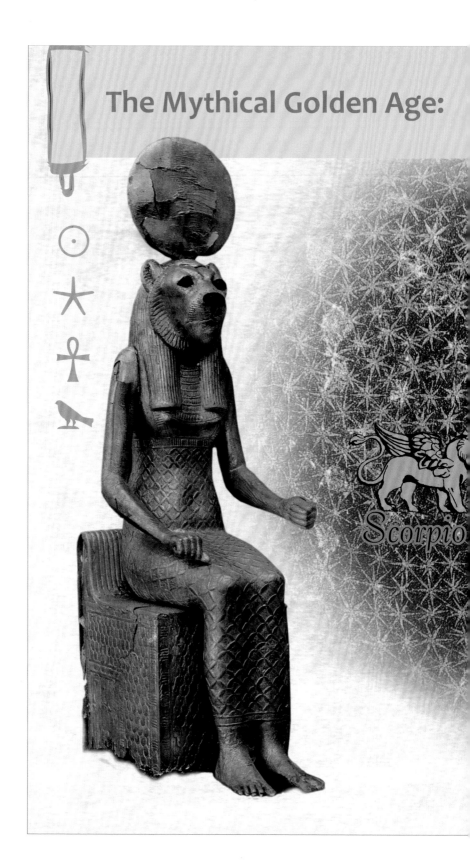

The Mythical Golden Age:

When divine order reigned, the globe was held in perfect balance and the Children of the Sun God ruled over the earth in peace, harmony, and justice.

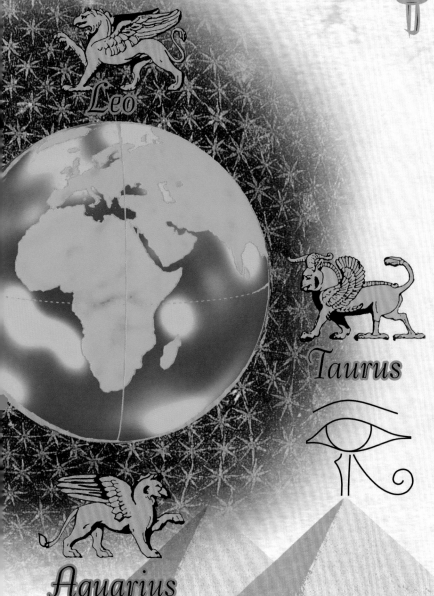

Leo

Taurus

Aquarius

Previous page: The Nile Meridian:
Zep Tepi – Line of First Time (first gold and first life on the planet)
And the corresponding East African Rift Valley – Birth Canal of the Human Species

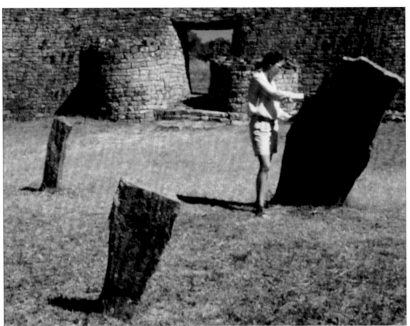

Great Zimbabwe: Linda Tucker standing beside an astrological stone gong. The sanusis are initiated into the ritual of communicating with certain heavenly bodies by sounding these stones

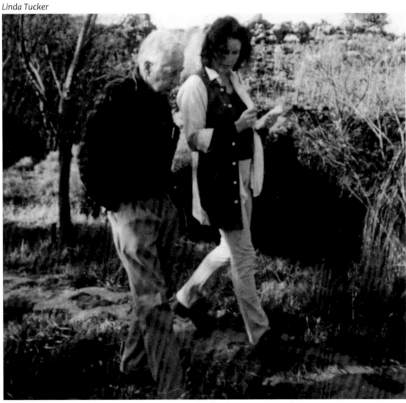

Swartkrans in the Sterkfontein Valley: Linda Tucker with Dr Bob Brain at the hominid site

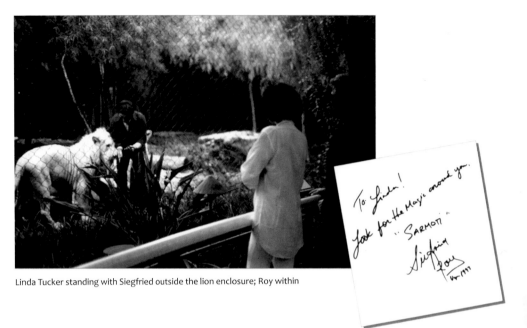

Linda Tucker standing with Siegfried outside the lion enclosure; Roy within

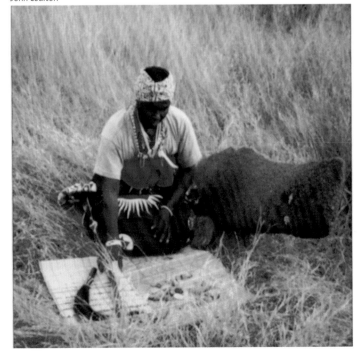

Timbavati: Maria Khosa, lion queen, divining with the bones, beside an astrological stone gong. According to Credo Mutwa, these astrological artifacts correspond with those of Great Zimbabwe, and are intended to demarcate Timbavati as a sacred site

Linda Tucker

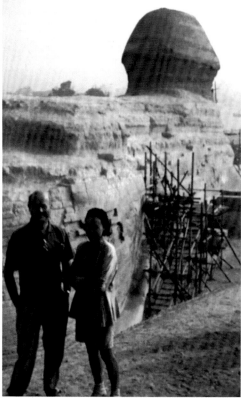

Linda Tucker

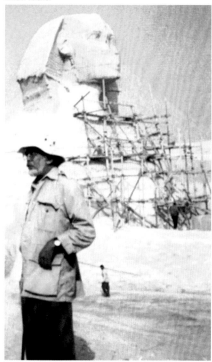

Linda Tucker with Adrian Gilbert

John Anthony West with the Great Sphinx under scaffolding behind

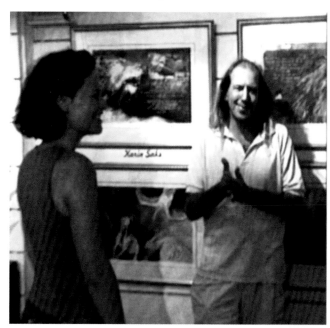

Linda Tucker and Gareth Patterson, at the exhibition of Karen Saks in celebration of Patterson's work

Richard Wicksteed

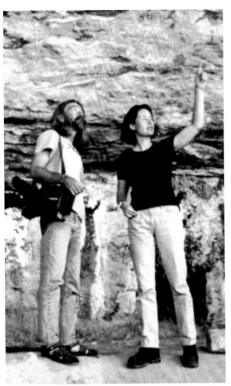

Linda Tucker with Richard Wicksteed, filming Bushman paintings of lions in the mountains near Bethlehem

Linda Tucker

The Coerland lion painting, Golden Gate, Free State. Bushman experts Lewis-Williams and Katz consider this depiction to represent the "hallucinatory combat between benevolent shamans and attacking shaman-lions." They note the "curious tusks that also appear on paintings of shamans." Could these tusked felines be representative of the now-extinct sabertooth?

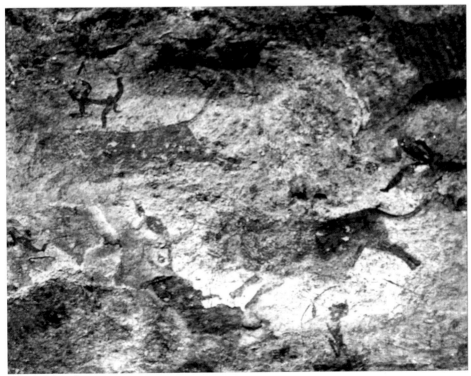

Richard Wicksteed

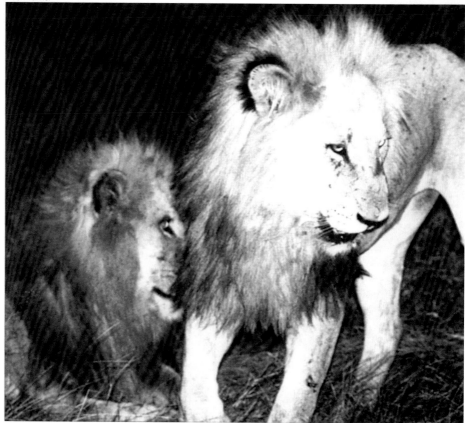

Some of the young lions of Timbavati are unusually light in color, suggesting they may be bearing the white gene

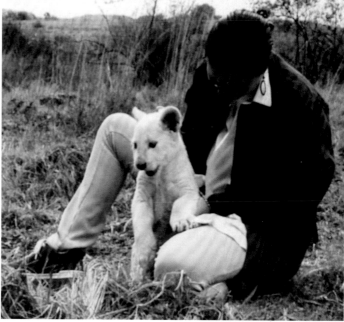

Linda with Tendile, born at Sterkfontein, cradle of humankind's evolution

Linda Tucker meets serious-faced Aslan for the first time, born in a "canned" hunting camp in Bethlehem

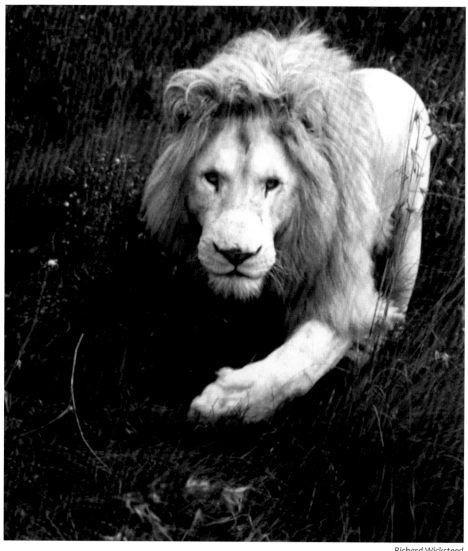

Aslan, born in Bethlehem (Free State). Pictured here as a sub-adult, not yet two years old

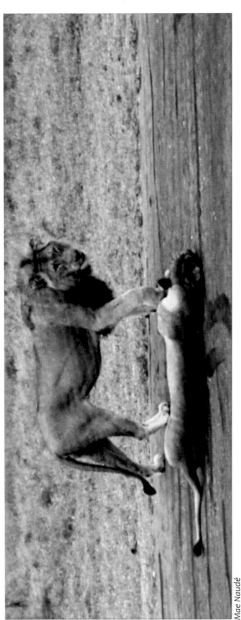

Mae Naudé

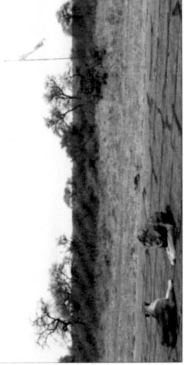

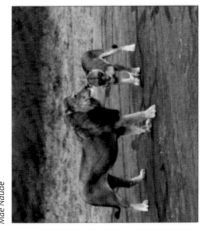

Winged Lion of Timbavati, Ingwavuma, with Maltese cross on his forehead, makes an appearance on the runway together with a young mate

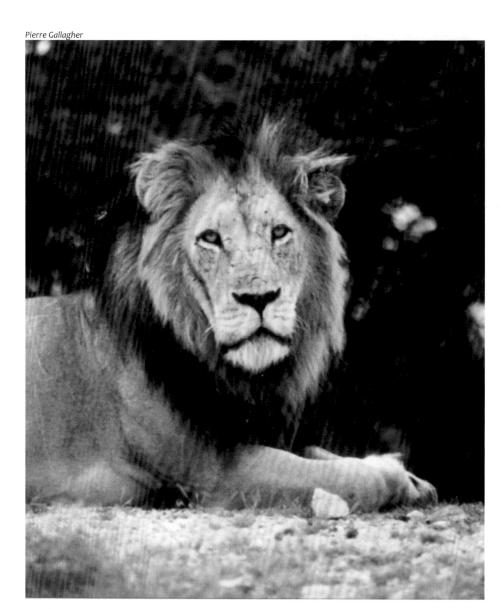

The wise face of Ingwavuma. This photograph was taken from the "identikit" compiled by rangers to identify dominant males, and later used by the hunter to approve his trophy

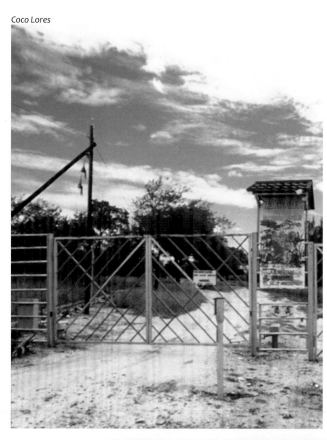

Coco Lores

On the outskirts of Timbavati, a White Lion "canned" hunting operation

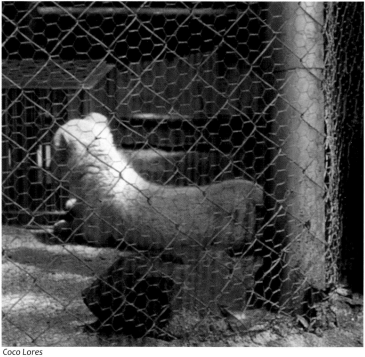

Coco Lores

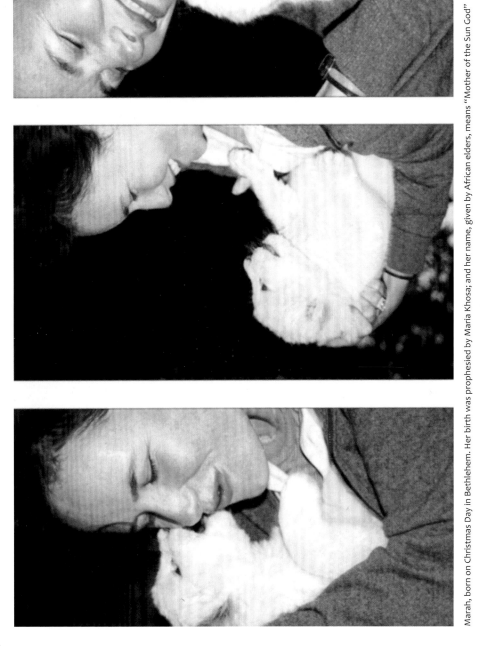

Marah, born on Christmas Day in Bethlehem. Her birth was prophesied by Maria Khosa; and her name, given by African elders, means "Mother of the Sun God"

Richard Wicksteed

"Gold has been the cause of great civilizations, and of deadly wars on earth," Mutwa told me gravely. "By mining gold, ma'am, human beings are enslaved to forces of which they are not even aware."

He gave a deep sigh, and I felt the chasm of knowledge that separated us.

"Amarava has instructed me that if I am to become this country's leader, one of my first tasks is to stop the mining of gold."

In that brief moment, I got a hint of the scale of the task that the Great Creator Goddess was demanding of this mortal. Close down South Africa's gold mines! How could any individual take on the sole responsibility for dismantling the powerfully entrenched vested interests of mercantile mining? Why would anyone want to?

"But Credo, I don't understand. Why should it be so important to stop the mining of gold?"

"Ma'am – if you only knew! Where do I begin?" he said, patiently.

He went on to tell me that gold's natural existence in the bowels of our planet is essential to life on Earth. Most specifically, it controls the existence and flow and purification of fresh water. Gold and copper (rather than gravity as we understand it) supply the energy that causes rivers to flow and be cleansed, since gold is not simply a physical metal but a spiritual metal with a profound metaphysical purpose.

"Gold is an 'entity,'" he explained. "Just as we have such minerals in us – gold, copper, iron – so has our earth. And they are not there to be mined by humankind," he added grimly.

Feeling the weight of ideas that I did not yet fully comprehend, I sat in silence.

I had now ascertained that the legendary Lulungwa Mangakatsi was not only a great river running beneath the earth like the shower of stars of the Milky Way in the heavens, but also appeared to be a vein of gold running beneath the African continent. Amazing as this revelation was, it made perfect sense. I thought of the Monomotapa empire linked by a chain of gold-bearing rivers, centered on the source of the Nile, and goldfields clustering around the 31°E meridian. In Zimbabwe, even today, alluvial gold panning is considered the nation's "rural alternative to subsistence farming."[6]

The accounts of the Portuguese historian Joao De Barros make it clear that the auriferous (gold-yielding) sites are centered on this specific meridian:

> All the land which we include in the kingdom of Sofala is a great region ruled by a heathen prince called Benomotápa; it is enclosed like an island by two arms of a river which issues from the most considerable lake in all Africa, which was much sought after by the ancients as being the hidden source of the famous Nile . . .

De Barros goes on to describe the Zambezi River, Limpopo River, and tributaries, "all of which water Benomotápa's land, and most of them carry down much gold which is yielded by that land," focusing on the gold wealth around the site of Great Zimbabwe, already ruined at that time.[7]

Similarly, the maps of the goldfields drawn by researchers at the turn of the 20th century also detail smelting sites clustered around the 31°E longitudinal line.

With this meridian in mind, I thought again of the metal-smelting sites in Timbavati, which Mutwa had said were of a "very sophisticated kind." In the late 19th century, J.M. Stuart recorded gold-mining operations ranging southward beyond the Limpopo into the then Transvaal. He himself had come across numerous old workings "showing that centuries ago mining was practised on a most extensive scale, and that vast quantities of ore had been worked, and that by engineers of a very high order."[8]

More recently, gold-rush sites such as Bourke's Luck Potholes and Pilgrim's Rest (where Victorian gold-mining structures may well be positioned over older indigenous sites) are concentrated around the 31°E longitudinal line, the most famous of these being the Victorian gold-mining town of Barberton. On the African continent, the distribution of gold is concentrated around this meridian, with the gold yield in and around this area in the Southern Hemisphere recently accounting for more than half the world's gold production.[9]

Could this geographic positioning around this prime meridian really be coincidence?

If there was a gold artery running through the entire continent of Africa, what had this to do with the Nile, which followed this meridian to its Delta in the north? I knew that the notion of gold linked this artery to the lion symbol. But what this lion–gold connection signified remained profoundly mysterious.

Subterranean River of Gold

These were the questions that remained with me after I parted from Mutwa and traveled the dark road back to Pretoria and my father's home. My father still lives in the lovely Victorian house in which I was born, about an hour away from where Mutwa was temporarily lodging in Johannesburg. This had become my base over the period I was working with Mutwa. Each evening as I returned home, I found it increasingly difficult to integrate the extraordinary information received during my days with Mutwa into my suburban surroundings. Only in those quiet moments at night, before I dropped off to sleep, did Mutwa's words find a way to settle into my consciousness.

Bearing in mind that at the level of highest priesthood, gold and sacred knowledge are one and the same (the one being the spiritual form of the other), I now saw how Mutwa himself, who had ascended through all stages of lion initiation, was the living embodiment of the gryphon, Guardian of the Great Knowledge (or "gold"). The *Encyclopaedia Britannica* specifies that the gryphon is "consecrated to the sun" and watches over gold mines and secret treasure. Yet, by sad contrast with Mutwa's description of this hybrid beast as "the Beast of Truth" and knowledge, the *Britannica* informs us that the gryphon is construed as the symbol of "human avarice and greed." This apparent misrepresentation of ancient knowledge gives intimations of the deep-seated corruption within human nature that has destroyed real values and replaced them with false ones.

When I alerted Mutwa the following day to our dictionary interpretations of the gryphon as the symbol of human avarice and greed, the Guardian of Umlando shook his head gravely.

"We have lost our soul essence, ma'am. You will remember that the Portuguese caught the last of the Monomotapa kings and skinned him alive to torture him to reveal where gold was hidden." It was a gruesome reminder of the lengths to which humanity will go for material gain.

"Listen to me carefully," Mutwa continued with the same gravity. "In our tradition we believe that in the center of the earth there is a very deep hole, and in that hole there is a sacred mountain made completely of gold or copper." He went on to explain how wisdom emanated from this golden mountain of hidden knowledge "like a great river, nourishing all places, all lands, and all beings."

He spoke prophetically about how it would be brought to the surface for all to see "at the end of this world and the beginning of the new world" and how "it will shine for all living beings." At this epiphanic moment in time, he told me, "all beings shall share in the great knowledge of the gods, and become as gods."

While I was mesmerized by the beauty of Mutwa's rhetoric, I was reaching a point in our exchanges when he was beginning to lose me. It wasn't that I did not want to know more but, wondering where all this questioning was heading, I had reached the edge of my capacity to take in further information.

On the Timbavati–Giza connection – and the vein of gold that appeared to link them – I was hoping Mutwa would help me reach some clarity, but I sensed that his words would only lead me further and further into the fathomless depths of a profound and unsolvable mystery. I had forgotten for a moment that all knowledge in the Great Tradition is intrinsically connected – unlike scientific knowledge that separates and categorizes.

Mutwa's answers perpetually uncovered deeper riddles. In pursuing them, I had come to deal with an increasingly unsettling sense that I was venturing into territory where even angels would fear to tread. Yet I could not stop. There was no question of returning along the route I had taken. It was simply too exciting to turn back.

14

WINGED LION OF TIMBAVATI

The first beast was like a lion, and had eagle's wings. Then the wings thereof were
plucked, and it was lifted up from the earth, and made to stand upon two feet like a
man, and a man's heart was given to it.
– DANIEL DESCRIBING HIS DREAM IN THE OLD TESTAMENT (DANIEL 7:4)[1]

While I regarded every minute of my time with Mutwa as precious, it was with some
relief that I was reminded of a commitment that drew me away from him for a while and
gave me a chance to assimilate the information with which I was wrestling.

Shortly after I parted from Mutwa, a strange thing happened.

Lion Guardian

I had been asked to give a lecture on the significance of the vernal equinox in ancient
African cultures. The vernal equinox is that time of year (mid-spring) when day and
night are equal. As it turned out, this notion would be of great consequence to the riddle
surrounding the Sphinx, as well as the related White Lion mysteries. It is important to
note, however, that at my lecture no mention was made of my interest in lions.

In the course of delivering a preview of this lecture in Cape Town, I had an
uncomfortable experience. Throughout my talk, I was aware of a slightly disheveled-
looking man seated in the front row, with his eyes closed. It was disconcerting, naturally,
for I could only imagine that what I was saying was effectively putting him to sleep.

After the lecture, when the audience had left, I was surprised when this man came
up to me and said, "There is something I need to say to you. You can choose to take this
how you like."

"Okay," I said, guardedly.

"I was told to give you two names," he said, and proceeded to write down on a
scrap of paper a couple of rather archaic-looking names – Count Saint-Germain and
Serapis Bey – neither of which meant anything at all to me.[2] He was "told" to give me
this incomprehensible message – by whom? I was at first entirely perplexed. But then I
found myself asking: "Are you psychic?"

"You may call it that," he said. "I do see things."

"Well, thank you for conveying this message to me," I said with a shrug, still uncomfortable at his intrusion.

"There is a second thing that you should know tonight," he continued. "All the while during your lecture, there was a huge male lion standing by your side. He looked like a king, and behind him were standing a number of tribal warriors."

Instantly delighted at the image, I thanked him and said good-bye, watching him retreat and shut the door without even thinking to ask his name. For some reason what he had told me now seemed completely natural. It was only when I turned to my husband and the others standing with me and saw the astonishment in their faces that I realized how uncanny this was. A regal spirit lion standing beside me all the while I was delivering my lecture! Remembering the images of lions as sentinels, or guardians, in world mythology, I could picture clearly how this mighty lion might have looked, and it thrilled me to think of him standing guard at my side.

I regarded this as invisible support for my work and left the venue feeling uplifted and encouraged, only regretting that I had not been kinder and more forthcoming to this unknown person who had relayed information of such significance to me.

Lion of the Ancestors

I returned to Timbavati soon afterward, bearing messages of goodwill for Maria from Mutwa. I had hoped that Mutwa would accompany me, but his health was failing. On top of diabetes, he had prostate cancer, which made long-distance travel increasingly uncomfortable.

The experience at my lecture had both disturbed and thrilled me. It was one of many unusual coincidences that had started to occur in my life. While in Timbavati, I spoke to Maria about it. Her response, through the interpreter, took me by surprise. "Maria says that the lion that stood guarding you while you spoke – that is the lion of your dreams."

Although, at a non-rational level, it made immediate sense, this was an entirely unexpected connection. "Does Maria mean that the lion that keeps roaring in my face in my recurring nightmare is the same lion that this man saw standing beside me when I gave my talk?"

"Maria says yes. That lion you have been dreaming of – it is not an ordinary lion. She tells me it is a Lion of God."

Once again, my first thought was how improbable this was, yet I could not suppress a sense of excitement.

"Please ask Maria to explain what she means. Does she mean it is a White Lion? Tell Maria that, in my dream, he is definitely a tawny lion – not white."

"She says he is the father of the White Lions. It is through him that they will return."

"The father? Does Maria mean that he is carrying the white gene?"

"Maria says yes. One day he will give Timbavati back the white cubs."

Although barely comprehensible to my rational mind, this information felt electrifying. "Please tell Maria I don't really understand. That lion is part of my imagination – part of my dreams. Now she seems to be saying that it is a real lion – a flesh-and-blood lion."

"Maria says it is a real lion. She says that you will come to see him soon – before you leave Timbavati this time. He is here to greet you, he knows you are here. He knows who you are. He knows where to find you." The interpreter paused and listened to Maria's further explanation. "She says that this lion already knows that you and Maria are speaking – but she asked, 'Do you know where to find him?'"

I told Maria I had no idea where I might find him. In fascination, I mused over what she had told me. "So Maria is saying that the lion in my dream is a real lion – and he is around here in Timbavati somewhere?"

"Maria says that he is a real lion. She says that you will know it is this lion because this lion has wings."

Although captivated by the idea unfolding in my imagination, I was now thoroughly perplexed. From what I had learned from Mutwa of the elevated spiritual overtones of the White Lions, it did not surprise me that these legendary beasts might be associated with the mythical winged lion – symbolic bearers of spiritual enlightenment. Maria's present comment seemed to suggest the same. It was easy enough to understand this in symbolic terms – as angelic lions or spirit lions with wings – but what a "winged lion" might mean in everyday flesh-and-blood reality puzzled me. It took me back to Mutwa's discussions about the four stages of spiritual evolution in lion shamanism. When Mutwa had described the notion of a lion with the wings of an eagle, I had seen it as an idea. It did not occur to me that, in my quest to find the truth behind the White Lions, this mythical creature might make an appearance in real life. Returning to camp after my discussions with Maria, I walked down the sandy path, my mind filled with incongruous visions of the winged lion of Saint Mark, or the heraldic gryphon-type emblems I had studied in books: part lion, part eagle. The idea of meeting such a creature in real life was so implausible that, although I did not exactly dismiss it, I attempted to put it to the back of my mind and steep myself in the tangible reality of nature all around me.

As my visit to Timbavati drew to a close, I was no nearer to understanding Maria's cryptic message. Although I had not again been plagued by my lion nightmare, I recalled that the first time I had experienced it was in Timbavati. The night before I departed this time, a dominant male kept me awake roaring quite close to camp all night long – a sound that, like Maria, I had grown to love. Rather than terrifying me, it felt deep, earthy, and heartwarming, and I was inspired by the *sangoma*'s assertion that when she heard the lions roaring, she felt "happy."

At dawn the next morning, I went out with trackers trying to trace the lion – unsuccessfully. We found his pawprints and followed them, but after a distance, the trail suddenly disappeared. Again we picked up tracks, and yet again they seemed to evaporate into thin air. This was not an unusual experience in the bushveld – tracks, of course, are not cast in concrete, and are susceptible to any number of corrosive influences. But the recurrence of this pattern of hide-and-seek began to frustrate the tracker.

Eventually, defeated, we decided to return to camp, anticipating a hearty breakfast. We took a short cut back in the Land Rover, via the landing strip. Normally, rangers guiding tourists avoided this route, because of the unsettling incongruity of encountering a tarred runway in the middle of the wilderness. As we had no guests with us, however, we decided to opt for the quickest route back.

On the runway itself was a monumental male lion and his utterly gorgeous lioness! This was the very male we had been tracking, and the ranger could not believe his luck. As for me, there it was. A couple of meters (roughly six and a half feet) away, a perfect view of a lion and his mate on the landing strip, right in front of the wind sock. No better symbol of the winged lion of Timbavati.

He was in immaculate condition, truly magnificent – a lion in his prime. When he lowered his head his crown parted in such a way as to create a perfect Maltese cross. It was the distinguishing feature by which I came to know this particular lion. He looked up suddenly, as lions do in the wild, making razor-sharp eye contact that cut to the quick. I felt an instant connection. Was this really my totem? Was this the same lion who came to me in my dreams? The truth is that his real interest was in his female companion, an exquisite lioness (although slight in build) with slanting eyes framed in coal black, like those of an Egyptian goddess. The trackers identified this young female as one of the lionesses from the Caroline pride, a female who had been pregnant several times but miscarried time and again, and so never produced cubs of her own. Seeing them together in this context felt magical, all the more so once I remembered Maria's allusion to this lion as a bearer of the white gene. This implied something prophetic in their union.

Feeling jubilant after this unexpected surprise, I impulsively canceled my return trip and stayed in Timbavati.

After hearing my news, Maria told me that this was the sign she was looking for. The rangers themselves had identified this lion as Ingwavuma, the name he was commonly called in that region, but Maria gave me another name, which she called his secret "spirit name." I was not at liberty to disclose this name to others, but its meaning was "wise one, the one who carries great knowledge." As a consequence of my sighting of this winged lion of wisdom, Maria now revealed to me that the ancestors had long since instructed her that I, too, had a title. It was *Mulanguteri wa Ngala yo Basa*: "Keeper of the White Lions."

Keeper of the Sacred White Lions

I began to realize my increased status in Maria's eyes when she invited me to accompany her to a gathering of lion *sangomas* in the territory. Over the past couple of years, I had grown increasingly familiar with the bones-throwing technique of divining information from the ancestors, and spent many afternoons with Maria refining my interpretations of the art. Another technique of reaching the mystical dimension to which traditional healers have access is through the use of ceremonial drums. At the gathering of *sangomas,* I would have a chance to witness the power of drum rhythms in inducing altered states.

The ceremony was held in a mud *rondavel,* where several women sat on the floor, legs outstretched, each with a different-sized drum between her legs. Maria, in her full *sangoma* regalia, was joined by several female *sangomas* on grass mats on the floor. I was accompanied by an interpreter and was seated slightly apart, near the entrance.

From the moment the first drum was sounded, I felt an energy run through me. I had naïvely imagined I would be able to observe the procedure with journalistic detachment, but I soon felt the waves of rhythm overcoming me. The perfect acoustics of the confined circular space seemed to intensify the powerful pulses. I tried to stay grounded.

The second, third, then fourth drummer sounded her rhythms – each a different syncopation, but seeming to converge at peak moments. The vibration was resounding in my bones. The drummers reached a particular pitch, and then stopped dead. In this protracted silence, I watched the *sangoma* named Sarah Khosa, and the transformation that suddenly overtook her. An energy convulsed through her, and her expression glazed over. Then she started speaking in an urgent masculine voice.

This, I later learned, was the "formalized greeting," the spirit of the ancestor who worked through her, Gegege, announcing himself to the company. A little disappointed at first, I noted that the sound that now came from Sarah's mouth was not the roar of a lion but distinctly an old man's voice.

The drums sounded again and the rhythm chased around and around the *rondavel* – then stopped dead as suddenly as it had begun. Sarah's ancestral voice started up again. Her hand was flicking a tailed, beaded whisk across her face and her body was filled with a vibrating energy I had never witnessed before. It was so intense it seemed more than the human frame could tolerate, and I felt serious concern for her health.

Suddenly I grew aware that the spirit was addressing itself directly to me. The interpreter explained that the message had to do with my long and hard search to find the sacred White Lions, and failure to do so.

"The ancestor tells you they are not dead," he explained emphatically. "You must keep going with your journey. The White Lions urgently need your protection."

Again the drumming resumed. Maria herself was now drumming. I suspected that at any moment she, too, might leave us and be overtaken by ancestral forces. But instead she seemed in complete command of her energies. There were moments when I felt it was me, instead, who was at risk of losing my senses and becoming the center of the rhythm, the heart of the drumbeat.

I tried to focus on Sarah, who was gyrating in an alarming fashion. It was not only that she was speaking with another voice, but her whole being was infused with another energy entirely. The frequency of sound emitting from her lips did not coincide with the woman voicing it. Her gestures, too, were entirely transformed. She was beating her brow with the long-tailed ritual whisk as if swatting flies and wiping the sweat from her forehead with her other hand, as an old man might do in a gathering of tribal elders. She was not the plump youthful woman she had been moments before; she was transformed by the ancestral male energy coursing through her body.

The spirit message that came through now was again addressed to me, saying that Maria was "Lion Queen of Timbavati" and that any question that needed answering in the Timbavati region could be addressed by her. It went on to instruct me that I, too, was destined to become a *sangoma*.

Again, this information – which had already been conveyed to me by both Maria and Mutwa himself – felt deeply ambivalent, like a mixed blessing: excitement and honor mixed with dread and fear of change.

The message continued. In translation, I was told: "Remember, you are protected. The White Lions lie down beside your path. The light shines on you. Remember, you do not walk alone!"

Although they did not make immediate sense, these words stirred me deeply. They conjured up a sublime image of a row of White Lions lining my path, like an endless avenue of carved sphinxes. It proved to be an image I would never forget. Even today, at times when I feel fearful or confused, I take strength in calling it up again and again.

I returned from Timbavati with messages of goodwill for Mutwa from Maria.

Sitting beside the window in the stark Johannesburg room, the curtains half drawn, I observed my great Sanusi friend.

Today his mood was desperately low. He had seen a recently published article in which the journalist had misunderstood and actively misrepresented the spirit of his words. In a bleak state of despondency, he questioned what good any of his efforts had achieved, and lamented how his words were misused, or even actively employed toward destructive ends, by "misinformers." Sensing that ineffable death wish I had felt before, I tried to comfort him as best I could.

"Credo," I said, "you need to remember all the great sacrifices you have made for humanity. Never forget these. Your words will always stand. What people decide to do with the knowledge that you have handed over is their choice."

Although I felt inadequate in relieving his suffering, he seemed soothed by my comments. We spoke about Maria, and I recounted my exhilarating experience of discovering my winged lion of Timbavati. Mutwa nodded slowly throughout my account, and when I got to the end I was pleased to see him smile with pleasure. I showed him a photograph that I had taken of this lion on the landing strip, and he scrutinized it closely.

"That, I believe, is the son of the great lion that the hunters wanted to kill. You can see the likeness in his muscles, and in his face and mane, ma'am."

"There are many lions in Timbavati, Credo," I pointed out. "Do you mean to say he is the son of Ngwazi – the very lion that you protected?"

"I believe so, ma'am."

"Do you know that Ngwazi is still alive, Credo? All these years later . . . He is old now, and no longer the dominant male of the territory."

"I know that he still lives, ma'am. This I know."

Even under natural circumstances where a lion is not threatened by hunting, it is unusual for it to survive into old age. Thinking over Mutwa's achievement, I confessed, "I want to be able to protect animals in the way you protected Ngwazi."

Mutwa gave a short exhalation of breath, something between a snort and a scoff, but his tone indicated that he had no intention of being insulting.

"You cannot call a lion out of the bush until you become One. You cannot call a dolphin out of the water until you become One, ma'am." This was followed by one of his characteristic sighs. "You cannot summon a creature unless you become that creature, and all creatures . . . I wished to pass on this knowledge, ma'am. Unfortunately, I have not found a student who can do this, ma'am."

Feeling that primal urge rise in me again, I confessed that I truly wanted to learn these arts.

"No, ma'am, no," he responded. "What I have to teach might endanger your life, and I will not risk that."

Hesitating a moment, I then revealed to Mutwa how the Timbavati ancestral spirits had instructed that I was destined to be a *sangoma*. Scrutinizing me closely, Mutwa inquired, "Did you not have an illness some years ago, ma'am?"

"Yes, in fact I did, Credo," I answered, thinking back. Having been one of those lucky individuals who enjoyed perfect health, I recalled only too well the uncharacteristic health crisis that had brought my life to a standstill.

"This was in fact no ordinary illness," Mutwa concluded. "This was the path of the shaman."

It was then that I realized with a shock that what I had been through was allied to the mind-expanding experience that the shamanic initiate would call *twasa*. Although I had little inclination to recall the suffering that I experienced during this time, the vivid memory of each detail came back to me at Mutwa's prompting. Since it was pre-empted by a manic six-week period during which I had snatched no more than a couple of hours of sleep a night, staying in several different hotel rooms in several different countries each week, I had put my unexpected nervous collapse down to sustained high stress, high-adrenaline advertising activity, and the attendant sleep deprivation. I remember how, all of a sudden, normal functions began grinding to a standstill. I stopped eating, I stopped sleeping, I stopped functioning. It was a terrifyingly unfamiliar condition, from which I feared, at the time, I might never recover. As it happened, I regained physical health surprisingly quickly, but I doubt that I will ever forget the extraordinary mental states that I experienced during that period.

Despite coming into contact with drugs in the fashion and advertising industries, I have never been tempted to take any form of hallucinogenic or narcotic drug. It may sound coy, but I've never smoked substances of any kind (including tobacco), or experienced what it is like to be drunk. I also can't remember when last I needed any form of medicinal drug. Now, in light of what I had learned through the study of shamanism, I suspected that I had naturally avoided these things because I might be particularly susceptible to them and their mind-altering properties.

For this reason, the unfamiliar loss of control that overtook me during that time of physiological collapse was all the more disorienting. Although I avoided mentioning this to others at the time, I was also suffering from hallucinations and strange out-of-body experiences. I distinctly remember how I experienced the disconcerting perception of hearing people think, which often differed from what they said. Sometimes I could hear their thoughts from across a crowded room, or even simultaneously as they spoke, and I had no difficulty in hearing two individuals thinking at the same time. I also remember how time changed its quality entirely. A single minute became an agonizing hour in length – I remember believing that the clock's hands must surely have stopped, frozen in place, but then I realized that it was I who had apparently stopped time. I also remember the vivid images and symbols that flashed before my eyes. One repeated image was that of an hourglass spinning backward, another was a lion's head from which the sun's rays radiated. While the mind-altering experiences can be compared with the kind experienced by drug users, the shaman knows that taking artificial narcotics ultimately weakens his powers of connectedness to the magical workings of God in nature. Alarming as these unfamiliar experiences were at the time, through Mutwa's kind words, I now began to view them as glimpses of heightened powers that I would be a fool to turn my back on – a far cry from what Western psychiatrists might term a "nervous breakdown."

Apparently, in many cases of clinical breakdown the individual is left with little or no recall of the experience he or she has undergone. I find this surprising. It implies that little may be gleaned from a temporary malfunction, or that what may be gleaned is not easily applicable or translatable into normal life. For me, each unusual detail that I experienced was clearer than normal reality. So much so that it actually put the overhyped modern city mania of my life and my job into proper perspective. While most of us call this frenzied self-centered condition "normality," I now understood how the shaman would view such living conditions as abnormal and unnatural, and seriously out of touch with the true realities of humankind's existence on earth.

This was perhaps what Mutwa had had in mind when he inquired of me whether I remembered the period of my illness clearly.

"As if it happened yesterday, Credo," I explained, thinking back. "Not only that, but it is as if I can remember every single second of what happened during that period."

As I recounted the experience for Mutwa, he simply nodded, with understanding, explaining that what I had experienced was "time travel." "Astral travel" is one of the qualities of the "star thing" to which Mutwa so guardedly alludes.

The shaman believes that the linear way we perceive time is not necessarily the true reality. Time can be experienced as simultaneous, which helps explain why shamans are able to "foresee" the future.

The lead-up to my health crisis had been much like the experience of running, running, running, being unable to stop running. And then, suddenly, everything stopped, and time changed. Now that I had experienced the drum ceremony, I identified similarities in the endurance drumming technique of the *sangomas*. In my case, along with the other bodily functions that had ground to a halt, I had lost all desire for food, drink, or sustenance of any kind. This condition continued for almost six weeks. I must have been very close to death. In fact, I experienced what clinically dead patients describe as "the tunnel": like a rocket, I was racing down a dark tube toward a radiant light. But just before I reached the white light, I was wrenched back, with a clear message: *You have work to do*. I knew I had to return to Earth, and I recognized for the first time that I was a spirit being, not just a person with a rational mind and a physical body. I also knew that I had a clear reason for being here. It is difficult to describe, but it was at this point that life became purposeful. The "illness" that accompanied the trance state (*twasa*) that had nearly killed Mutwa had kept him bedridden for more than three years. I was lucky enough to recover from my condition after less than three months. Looking back on it afterward, rather than a breakdown, it represented a breakthrough. It felt like breaking through the four seasons of our everyday existence on Earth into a magical fifth season, where other principles of reality applied. Only after recovering from this experience was I strong enough to face the questions Maria's lion action had prompted in me, to face up to the truths that had existed all along without my even noticing them.

All this was excruciatingly awkward to own up to in my middle-class academic and advertising context. But having been brave, or foolhardy, enough to cross the great divide and enter the spiritualized world of shamanism, and having discovered that somehow it all began to make sense, there was no chance of backpedaling. I took great comfort in the physical presence of Mutwa and Maria, who represented this other way of seeing: I felt soothed by their power and reassured by the meaningfulness of their utterances – which somehow were sensible, despite operating at a level so far removed from everyday Western sensibility.

Up to this point in my quest, I might have been content to return to my comfortable former existence, in the knowledge that the White Lions, as a mutant subspecies, were not intended to survive – along with any other species born at the wrong time and in the wrong place. Instead, I now knew in my heart of hearts, from my experiences with Credo and Maria, that the reverse was true: the White Lions had declared themselves at this time and precise place for a reason. In the ancient Great African Knowledge, they are messengers, or harbingers, and the message they carry is critical for humanity at this moment in its evolutionary history. I could hear the voice of the lion ancestor speaking loudly and urgently through the female shaman, instructing me that the White Lions urgently needed my protection. I had only just begun to know of my personal role in the

White Lion mystery, as the Keeper or "Protector" of the White Lions, and it remained unclear to me how I might personally be able to protect them.

To be called as the White Lions' protector was an awesome, frightening concept. The title had the inexorable ring of destiny about it – almost as if I wasn't actively choosing my new role in life; instead, it was choosing me. I knew it was not something to take lightly, but I did not know at this time just how seriously I would be compelled to take it. I did not know that I would have to challenge the power of landowners and trophy hunters, which ultimately rests on the power of money and influence, and the guns wielded by ruthless men (and women). All I knew was that I felt profoundly honored by this message, and in return I needed to profoundly honor the message – as sacrosanct, unimpeachable, a sacred contract between myself and the ancestral White Lions of Timbavati.

15

PLAYING WITH THE SUN GOD'S CHILDREN

It is an African belief that the wild animals do not belong to man, but to God. To kill them for so-called "sport," I believe, is a crime against God. In contrast, to protect the wild animals . . . we reflect God within us.

– GARETH PATTERSON

While Mutwa's despondency at the human condition weighed heavily on my own spirits, there were many occasions when I felt uplifted and inspired, overcome by an intense sense of pride. Unexpectedly, one day Mutwa told me that he would "begin to inlay the three arrows of green, red, and pure transparent and pluck the feathers of the eagle" in preparation for my introduction to the ritual of the sacred bow sometime in the future. I had never had any leanings toward priesthood or a religious calling of any kind, yet I was being drawn further and further into the mysterious world of lion shamanism. I felt deeply honored by his words, but they scared me, too. I remembered how the lion-heroine figures from world mythology were often depicted with bows of spiritual armament, and wondered what battle lay ahead.

"I am history, ma'am, you are the future," he said poignantly. "Sharpen your sword and *assegaai* [spear] of the spirit . . . Sharpen the gifts which God gave you, so that you can help to liberate mankind from his mental imprisonment."

"But how might I do this?" I asked, feeling inadequate and uncertain of the role he was bestowing upon me in respect of humankind's "imprisoned" condition.

"Begin by sharpening your natural powers of prophecy," Mutwa explained further. "Prophecy is not a supernatural force – it is a gift we all possess. As you should know, ma'am, wild animals possess great powers of prophecy. When everything looks fine but we know in our hearts something is wrong – what we might call an "early warning signal" – that is prophecy."

I listened quietly.

"Seers all over the globe have been picking up the warning signals for a long time, ma'am. Today, we live in the most important time for human beings. We live in a time of catastrophes and real miracles."

These words reminded me of Mutwa's observation that, for the first time in human history, the various religions of the world are agreed on one thing: the anticipated return of a god or gods. In Zululand, he had told me, his people, the Zulus, are expecting the return of Mvelinqangi, the one-legged sun god.

He had also told me of the prophecy made by King Shaka a few years before he died, that the seventh king of the Zulus ruling after him would be the last king of these people. Explaining that his heart ached for his people, he pointed out that "today's King Zwelethini is the seventh."

On being asked whether this prophecy meant that things were coming to an end for his people, he responded with a grim nod of his head. "Yes, ma'am, that is true," he conceded. "But listen to me carefully: a prophecy does not have to be fulfilled. It only comes about if we are blinded into believing that we can do nothing about these warnings. This is the truth that the White Lion messengers bring us: we should not forget that we as individuals and as human beings can do something."

"Are you saying that we can control our destinies?" I asked – the oldest question of humankind.

"Yes, ma'am, yes! Sometimes I get hopping mad," he said, and I could feel his bitter frustration, "I feel so lonely like a fool, a *mampara*. But all I can do, ma'am, is try..."

"...try to help humankind understand?" I asked, completing his sentence.

He gave a deep sigh, and I could only guess at the accumulated efforts of more than half a century of unerring service to the enlightenment of our species.

"I am glad I will soon kick the bucket, ma'am," he concluded, with a wry lightening of tone. "That way I will not have to witness the grave which modern man is shoveling out for himself!"

Digging Our Own Grave

Alarmingly, I had determined on my most recent visit to Timbavati that, in real terms, the spirit ancestor's warnings about the White Lions needing "protection" were urgently applicable. The White Lions of Timbavati – the "Children of the Sun God" as they are known among the shamanic orders – are, appallingly, not a protected species. They are not even offered the most basic rights of protection. Worse still: they are actively hunted, and skinned for trophies.

Knowing Mutwa's gloomy proclivities, I had hesitated at first in transmitting this news, but then, with regret, I finally decided it was important to inform him of the circumstances at the outskirts of Timbavati, where a trophy-hunting program was still operating. Upon hearing this, the old lion shaman showed deep pessimism about the nature of humanity. Exhaling his breath with a deep sigh, Mutwa delivered words I shall never forget: "We live in a prophetic time, ma'am. Some human beings are becoming godlike. But when you bring me this bad news, it makes my heart despair for us all – each one of us – and for the future of this planet."

The trophy-hunting operation has been appropriately dubbed "canned lions" since the lions are farmed, drugged, and then shot at close quarters in enclosures. Although this information is veiled by a great deal of secrecy, I have it on good authority that lions from Timbavati have been captured and relocated, where they are bred for the white gene for hunting purposes. The fact is that White Lions are being sighted in the hunting camps and form the basis of a lucrative industry.

In South Africa, there remain fraternities of men who are associated with apartheid crimes, and it is such men who generally operate the hunting programs. In investigating the background to the hunting story, I have been in touch with Gareth Patterson, the lion man who was brave enough to uncover the activities of the game hunters, and went some way to exposing their activities in his book *Dying to be Free*. This remains a risky venture against strong vested interests in the private and state sectors.

It is to his great credit that Patterson has not been stopped by the death threats he and other conservationists have received, although it has cost him dearly. He does not sleep easy at night, and his every cent is channeled into this cause. His ceaseless and fearless fight on the side of the king of the beasts has earned him the title *Ra De Tau* – "Man of Lion" – in the African community. Another brave and enterprising man, lion breeder Simon Trickey, who against great odds managed to reintroduce two white-gene-bearing Timbavati lions back to South Africa after they had been discovered in zoos in America, had hoped to produce white offspring. Devastatingly, his prize gene-bearing male was killed. This truly magnificent lion, which I had filmed and very much admired, was disemboweled to remove the evidence lodged in his stomach, which appears to have been the arrow of a sophisticated laser crossbow. Having suffered repeated death threats himself, Trickey finally sold his lion sanctuary and left the region. When I last spoke to him a few months after the killing of his lion in December 1999, he sounded devastated, his dream of saving the White Lions shot to pieces.

I have heard it argued that the hunters' speed-breeding program is beneficial in preserving a strain of lions that would otherwise be extinct. This argument is cynical and self-serving. White Lions born under these artificial conditions suffer serious genetic malformations: lions without manes and tail tufts; cubs needing open-heart surgery. White Lion trophies command figures of between $65,000 and $120,000. The truth is that the big-game hunters' intention is not to save the white breed but to ensure that it remains a great rarity, on the brink of extinction – for the highest commercial profit.

I've often wondered what kind of man shoots a defenseless animal at close range in an enclosure with a shotgun or laser technology. And this in an attempt to prove his "manhood." What kind of man kills for fun? Where's the heroism in such a purposeless and cowardly act?

Shamanism, which honors the soul connection between different species, was beginning to teach me the true meaning of courage, which is ultimately heroism of the spirit.

A true hero is ethical. Maria Khosa and Credo Mutwa taught me that heroism is, first, the ability to see the connection between humankind and the most fearsome predators on earth. Second, it is the ability to honor that connection. In doing so, the lion shaman reaffirms his faith and trust in nature itself.

If it is difficult for us to understand this way of thinking, it may be that we have long since lost our sense of ethics and our spiritual values. If African shamanism seems obscure, we should draw on our own Christian Bible to show us the lesson. We could hardly have a better example of the true spirit of heroism than that of Daniel in the lions' den.

Daniel is hurled into the lions' den and a huge stone is rolled over the entrance and sealed with the king's own signet to prevent escape. Here is an echo of the practices of lion shamanism, in which the initiate is forced to face a life-threatening ordeal. In Daniel's case, he is left all night, incarcerated with the lions. In the morning, the king gets up early and hurries to the den to see what has taken place overnight. Miraculously, Daniel is unharmed: "No manner of hurt was found upon him, because he believed in his God."[1]

The Old Testament tale conforms to the principles of lion shamanism at the deepest level. Daniel has survived his terrifying ordeal by upholding the primary law of lion shamanism: overcoming fear though the power of faith. In respect of trophy hunting, it seems to me that the question is not so much why a number of morally bankrupt individuals get pleasure out of killing beautiful animals; the real question is why the rest of us let them get away with it.

Contact with African shamans has helped me understand that trophy hunting is not only a cold-hearted blood sport, it is a crime against humanity. The hunter might pay the lion farmer the current going rate for the lion he kills, but the real cost is to us: to our earth, our heritage, and our future.

Persistent mercenary exploitation of this kind has all but destroyed our own natural inheritance. This has grim consequences. While the trophy hunters do the killing, we, the oblivious bystanders, will live with the consequences.

In standing by while the earth's most precious animals are killed for money, in silently condoning material values at the expense of our own natural environment, we humans have all but lost our spirit. I was coming to see that there is a natural and perfectly logical wisdom in the words of the lion shamans in respect of harming the White Lions and devastating our earth. A world without spirit, without its very life-force, will ultimately perish.

Existing on the brink of catastrophe, as prophets such as Mutwa and great shamans on other continents warn us, it should be clear to us that our attitude to our earth and its wildlife is directly related to our own future. Having spoken of the grave we are digging for ourselves, Mutwa went on to give me an unexpected piece of information in respect of the plight of the White Lions.

"Ma'am, there is something else you should know," he said. "The White Lions are not dead. They are alive, but are confined in a remote part of the globe."

"You don't mean at the outskirts of Timbavati?" I asked, thinking again with abhorrence of the hunting camps.

"No, ma'am, I do not. Another continent entirely."

Unsure whether this was good or bad news, I asked him to explain further.

"Let me tell you a story, ma'am. One day in Mafikeng, in our village, there came two very handsome white men. Real Nordic warriors. When they gave me their names, I told them: 'You are not who you say you are.' It was then that they told me that they were in fact the most famous magicians in the world. Well, ma'am, these men started playing tricks upon us. Ordinary tricks involving money, for example, showing us how the note was being lifted off their palms and suspended between their hands. Now, some of the *sangomas* were impressed, but I was not. I had seen this trick many times before. But then these Americans showed me photographs of themselves with white tigers, and that impressed me deeply, and saddened me. These men had come to South Africa to collect White Lions from Timbavati to take to their faraway city."

Mutwa looked perturbed at the memory. "I must confess to you, ma'am, I really blasted them. I asked them: 'How would you like to have your God taken away from you to an alien land where it will be treated as a spectacle for gawking tourists and gamblers?' I said: 'Gentlemen, what you are doing is wrong and immoral.'"

Mutwa must have noticed my concern.

"There is an old Zulu saying, ma'am, which goes: 'If you abandon your own children, do not be surprised to discover that a cannibalistic giant is guarding over them.'"

"So what did the magicians do, Credo?" I asked.

"I do not know, ma'am. They would not say," he observed grimly. "The moment you take a thing from the wild, a thing that belongs to the bosom of nature, you no longer have a wild animal, you are killing the spirit of the animal. You are debasing it. My heart aches for those lions, ma'am."

My heart ached, too. And I decided that I needed to get to the bottom of the story.

On further investigation through the Johannesburg Zoo, I learned of the background to Mutwa's information. A couple of decades ago, a tawny lion that had been shot in Timbavati was taken to the zoo in a bid to save it. Having fully recovered, the lion fathered a litter of pure white cubs, so it was discovered that he carried the special gene.

Noticing that the "visitor value" of the White Lion cubs was unprecedented, the zoo decided to set up a dedicated project aimed at preserving the White Lions. But, given the prohibitive expenses involved in a big carnivore breeding program, it was soon clear to zoo director Dr Pat Condy that a partner was desperately needed to help carry the financial burden: a partner for whom (to put it bluntly) money was no object.

This search led them to Siegfried and Roy, styled as the "world's greatest magicians." Under Condy's directorship, a joint breeding program was set up between the Johannesburg Zoo and the celebrity magicians in Las Vegas. Siegfried and Roy have animal holding facilities on a scale second to none. Condy's idea was to create a hospitable base where the White Lions might safely breed quite apart from the zoo itself, to avoid inbreeding.[2]

My immediate feeling was consternation that these majestic beasts had been relocated to such a foreign and unnatural context. But that they were alive at all was the first miracle. What exactly was going on here?

Leaving Pat Condy's offices at the Johannesburg Zoo late on a winter's afternoon in August 1997, I decided to prepare for a trip to Las Vegas. I wanted to meet the world's most celebrated magic men and see the situation for myself. More especially, I wanted to meet the magical White Lions of Timbavati.

16

WHITE LIONS AND MAGIC MEN

When any creature becomes extinct and vanishes from the earth, all of us are
diminished. We are all connected. We are all – every one of us – stewards of a precious
legacy, a wild legacy that is dying.

– SIEGFRIED AND ROY

In September 1997, after crossing the Atlantic and several time zones, I landed at Los Angeles Airport, and spent the night at my cousin's apartment. The next day, in a hired car, I set off on the long drive through the Nevada Desert to the glittering oasis of Las Vegas.

After six hours, the last light began to fade over the pink desert and I picked out Vegas glittering in the distance. A giant mock-up of Sleeping Beauty's castle greeted my arrival, and, above the high-rise constructions, a rollercoaster hoisted new arrivals into the heart of the world's biggest shrine to gambling. Casinos lined the city center, and giant billboards, either side advertising nightly shows, were illuminated by gaudy neon fairy lights. It was not long before I picked out Siegfried and Roy's billboard: one blond man, one dark, both surrounded by snowy felines – the brightest of all the stars on the Strip. Vegas was precisely as I expected: a fabricated world of dreams and illusions. When I arrived at the aptly named Mirage hotel, a valet took my keys and a porter collected my bags. At check-in, I was issued with a map to my room, which took me through the so-called Tropical Rain Forest straight into the gambling emporium. Looking for a way out, through the highly decorated army of the clinking and flashing one-armed bandits, I discovered that I had been walking in circles. I finally enlisted the assistance of a uniformed usher who led me through the maze of marbled corridors to an atrium of platinum elevators. My room was on the 16th floor.

Once in my room, I tried to collect my thoughts, which were spinning like a roulette wheel unable to fix on a lucky number.

The World of the Magician: A Secret Sympathy

Later that night, in a slightly calmer state of mind, I experienced the spectacular sensation of watching the most celebrated magic show on Earth. For the most part it

153

was a typical Vegas affair: thunderous music; fabulous fanfare; an intergalactic battle between designer-clad aliens and the forces of good, Siegfried and Roy. Around me, the vast darkened auditorium was packed with diners drinking cocktails, their faces occasionally flashed into illumination with the explosive special effects. No White Lions to be seen. I was beginning to feel disoriented again, when, all of a sudden – the felines appeared!

The show stopped, and a calm descended. Amazingly, there were no cheap circus tricks, no hoops of fire – the audience was suddenly enveloped in the presence of the great cats. At this moment all the fabricated apocalyptic visions, the end-of-world scenarios, and the high-tech Martians and metallic monsters belching fire and brimstone dissolved, and silence reigned. My heart leapt – it was a truly magical moment.

There is no doubt that the cats stole the show. During that suspended moment, when the tremulous music skipped a beat and the White Lions made their stage debut, I sensed the entire audience holding its breath. Radiating sublime beauty, the lions merely existed. That was enough. They simply appeared, and well, yes, this being a magic show, they disappeared as well.

At which point Siegfried's voice resounded over the microphone: "Look for the magic that is around you. In nature, plants, flowers, and all the animals that share the planet with us . . ."

I began to see what the conjurers were up to. Their magic attempted to serve a higher purpose. Ultimately, the spellbinding devices and perfectly manufactured special effects paid homage to the all-encompassing magic of nature. The audience was encouraged not to forget that the snow leopard, the Siberian tiger, and the White Lions of Timbavati originated in nature's own secrets. Ultimately, the show was saying that the magic of nature superseded all fabrication.

After the performance – their second show that evening – Siegfried and Roy's publicist came to collect me. It was one in the morning. I felt exhausted, and increasingly apprehensive about the imminent interview. Doubtful about my ability to present appropriate questions and get genuine answers in this showbiz context, I followed the smooth-suited figure through the velvet curtains of the stage door. Backstage, the performers' walls were plastered with autographed celebrity photographs: Michael Jackson (who wrote the music for their show), Elizabeth Taylor, Barbra Streisand, Liza Minnelli, Muhammad Ali, Elton John (all personal friends, it seemed), Andrew Lloyd Webber, Brooke Shields, Bruce Willis and Demi Moore, Sylvester Stallone, Arnold Schwarzenegger, Eddie Murphy, a limitless Hollywood Who's Who. I also recognized politicians and royalty: Bill Clinton and Prince Rainier of Monaco. That was about as much as I could take in before being swept up the stairs and ushered into the lush backstage premises.

There was an awkward hiatus while I waited. Then the showmen entered, radiant after yet another successful conjuring spectacle. Disconcertingly, I realized all my memorized questions had dissolved in my head. They were shaking my hand and introducing me to various minders and publicists and *artistes* from their show.

I was at a loss. The earnestness of the script I had prepared was entirely inappropriate. How could these manicured men shed any light on the profound evolutionary questions that had begun to emerge in the course of my research? What was I doing here?

I gained some comfort at the thought of Mauritz Basson's flattering letter, sent to the showmen by way of introduction, in which he had written in South African English that he "would like to take this opportunity to introduce [them] to a lady that is almost as passionate about the big cats as Roy is! She is a South African with a Paris fashion modeling background and a Cambridge education and is at present writing a book [on] the White Lions of Timbavati which deals with the 'magic' of those white individuals . . ."

"White individuals!" Bless him. I had soon detected that the Johannesburg Zoo's animal handler never quite distinguished between animals and humans. And it was on this level of mutual passion that Roy and I reached an immediate rapport. I had been warned I had only fifteen minutes. Fifteen minutes? We could have spoken all night and all morning – this being Vegas – of our most passionate topic: big white cats.

We spoke about his visit to Timbavati, and how the wild felines had come to greet him and apparently kept guard outside his tent; we spoke about his introduction to Credo Mutwa, and how the shaman had seen straight through his and Siegfried's pretense at being anything other than showbiz personalities, and we spoke about his goals and visions for the White Lion breeding project.

At 2:30 A.M., over an hour later, we parted – after Roy had invited me to his and Siegfried's "Secret Garden" later that same day.[1] Feeling elated, I retired to bed, hoping to catch some White Lion-filled dreams. Standing outside the enclosure at around noon, I watched in rapt delight the first White Lions I had ever seen – an entire pride. The performers' collaboration with the Johannesburg Zoo had resulted in three generations in their possession, and today the delicate exercise was to introduce these to one another. I was so overwhelmed at seeing the White Lions close up that my first request was to be allowed into the enclosure, but this was refused. Understandably, Roy was reluctant to allow a "new element" into the arena.

The names of the lions were well chosen. Mystery had just pounced on Pride's back, and was being taken for a ride. Pride was the largest of the white pride and, at two and a half years old, was showing the first signs of a mane. He was padding along with his sibling attached to his rear, then suddenly shrugged him off. Above him, Vision was surveying the scene from atop a rocky outcrop. His eyes were narrowing in predatory mode. Following his gaze, I spotted a white turkey on the far side of the Secret Garden, safely behind wire netting. Below him on a gravel pathway, Secret flopped about on giant paws that looked like oversized fluffy slippers which, one day, he would grow into.

There were men standing among the lions, dressed in designer jeans and wearing sunglasses, watching attentively. One of these was Roy. Well into his fifties, he still moved like a panther. I had observed his intense bright eyes the night before, and a delightful lightness of spirit that only those in touch with an inner life-force exude. I watched as Mystery approached him and rubbed his cheek against Roy's leg in passing – *en route* to tackling his sister from behind a palm tree. Unshaken by the surprise tactic, his sibling returned the onslaught by chewing his ear. Vision tumbled off his rocky perch to join the fray. He had Mystery's tail in his mouth while Quest had hold of his tail. Mesmerized by this scene, I saw him bound over a rock, then stop short – while the daisy chain behind him collided in a mound of cavorting snow-white fur.

Through all this frivolity, the full solemnity of the moment suddenly dawned on me: I was watching the world's last surviving White Lion pride at play.

Las Vegas: home of Siegfried and Roy's Secret Garden, a Disneyesque fantasy playground of living legends. In reality, a grotesquely inappropriate context for African beasts of prey.

Observing the scene, I watched Pride dart one giant paw into the water, suspended on three legs, intent on reaching a bobbing log. His golden eyes were laser-bright, boring into the timber innocently floating toward him. Precariously perched at the edge of the pool, he kept an uneasy balance thanks to his serpentine tail until Passion strode past, tipped him over, and they both tumbled into the fountain. He emerged with his pride barely intact, and his tail flicking indignantly. By contrast, the young lioness shook herself off, cuffed him playfully, then dropped the game and headed off to Roy to get her nose tickled.

In his and Siegfried's joint autobiography, *Mastering the Impossible*, Roy admits that "no matter what happens between me and the people I care about, the real love affair in my life will always be with my animals . . . Although it is hard to discuss, the reality of my life is very simple: my animals are friends who will accept me always for what I am – rich or poor, fat or thin, dumb or intelligent."[2]

Watching his interaction with his animals, I could no longer doubt him. The affection between man and lion was unconditional. The exchange was as natural and warm as that between mother and child, husband and wife, friend and confidant. I couldn't help wondering where and how this Vegas showman had developed his fearlessness, his ease in the company of dangerous predators, his perfectly relaxed sense of power and understanding.

Beside me, watching the lions from outside the enclosure, was Siegfried, Roy's partner in magic – a performer from the tips of his diamond-encrusted fingers to his rhinestone-studded toes. From his publicity agent I had learned that his performances included a cast of more than 100 in front of 3,000 spectators, twice nightly, six days a week, eleven months a year. There was only one day a week when the show stopped – when the Mirage was "dark," in theatrical lingo – and that day happened to be today.

The night before, after the show, Siegfried had appeared in a designer coat that combined a magician's cape with the metallic garb of a *Star Wars* android. Yet, beneath this mantle, I had imagined the man displayed just a hint of frailty. I felt that if one got to know him one could genuinely grow to like him.

Roy had first met him on an ocean liner, where the young Siegfried had started performing magic tricks for the passengers. Audacious even at this early age, Roy had succeeded in smuggling Chico, his cheetah, on board ship, primarily for companionship but as a later afterthought, he claims, as a live feature in Siegfried's magic show. I was interested to see the words with which Roy described the connection: "Chico was my first soul mate while Siegfried was the best 'two-legged' friend I ever had."[3]

In their private lives rather than their hyped stage personae, I detected signs of their age-old shamanic connection with powerful animals. Observing these still-young "power animals" – as shamans call them – I saw that Mystery had arisen from his doze. Padding along innocently, he was suddenly ambushed by a sinuous twist of virile feline, who grabbed him by his scruff and pulled him down. Pride had Mystery pinned beneath him. The smaller cub was invisible beneath his big cousin, his paws curled up protectively to shield Pride's full weight. At this point, I watched Roy give a decisive nod, and a minder moved curtly over to the entanglement. Pride wasn't letting go. Mystery couldn't be seen – a repentant paw curled up under his cousin's belly.

"Oi! Pride! Leave off now!" one of the men issued a curt slap on the lion's haunch, and the beast relented, allowing Mystery to spring to freedom. The minder gave a more affectionate slap on the cub's flank now, and Pride, still irritable, tore an impressive chunk – the size of Mystery – out of the roll-on lawn he now dragged around with him.

Approaching me from inside the enclosure, Roy let out one of his delightful chuckles and, in his German accent, explained, "I'm staying in between. Vat can I do? Boy, Pride sits on you and you a pancake! I feel responsible. I cannot let anything happen to everyvun who is here! Little me: protector of za African roots!"

He was referring to the White Lion breeding project, and I was amused to note that the "everyone" to whom he alluded was his pride of Timbavati lions. He made a sweeping gesture toward the playground of cubs of different ages. "And I zought za tiger project was more than enough for one lifetime!" Clearly he doted on them. He was relaxed, content, glowing with paternal pride.

"Za lion is za ruler, za ultimate dictator. He is not like za tiger. You see, mit lions I only learn my ways now – because za White Lions of Timbavati learning me everything I know about lions."

"Is it more difficult to live with lions than with tigers?" I asked of a man who had cohabited with great cats ever since he wormed his way into Chico's cage because he felt the cheetah's loneliness. This primal understanding with felines had evolved into the most powerful defining force in Roy's life: partners in magic, soul mates in private.

"Well, za tiger is a very noble creature," he responded to my question. "He is a prince. Very aloof. A loner. He's one on one. If you do it right, you either can romance him, be his partner, even his friend. You're never going to own anyzing of him. His whole social structure is so different than from a lion. If a lion says this is the way how it goes: there is no other way. He is za patriarch, za king." It was regal terminology, but this was Roy talking about his "kids." He looked affectionately around the playpen. "I'm going through all of this now with my boys – Mystery and Secret – who are becoming adults. Zey're growing their manes and all zat, so zey're going through their maturity and fighting over za females."

The three smaller cubs had got hold of each other's tails again. Quest leading, Vision following, Mystery tagging along. They bounded over a fallen log and headed for the waterfall.

In attempting to unravel the White Lion mysteries, I had been considering the age-old relationship between the lion, "king of the beasts," and human, "ruler of the earth." In the wild, lions once hunted and ate us. Now I was witnessing the contemporary world's best-publicized example of the intimate and loving relationship between man and lion. Even in our day, lions have occasionally been known to kill and devour humans. As for the tiger, it is considered the most notorious killer of zookeepers. Game rangers with whom I discussed Siegfried and Roy's liaison with the big cats expressed the conviction that the showmen were dancing with death; some going so far as to say they awaited nothing less than a bloody outcome.

Roy knew the story but was unwavering. "Change anyzing in their nature? Vouldn't dream of it!" he spoke to me from within the wire caging. "And if I am in za wrong place at za wrong time – if I am treating zem disrespectfully like certain zookeepers do – I would expect to die, too."

This from a man who sleeps with his cats, who cares for them when they are ill, who was present when his tigress gave birth. Experienced conservationists know that not even the father of the cubs would dare to venture near at such a moment.

"One zing you don't do – go near a tigress when she is giving birth." Roy agreed when I reminded him of the well-documented occasion of the delivery of his tigress's cubs. "But me – I'm ruled by instinct and my heart. Noëlle vas so tired, she had left za last-born suffocating on its umbilical cord. I had to intervene – it didn't occur to me I vas risking my life."

The previous night Roy had shown me a videotape of the birth which, on consideration, must count as some of the most riveting footage in animal documentary history. Man and cat together after her labor. Roy holding the last-born, scrunched-up mitten of striped fur to his cheek, while behind him Noëlle, the tigress, watched: intently, ferociously, protectively – lethal incisors bared – yet, it would seem, serenely comfortable in his presence. Spine-tinglingly, Roy has his back to her! Facing the television camera, danger is the last thing on his mind.

Thinking about it now I realized, of course, her teeth were bared at the cameraman who was venturing into their territory – she and Roy's sacred space.

"That was truly amazing," I marvel to Roy. "Your assisting the tigress in the birth."

"Assisting?" he shakes his head. "I vas just tolerated."

His modesty shrugged off an extraordinary gift: the natural achievement of mutual trust between species. The gift that once might have been available to the rest of us, but which modern man has undeniably lost.

I was reminded of Roy's attempt in his biography to define this ineffable interspecies liaison. "When people ask, as they often do," he wrote, "how I developed such harmony with my animals, I rarely give a complete answer. I'm shy about describing my relationship with animals as a living karma, as a destiny, as the sum of my aura . . . How can I explain to well-meaning strangers that . . . my certainty of unconditional trust, unconditional emotion, and unconditional strength comes from my animals? Would it be interpreted correctly if I admitted that my animals and I are like partners in crime?" [4]

The shamanic approach to animals acknowledges them as equals, in clear contrast to our modern attitude toward pets, which may be doted upon but not treated as equals. In so doing, the shaman establishes his own kinship with the beasts. Clearly, this mutual respect and kinship is the key to the "magical" powers that Roy, like shamans before him, display with dangerous predators. It was precisely this attitude that characterized Maria's respectful approach to the Timbavati lions during my own near-death experience. Winsome as they might be on occasion, these are not fluffy teddy bears, but lethal predators that are quite rightly prepared to kill if they are mistreated.

As a tidy reminder of this, Pride chose this moment to pounce upon one of the attendants, and had to be separated by Roy, who gave the troublesome lion a curt reprimand while the minder dusted himself off.

Siegfried and Roy's liaison with the big cats rang with age-old Androclean dimensions, in which predators are ultimately understood as man's protectors or guardians. In Roy's autobiography, for instance, he describes how he owes his life, several times over, to one or other of his animals.[5]

Watching Roy in his lions' den now, I couldn't resist asking through the fence: "You more than anyone know the risks. Have your animals – your predators – really protected you in times of danger?"

"Oh, ja. Many times. Many times."

"Lions as guardians?"

"Precisely."

Clearly, Roy's life – as well as his million-dollar stage show – depended on such an understanding. One swipe from a big cat would knock a linebacker across a room. Every time Roy performed one of his split-second magical feats, he was putting his life in the mighty paws of one of his formidable felines. Those who are not familiar with the immense power and size of these felines tend to see it as sheer showmanship, and forget that all the while a trust exists between these two species that makes the magic happen. In Roy's autobiography he had written that "the harmony that I felt with an animal would be the strongest – the most magical – connection in my life."[6] For this real-life lion tamer, it is not danger but protection that the big cats offer. Such communication across the species barrier defies our imagination more than any illusionist's trick. This is true magic.

"But we can't take it for granted," Roy added, smiling at me from his den of lions. "You should never take a friend for granted."

Roy was a living example of an old family tie between man and beast. "So you respect their rules and their customs?" I questioned.

"Of course. Who am I to tell zem how it is?" He shrugged. "How can you gain respect if you don't respect zeir ways? My understanding of life comes from zem. My animals can sense my thoughts before I have zem. People think szis is mysticism. For me it's simply a fact. I don't always have to tell zem what to do. They know. Simple." Interspecies communication. No conjurer's trick here.

"And sometimes we don't even have to talk," he added. "Some days ve just sit together, me mit a little cognac, and ve just be."

"You and your lions . . ."

"Me and all my cats. All my animals. Ve just be ourselves. I'm a magician. But I never had a teacher or training. Mit me, I always saw za magic in nature: za greatest magic alive! When I vas a kid, I vas a rebel at school. Zey were asking us to describe God, zo I said: trees, rivers, mountains, animals . . . Zey put me in a corner. Zey called my parents to take me home!"

We both laughed.

"Zey thought I vas mad. But I don't zink I'm that mad. I vas alive. I vas awake. I wasn't sleeping, I vas aware of za living magic, za life of our world around us. That awareness is one day going to save all of us."

Roy exhibited the principles of the lion priest, the very same principles we find in the records of pharaohs, high priests, and great spiritual leaders the world over. Seeing the connections, I had to admit that Roy delighted me.

His assertion – "awareness is one day going to save all of us" – carried powerful resonance. The first great lesson of the shaman is heightened awareness. An awareness of the communication between species, which assists humankind to overcome fear and ultimately offers us protection by the very animal kingdom we ourselves have debased and all but destroyed.

Siegfried, who was still beside me, looking into the Secret Garden where Roy and the Timbavati pride were playing, explained: "That was it, you see. We realized we didn't need to make magic – it was there before our very eyes, in nature."

In Roy's special ability with carnivores, I detected a sympathy between different life-forms – which is ultimately what the real "magic" of nature is all about. Marveling at Roy's uninhibited interaction with his boisterous companions, I thought of Maria, and her mastery over the untamed Timbavati pride; except that, rather than "mastery," what existed between the species was a sacred contract and recognition of kinship. Like the hunting magic of the Bushmen, real magic is gaining access to the deeper interrelated connection between all things.

"Have you seen wild animals ever look so happy?" Siegfried broke into my thoughts – and suddenly I felt my defenses go up. Wild lions in captivity: happy?

For several hours I'd been watching the leonine antics, the playful frolicking and – dared I use the term in Las Vegas? – the boisterous gamboling of the cubs. In the wild, in Timbavati where I'd spent so many rare moments over the years, lions can be playful, too. Being social cats, the lions are infinitely tactile; they adore cuddling and caressing and game playing. They spend hours at a time, during the hot hours of the day, lounging in each other's company, basking under marula trees. Then, all of a sudden, the fun stops, and the hard, brutal business of survival begins. Nature lives by uncompromising laws. In Timbavati, a lioness might narrow her gaze into a golden arrow, twitching her ears for the sound of a passing herd of impala. Alert, primed, intense, anxious, and – if the kill has been unsuccessful – wretchedly hungry or abjectly suffering. For a hunting lion, only one out of every seven attempts is successful.[7] And a mismanaged kill can mean death for a predator. With one thrust of its rapier horns, an impala may rip open a lion's belly. Even a superficial wound – the torn tip of a lion's tail – may fester and work its way up the living flesh to infect a perfectly healthy specimen. I have watched this slow death infect a lion, whose suffering would have met an undignified end – gangrene of the rectum – had not my ranger friend, Leonard, intervened and sterilized his tail. I have seen documented material of a lioness, whose jaw, broken by the kick of a zebra, dangled pitifully beneath her majestic face. The others from her pride attempted to coax her to eat from the zebra carcass she had helped to take down. Unable even to drink, she followed them for agonized days, suckling her perplexed cubs before disappearing into the wilderness to die in solitude. The cubs were left to their fate.

As to Siegfried's question of whether I had ever seen happier lions, I replied cautiously that he might be right. The critical difference between these lions and the ones one cannot bear to watch in zoos or circus cages was that they were nurtured, cared for, and constantly stimulated. The showmen's lions were a picture of health and contentment. They appeared even larger than wild lions of the same age. I wondered whether it was my proximity to the lions in the enclosure, but certainly the 9-month-old Secret resembled in size 12-month old cubs I knew from Timbavati. Later, in a quiet moment, when Roy was showing me the holding facilities behind the scenes, he confessed that the bid to save the white felines had begun after he experienced a recurring dream in which his golden cat turned snow white. This premonitory vision represented a turning point in his life. He also admitted to his belief that he himself might once have been a feline in a previous incarnation, and I could only smile at the shamanic echoes.

"You know za oldest rule in za performance industry?" Roy asked me with a theatrical gesture. "Never share za stage with a child or an animal – zeir innocence steals za spotlight."

And boy, was he right. I couldn't resist reminding him that the big cats did in fact steal the show from him. At which he responded, with a knowing twinkle, "Ja, it's true. But zey are me, I am zem."

He went on to talk about his project to save the white felines in terms of a "higher purpose," "a life's work," "a legacy" that would remain long after Siegfried and he himself had disappeared to never-never land and, for once (as magicians), not returned.

"Siegfried and me," he explained, "'ve are looking after zem. Mandela and Mbeki have so much to do. They sink of ze people first – all za homeless. And only zen come za animals. But by zen it might be too late! Ve try to preserve za White Lions – a big responsibility, ja. But zen," he concluded with inherent showman's flourish, "when za time is right, ve give zem back!"

I had come to Las Vegas, prepared to condemn their glitz and fakery, ready to dismiss their dealings with these most precious of animals as mere commercial exploitation. Now, I understood that we shared a mission to conserve the White Lions.

"But our work is not over yet," Siegfried contributed, once Roy and I had returned from our walkabout. "I know we have been blessed spending our lives exploring magic and illusion – but through this Secret Garden, Roy and I can show others the greatest magic of all – the magic of nature. It's a 'living classroom,' open to everyone. That is our objective."

In our times, no wildlife documentary fails to end with the grim reminder that, if urgent measures are not effected, yet another species will become extinct, and yet another wilderness area will be eradicated from the face of the earth. And humanity itself will be the loser.

I took a lingering look at the world's last white pride in the Secret Garden. The lion, king of the beasts, symbolic guardian over the earth and its creatures. Sovereign messengers of the legacy that humankind inherited. Mystery caught my eye as I stood staring into the enclosure – boring into my retinas, electrifying me. His scruffy mane designated him a teenager, but he had the muscular body of an almost fully grown lion. His slightly yellowed scruff resembled the scraggly rays of dawn, but one day, I knew, it would radiate around his head like Africa's midsummer sun.

Magic Lion Drawings

Retracing my route to LA, through the seemingly endless desert sands, my thoughts returned to Mutwa, and that particularly touching moment when he spoke of the loss of the White Lions of Timbavati, and of how the Las Vegas magic-men had taken "our gods away!"

The idea that Africa's most precious animals – Africa's "sun gods" – have been relocated from their holy land of Timbavati to the world's gambling capital indicates something profoundly disturbing about humankind's loss of real values. Instead of roaming free in their spiritual homeland, Africa's White Lions are the center of attraction in the world's gambling Mecca.

Yet, given the cold-blooded hunting practices that threaten their very existence at home, this bizarre state of affairs seems, for the moment, the lesser of two evils. In Siegfried and Roy's hands lies the fate of Timbavati's legendary White Lions. Inappropriate as it had at first appeared, I now suspected that these men had been allotted the task of disseminating the White Lions' precious message to the world, mastering today's leading-edge techniques – virtual reality, mass media, IMAX and worldwide communication – as the means to this end. I saw that the White Lions were safe – until such time as it was safe for them to walk in the sands of their sacred homeland once again. In practical terms, it was by no means clear how they might successfully be returned to Timbavati: other attempts at reintroducing lions to the wild have shown a success rate of close to zero. But, for the moment, the important point was that they were in a sanctuary, far away from the hunter's bullet.

Alone in the Nevada desert, I became aware of a new kind of hope taking shape in my consciousness – might these magicians be part of a bigger plan, a kind of master plan beyond their own making? What corroborated this view for me was the secret message encoded into the Nevada desert at an outpost called Blythe, California, west of the Colorado River.

Less than half a day's drive from Las Vegas, ancient engravings at Blythe delineate the secret liaison that links our species to the king of the beasts. So large they were only discovered by aviation, of unknown origin and unknown date, these ancient shamanic line drawings etched into the desert sands speak of lion–man mysteries.[8] Their message is the same as that encoded in the riddle of the Sphinx, or that conveyed to us in the fossil evidence of Sterkfontein. Depicting humans and felines in ritualized interchange, it originates in the remote bedrock of our hominid beginnings.[9]

Not surprisingly, Las Vegas has its very own sphinx and fake pyramids. I had also spotted a giant Statue of Liberty, and even a "live" volcano that erupted and spewed out fiery smoke 30 meters (100 feet) above the lagoons every 15 minutes from dusk to midnight. A glittering oasis of virtual reality on an unreal scale. Yet on the question of Timbavati's real flesh-and-blood White Lions, my feeling was: at least they're in safe hands.

That was the message I would take home to Credo Mutwa.

17

LION, STAR BEAST

When at my grandfather's, I listened to the stars.
I could hear the sound, the speech of the stars. . . .
Later, when full-grown, and a hunter as well,
I was the one who listened, still listened.
I could sit there and hear it come very close:
The star-sound Tsau, sounding Tsau! Tsau!

– /XAM BUSHMAN SONG

Back in South Africa, I relayed the Las Vegas situation to Mutwa in detail. Although cautious, the shaman expressed profound relief. "At least they are safe," he said slowly.

Then he asked me to convey his heartfelt gratitude to Siegfried and Roy, with the following words: "Please tell them, ma'am, that I had believed them to be God poachers; I see now that they may be god savers. May the Earth Spirit bless them with long life!"

Although I was alarmed to see how unwell Mutwa looked, at least he appeared lighter in spirit. We sat in the same Johannesburg room, drinking weak tea, while I described the shamanic catlike line drawings in the desert in Blythe, less than half a day's drive from the White Lion sanctuary at Las Vegas.

"They really are amazing, Credo," I said. "It's almost as if excited children visited Siegfried and Roy's magic show, then drew enormous pictures in the sand to tell the stars the story of the magical relationship they had seen between lions and men."

Drawing on my knowledge of shamanism to understand the giant etching plate of Blythe, I realized that arguments about whether the ancients had the technology to build flying objects missed the point entirely. It is unlikely that these symbolic geoglyphs were created by people who required aircraft to provide them with an aerial perspective. They rather seem to be the work of rare individuals whose ascendant spirit gave them access to this view of life. Like the lion shamans of Africa, the Native American shamans were believed to go on "flying" expeditions, sometimes induced by psychoactive drugs, in which the shaman left his body and made a "soul flight" to speak to the gods or ancestors. In the form of a bird, or flying feline, the shamans were able to view their universe from a bird's-eye perspective.[1] This would account for the shamanic line drawings' being designed to be viewed from above.

In our discussions up to that point, Mutwa had described a number of acutely exacting rituals performed by the initiate in the evolutionary process toward the astral condition. The initiate, who starts as a mere human, makes various attempts to pass through each of the four successive stages of ascension (known as "tree branches"), either through shamanic ecstasy trance or, as in Mutwa's case, through acute suffering. Having reached the winged lion (or pure hawk) condition, the initiate attempts entry into the star condition.

"It is not easy for us humans to achieve star knowledge on Earth," Mutwa once confided in me. "It involves much suffering and discipline. But if, as Sanusis, we are able to do so, it is our God-given duty to bring the enlightenment back to Earth for the benefit of all living beings on this planet."

This admission clarified a question that had puzzled me. I understood that the Great Knowledge was not simply information inherited through shamanic lineage but also a condition of enlightenment achieved through spiritual development. Mutwa referred to this spiritual enlightenment as "star knowledge," alluding to this subject with a great deal of circumspection.

Observing my dear shaman friend now, I wondered how far I might venture into these sacred territories. I had come to see him as a sounding board, a giant ringing stone of sorts, whom I would approach to test an idea, and see if it rang true. With some boldness, I asked Mutwa now what he imagined to be the meaning of the line drawings in the American desert.

"How large are they, ma'am?" the Sanusi inquired.

"So large, you can't see their shape from ground level. You need an airplane to pick them out."

"Do you indeed, ma'am?"

I sensed he was insinuating something. "They need to be viewed from above – from a bird's-eye perspective," I explained further.

"Perhaps, ma'am," he said with a knowing twinkle, "we should call it a 'winged-lion' perspective."

Star Knowledge

The secret orders of the Sanusis do not fear connections with the wider universe; instead, they are initiated into rituals of communication with certain heavenly bodies. This, after all, was the function of the astrological stones in Great Zimbabwe and Timbavati.

Mutwa referred to this intercommunication between the earth and the heavenly bodies as "the song of the stars." It reminded me of the Aboriginal term for sacred lines on our earth: songlines. Thinking over the Blythe site in California, I began to wonder whether those great line drawings of man–feline metamorphosis represented songs to the stars: lines of communication between earth and heavenly bodies, much like the ringing stones of Africa. As to their precise date of execution, I imagined this was less significant than the fact that they had been encrypted in a form that we are only now able to view in our age of aviation.

"I have not forgotten your words that we live in 'prophetic times,' Credo," I assured him. "Now that we can read these images, the challenge for modern man is to understand them, and learn their message."

"That is so," the Sanusi responded. It was one of the few occasions I had seen him glow with pleasure. "I see that the great spirit of Mbube has been speaking to you in your dreams."

"Who is Mbube, Credo?" I asked, feeling a sense of pride even before I knew the answer.

"He is the lion, ma'am, the star beast."

I considered awhile. "Is he the lion in my dreams? The same one that roams Timbavati?"

"Your lion comes from the stars, ma'am, he is a Lion of God," Mutwa said with a faint smile. After pondering a moment, he added, "Never forget that the story of the White Lions is connected to the stars."

I waited for him to continue, but he left these words to linger tantalizingly in the air. Then, reading my expectancy, he proceeded, "Let me tell you something. What do our people call a lion? Some call the lion *zimba,* which means "strength." Some call it *shumba,* which means the same thing. And Zulu people call it *ibubhezi,* which means "the one who judges." But the Great Knowledge tells us of another word. It is *Tsau!,* which means 'star beast.'"[2]

I did not know exactly what Mutwa meant by "star beast." All I knew was that my lion was magical for me. He appeared in my dreams, he guarded me from within the ancestral realm and he had even appeared in the flesh on the runway in the middle of the wilderness. I was uplifted by Ingwavuma's special power, even if I could not explain it. That was enough.

As for Mutwa's sacred word for lion – *Tsau!* – what little exists by way of records of ancient Bushman beliefs confirm the lion–star connection. *Tsau!* is very possibly

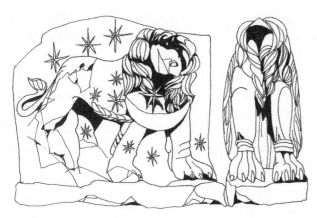

The Lion of Commagene, showing the lion as star beast.

the most powerful word in the Bushmen's highly complex vocabulary. A number of firsthand accounts by Westerners attest to this.

One is described by Laurens van der Post, who was working for the British government in the Kalahari Desert after World War II. He records how he witnessed the rescue of a group of starving near-dead Bushmen. They were saved by the telepathic powers of a Bushman tracker, who was able to intuit their distress many kilometers away. That night, van der Post witnessed a ceremony of thanksgiving, in which the rescued Bushmen held a baby up to the stars in gratitude, and called out *"Tsau! Tsau!"* He later learned that the Bushman mother was asking the stars to bless the newborn infant with a lion heart. Since the Bushmen believe that the stars are "Great Hunters," the human infant was blessed not only with a lion heart but also that of a star.

This experience was so significant for van der Post that it formed the centerpiece of his book *The Heart of the Hunter*. Ultimately, it led him to make observations about the nature of language, and the nature of genesis itself. "The revelation filled me with awe," he writes. "I felt as if I had been allowed to witness the coming of the Word in the darkness before time."[3]

Clearly, the Bushmen employ the word *Tsau!* in a very different manner from the way we commonly use the term *lion*. While this way of thinking was still foreign to me, I understood the Bushman usage was based on an affirmation of the interconnections between events on earth and events in the heavens. To sound the word *Tsau!* is equivalent to calling upon an elemental force. In Bushman culture, the sacred lion word may not be voiced under ordinary circumstances because, like the word *Yahweh* among orthodox Jews, it denotes "God."

This was my first attempt to come to grips with the great cosmic issues that Mutwa was raising.

"When you say that my particular lion comes from the stars, what exactly do you mean, Credo?" I asked, trying to determine whether this notion was simply poetic, or whether the Great Shaman was implying transmissions of some kind, from stellar sources.

"Your lion is a wise judge, a king," he replied. "Our people believe that lion kings are connected to the heart of the sky lion, which your astronomers call 'the little king,' Regulus."[4]

This sounded fitting, but it did not leave me any the wiser.

"If the lion mystery is connected to the stars as you say, Credo," I probed again, "how did this lion–star connection originate?"

"The lion is the star beast, yes," Mutwa confirmed. "But all life on earth is connected to the stars. We are not alone in this universe," he said with a short laugh, which implied it was ludicrous to believe otherwise.

Lion: *Tsau!*

Mutwa's clues led me up an extraordinary ladder of information – a ladder that spanned from Earth to the stars.

"The lion is connected to the stars, ma'am," my teacher informed me, "but not just any stars. The lion is connected, in particular, to Orion – the three stars of the belt of Orion. The Ndebeles call one of these stars Mbube, which means 'lion.' There are three belt stars, the middle one of which is Mbube. The Ndebele people believe that everything that happens on our earth is controlled by beings from the Mbube star. There is a song, ma'am, a song that people don't understand. It was a song that was sung by warriors long before the coming of the white man to South Africa. And today it is sung in America, its words shamefully distorted, where it is called 'Wimoweh' – which has no meaning. The song is really 'Mbube.'" [*Mbube* being a corruption of *ibubhezi.*]

Mutwa began to sing, and all at once I recognized the tune of the song I had heard chanted across America and Europe, where its popular lyrics go:

> In the jungle, the mighty jungle, the lion sleeps tonight!
> In the jungle, the migh-ty jungle, the li-on sleeps tonight!
> Wimoweh-Wimoweh-Wimoweh-Wimoweh ...[5]

But Credo's original version had a completely different ring. It was bold but lacked bravado, and his voice had a haunting and yearning timbre:

> Nansi imbube iyazingela iyanyonyoba, we Ma
> Emnyameni izinkanyezi sikhanya bha, we Ma
> Ye-ye-ye-yeyi uyimbube, Ma
> Ye-ye-ye-yeyi uyimbube, Ma

After a moment's silence, he went on to translate for me:

> Here is the lion, he is hunting under the stars.
> Here is the king, he is preying in the dark.
> Oh! You are the lion, you are the lion of the night.
> Oh! You are the lion of the darkness ...

"Now, ma'am," the Sanusi explained, watching my expectant face, "this song is sung not in honor of a lion but in honor of that particular star, the Mbube star of Orion's Belt. Our people believe that great kings are born under this star, ma'am, the Lion Star."

"So are we saying that the White Lions are connected to this Mbube star?"

"We believe so, ma'am. But they are also connected to the lion constellation in the sky, the one we call 'the Exiled Lion,' Mbubedingile."

"Is that the same constellation we call Leo?"

"Correct. In Africa, it is known as the Exiled Lion, because here on Earth a lion that roams on its own in the wilderness is old and has been exiled from the pride. In our tradition, ma'am, the zodiac with all its

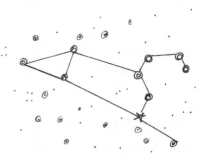

The lion as the constellation Leo.

creatures – the *Mulu-Mulu,* as it is called – is not just a band of stars. It is the band of constellations from which our animals on Earth have somehow originated. We are told that the lions came from the sky-lion constellation. We are told that all the sheep came from the ram constellation; all the cattle came from the bull or eland constellation; the birds from the firebird constellation that is also the two boatman of the gods which you call Aquarius; and all the animals of the sea came from the laughing dolphin constellation which you call Pisces; and the lobsters from the crab constellation. All the star families or constellations around the globe contributed living animals to the earth at the creation moment."[6]

"Are you suggesting," I wondered, "that everything on Earth has its equivalent in the heavens?"[7]

"That is the Great Plan, ma'am. The Earth Mother asked the Exiled Lion, I Mbubedingile, to send down great carnivores to Earth – lions, leopards, and wild cats – to protect humankind from negative entities. Man was too scared to live with lions, so he chose the wild cats to tame and live together with him in his houses."

Mutwa was seated beneath his impressive oil painting, now complete. While he was describing how the carnivores were brought to Earth, I realized that this very theme was vividly illustrated in the canvas above him. In one corner of the canvas, opposite the mighty eagle and the man-made rocket ship, was a powerful rendition of a sabertooth. Directly above this was depicted the constellation of Orion. This implied some kind of connection between the prehistoric feline and that specific constellation.

"Our people do not believe that human beings are native to this planet," he proceeded. "They say that humans also came to Earth from this central star of the belt of Orion: Mbube. They were brought here by the Mighty Hunter, Matsieng, who also brought lions (and all carnivores) to Earth.

"We are told that we human beings, like lions, are descendants of the 'Far-Walking God,' the god who goes very far, the god that white people call Orion. We call him Matsieng in Setswana: He Who Travels Very Far, the Lord of the Road, the Eternal Wanderer. He is also the Great Hunter.[8] But note, ma'am: he does not kill the animals that he hunts – he just outruns them, out-tricks them and captures them alive – then lets them go. That is

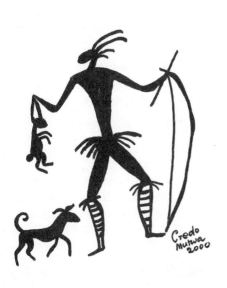

Matsieng, the African lion hero who came from Orion.

why he is also known as the Trickster or the Hero. This god is followed by two creatures: his dog and his friend Lion."[9]

He paused, while I waited in silence.

"In Africa, healers sometimes use the symbolism of the hero tracked by a friendly lion or a loyal brave dog, by which they are referring to the Sirius star, *Lii to lapiri*."[10]

I now realized that Mutwa had provided me with three different sources for life on our planet. The heart star of the Leo constellation, the central belt star of Orion, and Sirius.

"That is so, ma'am," Mutwa asserted, implying there was no contradiction here. Again I waited for him to continue. By now I knew that Mutwa's outrageous and sometimes seemingly unrelated disclosures were all critical clues to the mystery I was uncovering. With time, I would see how every disclosure pointed to the White Lions as vital portents to the future destiny of our planet. In the meantime, I had to accept that many of the cosmological references would seem obscure.

As a graphic illustration of Sirius's part in the story of origins, Mutwa now produced yet another extraordinary artifact from his secret collection: a huge rock of pure verdite in the shape of a skull, human-sized, but distinctly hominid in appearance. With its flattened cranium, it was not unlike an *Australopithecus*.[11] On the back of the cranium was engraved a symbol depicting an unusual cross within an elliptical circle that, Mutwa said, represented Sirius. Beside the circle was a smaller ring that represented Sirius B. On the front of the skull was a symbol representing the earth.

"This object, ma'am, is said to represent the root race of humankind that existed before our own," Mutwa explained.

Turning the giant verdite artifact over and over in both hands, I wondered about the message encoded in the stone. Mutwa told me that skulls carved from certain stones – diamond, crystal, rose quartz, verdite – might be invested with knowledge.[12] If a skull is carved of these stones it is capable not only of remembering, but also of transmitting memory. It is used to pass information from one generation of astronomer-priests to another, who would keep the skull on their heads under their pointed hats to absorb and transmit information from their brains. The hats themselves were designed in a pyramidal shape to point to the stars. Under certain circumstances and through certain rituals, skulls may be made to "talk" and reveal their hidden knowledge. This is particularly the case when 12 skulls of a kind are brought together. Holding the weighty artifact in my hands, it suddenly seemed as if I could tap into this knowledge. Sirius-earth-Sirius-earth-Sirius-earth. What was meant by the symbolic representation of a protohuman cranium with the Sirius planetary system on one side and Earth on the other was a transmission through interstellar space. Space would then be represented by the brain itself: the space between the back and the front of the cranium. The brain, after all, is the organ of the hominid most likely to have received such a transmission, leading to the evolutionary expansion in our species which scientists term "the brain explosion."

As I returned the sacred relic to Mutwa's care, I felt shocked at the revolutionary hypothesis that had formulated in my mind while handling it. It was unlike anything I had ever considered before. Whether or not this notion had any basis in reality, it suddenly highlighted the pathos of Mutwa's situation. Without a successor these sacred objects would go to the grave with the Guardian of Umlando – buried until some future time, when, he prophesied, they would be exhumed. With the burying of these artifacts an important part of our heritage would be lost to us.

As he offered more and more information, I wondered where the African tradition derived its astronomical knowledge from. South African astronomers with whom I had spoken were under the grave misconception that Africa had no astronomical tradition. From the evidence provided by Great Zimbabwe alone, in respect to strategic architectural alignments and key artifacts such as the zodiac bowl discovered near the site, this is plainly misinformed.[13] Yet it was not altogether surprising that the cosmological vision unfolding from the Great Knowledge had not found easy access into orthodox astronomical circles. All I could do was sit in silence, trying to come to grips with the star knowledge Mutwa was imparting.

"Ma'am," said Mutwa wryly, "if we were ever to write about the African folklore involving stars, we would write a book many volumes long, a book that would amaze people. For instance, there is a lot of talk recently about the Dogon people and their connection to the Sirius star system.[14] Somebody should wake up, please, because there are 15 tribes in Southern Africa alone that have even more dramatic connections to the stars. There are the Ndebele people. There are the Mashona people. There are my people, the Zulus.[15] The word *Zulu* does not really mean 'sky,' as anthropologists tell you. It means 'interstellar space,' but that is another story."[16]

As the silence lingered for a moment, I made a mental note to return to this question at a later time.

"How is Sirius connected with the great lion mystery, Credo?" I asked boldly.

Mutwa smiled. "Our people believe that the Great Earth Mother came from the Sirius star system. The Sirius symbol was used in the ground plan of Great Zimbabwe."

It struck me that the elliptical wall of the Great Enclosure with its tower closely resembled the diagram carved into the verdite skull.

In conclusion, Mutwa paused and drew a breath in his characteristic fashion. I waited in suspense for the usual masterful rendition of complex mysteries made childlike. I was not disappointed.

"Sirius is the 'eye' of the sky lion," Mutwa summarized, pronouncing each word with consideration and caution. "Mbube, the central star of the Belt of Orion, is the 'soul' of the lion. The star you call Regulus, in the center of Leo constellation, is the 'heart' of the sky lion. And then, of course, there is the sun. It is our belief that when the sun passes over this heart of the Mbubedingile constellation, a great kingdom will fall, or be born."

I sat in silence. While the symbolic picture he had painted wrote Timbavati's White Lion mysteries across the heavens, the message behind the symbolism threatened to expand into cosmic issues of which I had no understanding.

Praise Song to White Lions

These were revelations that I imagined I would have time enough to explore with Mutwa in due course. Instead of another day spent in lessons with my teacher, however, the next morning Mutwa and I put into effect an action plan that we had discussed at some length. Given the grim fact of the White Lions' extinction in the wilds of Timbavati, the lion shaman's only chance of making contact with a White Lion was in the Johannesburg Zoo. Although reluctant to see the king of the beasts behind bars, Mutwa agreed to make a rare public outing and accompany me to visit the creatures he described as the "holiest animals in Africa, the holy Children of the Sun God." The intention was to record on film for the first time the Great Knowledge behind the White Lions' appearance on earth.

When we arrived at the zoo, Mauritz Basson had arranged for a motorized golf cart to transport us. And then began an amazing experience that bordered on a surreal fairy tale. Adorned in his full Sanusi regalia, like a wizard from the pages of a lost storybook transported into the present day, Mutwa attracted a staggering amount of attention. He seemed at peace, with his hands neatly folded in his lap as all around us people stared and little crowds gathered. Having come to gawk at the exotic animals in the zoo, they now turned their stares on the gargantuan figure bedecked in giant sculptured rocks of crystal and verdite and ancient bronze symbols forged by Africa's blacksmith astronomer-priests.

But once we made contact with the White Lions, it was as if everyday reality dissolved and the storybook became real. I remembered what Mutwa had said in our first meeting, how he had gone to Timbavati hoping to see a White Lion walking free in the bush. If he had seen a White Lion, he said it would have helped him make "a very important decision which would have freed him from all nonsense." Now, as I witnessed the coming together of the lion shaman and the White Lions, I could only guess at what this meeting must have meant.

The White Lion and his two White Lionesses emerged from their den into the open enclosure, surrounded by a sunken moat. Watching them closely, Mutwa began reciting a eulogy in praise of the White Lions, and it moved me deeply to see the old lion raise his head, emit a thunderous roar of greeting, and then listen as Mutwa chanted:

You are the great beasts of the sun
You are as lovely as blooms that spring from the earth
You are as magnificent as the sun at dawn
Oh, lions that are white!

I remembered Mutwa telling me that, in the Great Tradition, if you sing songs of praise to animals (or even about them in their absence), you strengthen their position on earth and promote their chances of survival. Witnessing this larger-than-life figure delivering his salutations to the White Lions, the impromptu crowd had thickened around us. Mutwa had informed me he had not made an appearance in public for over a year. He had done so now to deliver into my hands the White Lion message, which would then be brought into the public domain. His gesture was an act of trust, which I appeared to have earned in uncovering the lion–human mysteries over the past seven years.

The unscripted speech that followed was the most powerful testimony I have ever heard. Accepting that this great orator's delivery is entirely lost on this sterile page – and the connection that I felt between him and the White Lions in the Johannesburg Zoo is in any event impossible to convey on paper – I have relayed Mutwa's speech word for word as it was uttered.[17] As always, he took a deep breath before he delivered the following words for the record:

> Behind me are the holiest animals in Africa: the White Lions of Timbavati. Our people believe that if these beasts vanish from the land of the black people, the whole of Africa will cease to exist.
>
> These animals are said to herald coming changes on this earth. The first White Lions, we are told, were born over 400 years ago, when a star-like object fell to earth in the place called Timbavati today. At first, not only lions were born of this color, but also leopards and other creatures as well – antelopes and even birds.
>
> These creatures ought to be preserved and protected, and the reason they are born of this color should be investigated. Africa has lost much of what is important and beautiful, through indifference, racism, and religious fanaticism. If it is right that the English people should preserve their ravens in the Tower of London, to shield and protect them, by military power if necessary, how can it be wrong to protect these sacred animals – the animals around which many prophecies have been uttered by some of our greatest seers?
>
> It is said that at the end of the world, a White Lion will roar for the last time – heralding the disappearance of the sun from the sky, for all time.
>
> The White Lions of Timbavati, the lions of the star that fell to the earth, must not be allowed to vanish from the pages of our country's history.
>
> I cannot say more. Thank you.

He was visibly tired, and I arranged for the golf cart to transport us back to the entrance. I sat beside him on the bumpy journey through crowds in the zoo, feeling too emotional to speak. In that brief encounter, I believed I had caught a glimpse of the "star thing" – the strange magnetism that the highest Sanusis are said to possess, which draws crowds, and moves monuments, and telepathically speaks to the king of the beasts in the secret language of the stars.

"Ma'am," he said, as we parted that afternoon, "do not forget that you have been given two faces: a black and a white face. The black face is the face that you turn to Umlando, the African Knowledge, while the white face is the face you must turn to the world."

"Is that a good or a bad thing, Credo – having two faces?" I asked.

"Ma'am, you are a bridge. Do not forget this. Perhaps you do not know that your personal story goes back a very long way in Africa – for many, many lifetimes."[18]

I had no intention of forgetting his words, and although I did not fully understand them, I imagined there would be plenty of time to uncover their true meaning. I did not know then that I would not be seeing my great lion shaman friend again for a long time.

18

BIRTHPLACE OF THE GODS

The tradition of the campfire faces that of the pyramid.
– MARTIN BUBER[1]

The next morning, when I arrived at the Johannesburg house ready to commit to further work with Mutwa, I found that the Sanusi had left. I felt disappointed and confused. Shortly after, I had word that his wife was desperately ill and that he'd suddenly had to return to Mafikeng to be by her side.

In the months that followed without contact with Mutwa, I had reason to ponder the knowledge the great shaman had shared with me. Mutwa's assertion that my own origins went back many, many lifetimes in Africa began to alter the way I perceived myself, and made the immediate black–white tensions in the country seem time-bound and almost superficial. His assertion that White Lions were star beasts compelled me to identify the persistent interconnections between the lion symbol and the star symbol in world symbolism. Most pressingly, his imperative for the White Lion's preservation forced me to recognize that not only did the lion shaman's words carry an urgent conservationist message, but also, I now suspected, a greater cosmological message.

Somehow, the White Lions represent the route to the survival of our planet.

Just as the famous winged lion of Saint Mark carries a message inscribed into his Book of Laws under his learned paw, so the White Lions of Timbavati are enlightenment-bearers bearing a message. This message has to do with the secret word *Tsau!*: lion as star beast.

Given the tantalizing clues provided by Mutwa and the connections that I had gone on to establish between Timbavati and Great Zimbabwe, it was now clear to me that my next step was a journey to Egypt. While Timbavati is the birthplace of the legendary White Lions and Zimbabwe is the sacred shrine of the lion, Giza is the site of the world's greatest and most enigmatic lion monument: the Sphinx. What is the thread that binds these three sacred lion sites? What profound secret did the ancients know, of which we have only the faintest inkling?

Shortly after Mutwa's departure, I heard that a group of prominent Egyptian scholars was due to meet for a symposium at Giza in November 1997. Among them would be the key contemporary figures in the debates currently raging around the Sphinx: John Anthony West and Adrian Gilbert. With a little inspired detective work and a number of phone calls, I arranged to join the group, and booked my ticket to Egypt.

Sphinx Riddle

When I landed in Cairo, it was midnight, two days after the Luxor massacre, and the city was shrouded in a sense of doom. Sixty tourists had been murdered in a shootout, turning one of Egypt's most-visited sacred sites into an unholy bloodbath. The British Embassy had issued a statement saying that it could not guarantee the safety of its subjects, and all the British tour groups were evacuated.

My concerned family and my husband, John, had been insistent that I cancel my trip. Indeed, the circumstances in Egypt had given me palpitations of fear and doubt. But having arranged to meet with people who might prove to be central figures in the mystery I was attempting to fathom, I could not possibly pull out. Besides, I argued that with the entire Egyptian Army mobilized in the wake of the massacre, it would be the safest time to travel.

The morning after my arrival, I awoke in my hotel room and walked out to my balcony, where I discovered to my consolation that my view looked out directly onto the Giza plateau. Above the smog of Cairo, above the apartment blocks, the palm trees and the haze, rose the pyramids: unadorned and uncompromising. I had seen so many postcard pictures of them, which had not prepared me for their overpowering presence. I had a full day to collect my thoughts before venturing out to meet these timeless monoliths together with some of the Egyptologists who had dedicated their lives to studying them.

At dawn the next morning, I was standing beneath the shadow of the Great Pyramid, asking the question that has haunted successive civilizations, and none more than our own, which prides itself on technological achievements: how were these unprecedented architectural feats achieved?

Standing beside me was John Anthony West, a lively 60-something man with a sharp wit and infectious vitality. After a quarter-century considering this question, he has become part of the Egyptological furniture. Several locals in turbans and flowing *djellabas* had already recognized him, and waved enthusiastically.

Beneath our feet were monumental paving stones, a mosaic on a colossal scale; an integral part of a higher message built to last. West's eye roved over familiar territory, from the gargantuan base blocks of the Great Pyramid to its towering pinnacle, and he put the question succinctly: "There are really only three possible explanations of how these incredible things were achieved. First, genius application of hard technology, such as cranes, pulleys, ramps – which we haven't discovered yet or correctly interpreted. Secondly, and I tend to go along with this one, the ancients may have used simple means to produce complex results, which is typical of the Egyptological approach: what we might call 'soft technology.' That is, by using a method of heightened consciousness, possibly of a sonic or acoustic nature. We are starting to get proof of this kind of thing: sound influences form; sound can move matter. This second approach would see these stones as a consciousness-raising exercise." He paused. "Finally, the third option is the theory of alien intervention." At which his eyes lit up playfully.

It interested me that West favored the "soft technology" option: acoustic or sonic technology. Call it an exercise in sympathetic magic: naked energy is sound – sound moves matter – architecture is music frozen in stone. Increasingly, these unfamiliar concepts started to take on concrete shape and form in the context of the monuments themselves. The power of sound to create form – a scientific field today known as "cymatics" – might ultimately explain the architectural mastery of technology as yet undeveloped by ourselves. Different materials have been shown at certain frequencies to take on specific shapes. Today's most advanced science is capable of levitating objects such as small rocks in midair using sound frequencies: a phenomenon known as "acoustic levitation."[2]

Listening to West's theories reminded me of Mutwa's assertion that man in fact possessed 12 senses, which included "the ability to influence not only animals but inanimate objects also." I remembered his veiled references to the "star power" harnessed by the hawk priests and lion priests, and how these enlightened individuals could move objects with sheer mind-power.

Judging from the current research of archeoastronomers on the sound emission frequencies of stone, and their proposal that the Egyptian obelisks were giant "tuning forks" used to "tune in" to the frequency of certain stars,[3] Mutwa's point about the ringing stones of Timbavati and Great Zimbabwe being used for purposes of communication with the celestial bodies struck me as a fitting echo, and reminded me of his sonorous phrase, "song of the stars."

Our small group was not allowed to travel a meter without military escort. Fortunately, once we arrived at the sacred sites, the soldiers remained outside, and we were left alone with the shadows and the acoustics. As we wandered through the temples, with their rhythmical rows of columns and resounding chambers, the deliberate use of harmonic principles in art and architecture forcibly asserted itself. Entering spaces enclosed in stone, I was caught up by the curious sense of being inside monumental musical instruments. I was beginning to see what West meant when he talked about the architecture as frozen music, a symphony in stone; each component part with its own constituent harmony. The great avenue of sphinxes that links the Temple of Luxor to the Temple of Karnak, for instance, struck me as musical notes, repeated rhythmically, statue after statue – drawing a chord of harmony between two sacred sites.

This avenue of stone lions is one of West's favorite places on earth, and I could understand why. For me, it was a picture-in-stone of the phalanx of lion guardians that had provided Maria with safe passage through the pride in Timbavati.

As we walked around the deserted acoustical chambers of the sacred sites, with our footsteps echoing behind us and our voices rising strangely at certain moments then dropping into ghostly hushes at others, West discussed with me the central notion of Logos for the Egyptians. The term *Logos,* the Greek translation of the Egyptian word *Maat,* meaning "the Word," is one of the most important concepts of ancient Egypt and, in fact, of all ancient cosmologies, including the Christian religion. Yet it remained a concept I had difficulty grasping.

"You could do with some lessons in Sanskrit or classical Greek," West instructed me, explaining that this sonic term did not translate easily into English. "You need to understand that the concept of Logos is more than simply 'the Word,'" he continued. "The best term we have for it in English is perhaps 'the verb,' or even 'the vibration.'"

We were passing beneath a stone archway into an empty chamber as he spoke and, as if to mock me further, his voice came echoing back in vibrato. "There we are!" he announced, looking delighted with himself, and placing my palm against the masonry by way of example. "It's almost as if one can *see* sound here, or *hear* form. Remember: *sound creates form.*"

His eyes were sparkling in his quizzical fashion, and he went on to remind me that Saint John's Gospel begins: "In the beginning was the Word, and the Word was with God, and the Word was God." This at least was familiar to me.

"Similarly," he continued, "the Egyptian Book of the Dead, which is the oldest written text in the world, contains the equivalent passage: 'I am the Eternal . . . I am that which created the Word . . . I am the Word,'"[4] This notion of Logos underlies virtually every sacred genesis text on the globe: "In the Beginning was the Word."[5]

The original meaning of "the Word" is identified with the notion of sound. *Logos spermatikos,* the "seminal Word," like the seed, gives form to unformed matter.[6] In this context, it interested me that ancient symbolism equated the lion with solar Logos: the Word of the sun. Although I could not rationally grasp the extent of what was meant, I could feel in my bones there was meaning here, of a primal cosmological kind.

Lion: Solar Logos

Wondering why "the Word" corresponded with the concept of creation, I remembered Laurens van der Post's story of the Bushmen who were rescued in the Kalahari desert. In Bushman culture, the word *Tsau!* – the lion word – carries the same vibratory power as the beast itself, a sonic resonance befitting a sun god. Observing the ceremony in which the Bushman mother held her newborn infant up to the stars, van der Post felt he had borne witness to "the coming of the word in the darkness before time."[7] Like van der Post, and First Man before him, I was beginning to understand that the ancient Egyptians viewed the energy of the sun – the solar Logos – as the cosmic law that linked lions, humans, and stars in our archetypal consciousness. Synonymous with "the Beginning," the solar Logos signals a primary moment of genesis in the human species: First Man's first word.

Given that our everyday language does not work in this way, "the Word" is a notion that is virtually impossible to put into words (as we normally use them). Rather than a highly organized system of naming things, which creates a copy of the real world, the Word is inextricably part of the real world.

In humankind's language, the word signifies the object. By contrast, in the language of divine causes, the Word *is* the object.

Signifier and Signified

Another researcher I had been keen to meet was Adrian Gilbert, a scholarly individual, both cautious and considered. We soon discovered we had much to talk about – not the least of which was our mutual fascination with lions, the lion symbol, and the constellation of Leo.

In his recent works, Gilbert writes a great deal about the lion symbol in ancient mysteries. It was over a cup of tea that he confessed, "Since I've discovered that my own astrological chart has five planets in Leo, I've wondered whether this has had something to do with my interest in lions." Then he added, on a more serious note, "The fact is the lion is without doubt one of the most important symbols of humankind. Certainly the Egyptians believed so."[8]

As Gilbert poured another cup of tea, I mulled over the central role enacted by lions in ancient Egypt. Numerous lion-humans or human-lions decorate the walls of sacred buildings, reminding me of rituals performed by shamans throughout old Africa.[9] In Egypt, the teachings of lion shamanism illuminated what would otherwise have been obscure to me. The ritual connection between priesthood and lions existed in dynastic times, with the Egyptian priests of the Late Period keeping sacred lions in the temple of Leontopolis.[10] On the stelae of sacred buildings, the pharaoh may be seen offering the hieroglyphic sign of a cultivated field to his lion, a clear echo of the harvest rituals throughout Africa.

Like the lion kings of Southern Africa, the correlation between pharaoh and lion is so close as to be virtually indistinguishable at times. One does not have to look further than the lion Sphinx with its pharaoh's face to find colossal evidence of this association. The lion–pharaoh association is borne out by fine wall reliefs such as the northern frieze of the Temple of Rameses II, where the dramatic four-part sequence depicts a great battle scene – the pharaoh in his chariot accompanied by his lion. In the penultimate scene of the frieze, Rameses is in full battle cry, and the lion beneath the chariot is at full stretch, his tail extended and jaws open, a horse in plumed headdress rearing above him. In the tradition of African lion kings, the royal lion of the pharaoh went with him into battle, pacing the royal chariot, ready to die alongside his human counterpart.

The beautifully realized depictions of these leonine monarchs delighted me, since I related the stories directly to Ingwavuma, who was both a lion and a king in my imagination. He also had associations with the sun or the sun god.

With these associations in mind, I questioned Gilbert more closely on the Egyptian tradition. "If the lion is the solar Logos in ancient Egypt," I asked, as we entered the solemn chambers of Dendera Temple, "does this imply that he is the vibration of the sun, hence 'the sun god'?"

"That would be correct," the archeoastronomer concurred. "In Egypt, the lion is associated with Horus, the heroic sun god, who represents the solar Logos, the 'Word' or 'Decree' of the sun, while alive, and returns to the stars upon death. Like other religions across the globe, the central thread in Egyptian cosmology is the bringing of civilization or enlightenment to earth. Horus is the bearer of solar intelligence or solar Logos to humankind, the incarnation of the sun's 'laws' at the moment of First Time." He paused thoughtfully. "The lion's connection with the sun is critical."

Horus King

In further discussions with Gilbert and the other archeoastronomers, it became clear to me that Horus was a key figure, the link between Egyptian ancient wisdom of the Great Tradition of Africa.

Like the mysterious occurrence at Timbavati, where something descended from the heavens "like a bird," the ancient Egyptian texts speak about Horus descending to the earth in the guise of a falcon or hawk. Once there, he begins to assume other qualities, most significantly those of a lion, as well as those of a human. In fact, the pharaoh himself is viewed as the living incarnation of Horus.

Proving himself to be a great hero figure, Horus has been compared to the Greek lion hero, Hercules (Herakles in the original Greek), by scholars. I was equally interested in the strikingly close comparisons between Horus and the lion hero figure of Africa who came from the stars, Matsieng. Significantly, the ancient Egyptian texts make reference to Horus being given a crown by the Leonine One – thus kingship is conferred upon him. While this appears to be a critical event in the evolution of the Horus king, the exact identity of the mysterious "Leonine One" has caused much speculation among Egyptian scholars.[11]

It seemed to me from the archeological evidence of the Sterkfontein Valley caves, when man evolved from the hunted to the hunter, that this evolutionary event was a fair explanation of the reference to the Leonine One handing over the crown. In humankind's evolutionary history, in a former Ice Age some million or so years ago, the lions handed sovereignty over to man, the newly evolved lion hero.

Yet, while the ancient Egyptian reference to the Leonine One giving the crown of the king of the beasts to the lion hero echoes the hunted-to-hunter evolutionary event, it takes the question of human evolution further. While the archeological evidence of the Sterkfontein Valley caves helps us understand physical aspects of human evolution such as bipedalism and brain expansion leading to language, fire, and tool invention, the sacred texts of the ancients are essential in creating awareness of the higher spiritual aspects of human evolution.

To me, it seemed significant that African lion shamans such as Maria Khosa and Credo Mutwa viewed this symbolic handover of the crown as a "gift" that the lions offered us, rather than our preordained right. The ancient Egyptian allusion to the Horus king assuming the crown from the Leonine One might, therefore, serve to remind us to question how humankind has managed his term of kingship or supremacy over the beasts. Unfortunately, the answer is that our management of our earth and its creatures leaves much room for improvement.

The reason for our mismanagement of our kingship over the earth may be that we have forgotten the higher metaphysical implications of the physical evolution that our species experienced. What makes the figure of Horus particularly interesting is that he not only embodies the lion-hero principle of physical evolution, he also seems to provide the key to the route to spiritual evolution. The key is literally a key symbol – for this is the way we are intended to view the ankh, which invariably appears in the hand of Horus when he is in his hawk-headed half-human form as Re-Horakhti. It also appears in the hand of Horus's female counterparts Bast, Hathor, and Sekhmet.[12] Again, it appears in the hand of Orion, when it is depicted as a constellation, one identified with Osiris, the sacrificial Christlike God and father of Horus. Most important, for our own consideration of spiritual evolution, it appears in the hand of the pharaoh himself. The last-mentioned may be of particular significance to us as evolving humans because, of all those figures mentioned, the pharaoh alone is mortal – or part mortal and part god, a human embodiment of the god Horus, whose godliness ultimately achieves its apotheosis in an ascension to the stars.

If we are intended to re-evaluate the spiritual aspects of the evolutionary leap that our species once made in a former Ice Age, it strikes me that the key may lie in the hands of the pharaohs of old, those lion kings of Egypt identified directly with the Great Sphinx of Giza.

It also lies in the hands of the Followers of Horus, a mysterious lineage of priestly initiates believed to have been custodians of the wisdom of the Sphinx.

Followers of Horus

In Egypt, I carried with me my most recent picture of Credo Mutwa: in full ceremonial regalia, singing the praises of the White Lion in the Johannesburg Zoo. After hearing my descriptions of the lion and eagle initiatory rituals enacted by this African lion-eagle priest and the Great Knowledge that he carried, Adrian Gilbert identified direct parallels with the Followers of Horus, the guardians of ancient knowledge who were depicted adorned in star-spangled lion regalia.

As I accompanied the archeoastronomers around the sacred Egyptian sites, I saw in the hands of engraved depictions of Horus and his "Followers" the symbol that hung as a centerpiece among the massive relics on Mutwa's chest: the ankh.

Once again, it seemed, my lion shaman friend was one of those select humans who held the key to spiritual evolution. It struck me as highly significant that the route toward ascension of the pharaoh's soul corresponded closely with the four-fold notion of initiation of the lion shamans of Africa. From the stories Mutwa had told me, and from the little I myself had been shown by way of initiation, I began to identify what this key signified. Mutwa's accounts of his trial as an initiate, buried neck-deep in the ground with predators sniffing his face, or hiding for days at a time in a trench hoping to catch the feathers of a great bird of prey, gave me an idea of the nature of this spiritualizing process. The key was to overcome fear.

This is well illustrated by the story of the Horus king, the hero. Horus heroically avenges his father Osiris's death at the hands of his evil brother, Set, and battles with various monsters.[13] Having taken on human and leonine attributes, the hawk-headed Horus, in my interpretation, comes to incorporate the serpent identity. Horus is now called Re-Horakhti: Horus-of-the-Horizon. As such, he has been specifically identified with the Great Sphinx of Giza, guarding the earth's balance and watching the sun rise on the horizon.[14]

Furthermore, as the Sphinx itself, Horus has been identified with the sun's passing through the Leo constellation, specifically the moment it joins with the heart star of Leo, Regulus.[15]

Living lion shamanism helped me see the relevance behind the Egyptian myths. Shamanism teaches that the route toward the spiritual evolution of our species is the path of love, light, and truth. These words are so familiar as to be almost trite. They have been so worn, abused, and misrepresented over time that they have lost much of their meaning. In the Egyptian context, however, they are invested with ancient and sacred significance that has new meaning for us today. Love, in shamanic terms, is the opposite of fear. The shamanic initiate does not kill the lion through fear, but rather honors it through love and faith. In ancient Egypt, I believe, this moment of overcoming fear through love is symbolized in the rare heavenly alignment of the sun touching the heart star of Leo. Symbolically, this implies the bringing of light into the lion hero's heart, thereby assisting humanity to overcome fear and darkness.

Truth (in lion shamanism, as in ancient Egypt) is represented by the Beast of Truth, the gryphon. Bringing together four hybrid identities, this multiple symbol is appropriate, since truth is knowing and understanding all things, incorporating

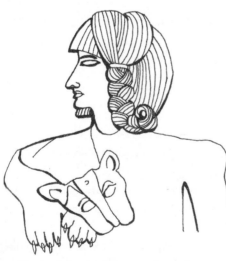

Detail from a relief carving depicting a Follower of Horus wearing a lion *kaross*.

opposites. In direct parallel with the four-fold aspect of Horus, the pharaohs wore breastplates symbolic of the outstretched wings of the hawk, with lion *kaross* over their shoulders, and the cobra on their headdresses. Having assumed the Beast of Truth status, the idea is that the Horus king, or pharaoh, can ascend to the stars. Yet, it is not any star, or any constellation, that is the intended abode of the pharaoh's soul, but specific constellations and specific stars within these constellations. The Horus king's status as star beast has to do with two constellations: Leo and Orion, constellations that in turn are the primary focus of Mutwa's Great Knowledge.

I concluded that, having performed the role of lion hero on earth, Horus must reconcile heroic consciousness with shamanic consciousness in order to return to the stars. Horus's reconciliation with shamanic truth is best symbolized by his ascension to the Orion constellation. As mentioned, Orion is identified with the sacrificial god Osiris, father of Horus.[16]

This seems paradoxical, yet there may be sense behind the myth. Horus is the son of Osiris; but if he achieves ascension, he becomes Osiris himself. Relating this notion back to the evidence at Sterkfontein provides an explanation. Hero consciousness grew out of an older shamanic type of Christlike consciousness (a consciousness in which all is one). In order to evolve spiritually, the hero needs to reclaim Christlike consciousness within heroic consciousness. The hero does so, it appears, by activating the lion heart (love, light, and truth) within himself. This was symbolized by the Egyptians, in heavenly terms, by the moment the sun passes through the heart star of Leo, lighting up these principles within the lion heart.

In short, in order to reach spiritual ascension, the lion hero has to reconcile with the lion shaman. Interestingly, this notion of reconciliation is not restricted to the Egyptians, but appears to be a central theme in other ancient civilizations. At one point, Gilbert produced a reproduction of an ancient Commagene stone tablet showing a lion priest shaking hands with a lion warrior, illustrating just this type of understanding between lion heroism and lion shamanism.

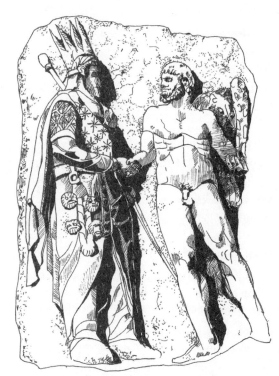

Commagene stone tablet indicating reconciliation between lion heroism and lion shamanism.

As Gilbert and I talked, the common base underlying the African tradition, the Egyptian, the Mesopotamian, and even the Mesoamerican traditions, began to astonish us both. It led me to reflect once again on the appropriateness of Mutwa's term: the Great Knowledge. While the man himself has been spurned in his own country, at every turn his wisdom is corroborated across the globe. While I had at first attempted to account for Mutwa's knowledge in terms of an inheritance that the shaman (as one of the guardians of old traditions) owed directly to the ancient Egyptians, my trip to Egypt began to reveal that this explanation was not good enough. Since other civilizations are based on the same traditions, it reminded me of Mutwa's explanation that the Great Knowledge is not limited to oral wisdom inherited by direct shamanic lineage, but is ultimately a condition of enlightenment (or "star knowledge").

Old Knowledge, New Meaning

Given the resonances across cultures and ages, the question inevitably arises: what are the implications for us today? To me, these timeless commonalities imply that there are essential truths that were understood and recorded by the ancients, the meaning of which may be vitally important for us to reclaim in our modern context.

The force behind the arguments of the new school of Egyptological thought relies on the understanding that these old mysteries should not be studied in isolation but should be seen as part of a global picture. The Egyptian edifices and sacred texts are understood to be deeply encoded with messages directly applicable today. The reason for the application of old knowledge to our specific age resides largely in the Egyptian notion of the beginning of time. While the ancient mysteries describe the moment of First Time on earth, it would appear from the new school of Egyptological thinking that these inscriptions are also prophetic: that is, they warn us about the approach of End Time.

The ancient Egyptian phrase for the genesis moment is *Zep Tepi*. Simply translated, *Zep* means "time" and *Tepi* means "first," thus First Time. By association, it comes to mean "the ancestors," those who came first. It is used in this manner in the Pyramid Texts, where *Tepi-aui* refers to the ancestral deities who prompted civilization in the Golden Age. The hieroglyphic sign denoting the *Tepi-aui* is the front half of a lion – which indicates that the first ancestors were leonine.[17]

This is a significant point. The lion-hero god, Horus, descends from a leonine lineage of deities traceable back to the original creator god, Atum,[18] whose first son and daughter, Shu and Tefnut, are born as lion cubs.[19]

Two further hieroglyphics identify the association between the notion of lion ancestors of the past and lion ancestors of the present. One is *xerefu* – meaning "the lions of yesterday." The other is *akeru* – meaning the lions of today.[20] By implication, this means that the gods not only at the beginning of time but also of today are leonine.

Lion Gods of the First Time

For me, the question remained why the key Egyptian gods and goddesses associated with the notion of the beginning of time should be leonine. As I wandered beside my male companions through these great wonders of world history, this question begged a satisfactory answer – one that I had an inkling might return me to the living mystery of the south: the White Lions of Timbavati.

The oldest figurine ever discovered (the leonine ivory carving in Höhlenstein-Stadel, Germany), reinforced my impression that this lion-god imagery was not exclusively an Egyptian preoccupation. As it had now become something of my own obsession, it was inevitably the subject of lion gods that formed the basis of my discussions with Gilbert the following evening. After a long day spent on foot in the echoing temples, we had settled down on a balcony of a strangely empty hotel lounge overlooking the Nile, with the Valley of the Kings on the opposite bank. The dusky sky was cloudless, and a single-hulled dhow, its sail billowing, carved its way upstream toward the southern horizon.

I finally decided to drop a provocative question: "Do you think it's possible that these enlightened beings actually existed?"

"Well," Gilbert smiled, "you tell me! Certainly, what makes the notion of 'First Time' so interesting is that the Egyptians were adamant about its *real* existence – and, furthermore, they prided themselves on being able to compute its epoch."[21]

The fact is that First Time itself has leonine associations. The Sphinx riddle hinges on this question of why the Egyptian calendar should depict the beginning of time as leonine.

Although this Egypt trip had not offered complete answers yet, everything pointed to the fact that I was on the right track. I now understood that not only does the *place* of the Golden Age have primary leonine attributes (symbolized by the Great Sphinx of Giza), but the *time* seems to suggest a lion epoch, very possibly the astrological Age of Leo.

Astrological ages, such as Leo, Virgo, Libra, and so on, are dependent upon an astronomical notion, still central to today's astronomy, known as *precession of the equinoxes*. This notion records the apparent movement of the heavens, or zodiac. It is determined by the prevailing constellation that forms a backdrop behind the rising sun, on the critical date of the vernal (spring) equinox each year. Due to the irregularity in the earth's rotations, this constellation gradually moves along the zodiacal path, changing from one constellation to the next approximately every 2,000 years. The entire cycle of 12 constellations in the rotating zodiac is completed approximately every 23,000 years.

Since the ancients believed that these leonine star gods were not only real and living figures, but arrived on earth at a specific leonine moment in time, the commencement of the Egyptian calendar of First Time leads to the idea that these lion gods were concurrent with a former Leo Age. Their association with the constellation of Leo prompted me to remember Mutwa's cosmological explanation that not only did lions come from Leo, but each and every wondrous creature on earth apparently had its origins in the stars. The fish came from the Pisces constellation, the crabs from the Cancer constellation, and so on. Like the fundamental belief of ancient Egypt viewing events on earth as connected to events in the heavens, Mutwa's deceptively childlike description of the African zodiac, the Mulu-Mulu, points to a Great Plan in the heavenly constellations that is manifest in real animals on earth. Despite the limitations of today's scholarship in proving such a notion,[22] it now occurred to me that what Mutwa was alluding to here was the transmission of stellar energy influencing living matter on earth, according to the founding principles of ancient astrology.

With this in mind, and knowing full well that it was probably an unreachable challenge, I came to a decision. Once I returned to South Africa, I would dedicate myself to learning the ancient knowledge of African astronomy and astrology, to see if I could prove, or at least illustrate, a causal connection between lions on earth and the Leo constellation. This astrological knowledge would prove significant in helping me understand past events – and events yet to unfold in Timbavati.

By now I should have anticipated what lion shamanism had been attempting to teach me all along. Instead of proving a connection between the lions of Timbavati and the Leo constellation, in due course, the seemingly magical lion–Leo connection would *prove itself* to me.

19

LION OF THE DESERT; LIONS OF THE BUSHVELD

The Sphinx has a genesis, and that was the lion.
— SELIM HASSAN, *THE SPHINX*

Almost two weeks after my arrival in Egypt, at the end of an extraordinary trip, I was standing beside John Anthony West, Adrian Gilbert, and a small group on the sloping alabaster-paved causeway leading up to the mortuary Temple of Chephren. It was before dawn. Resting in the giant trench below us, carved out of the bedrock itself, lay the Sphinx. Its famous lion's body was outstretched, with its reconstructed tail curling beneath its shanks and its upright human head, bedecked with a pharaoh's headdress, staring out over the desert.

The Great Sphinx of Giza: a huge monument to a lion. Why?

John Anthony West was leading discussions with infectious enthusiasm. "The Sphinx is an emanation of consciousness," he said, fixing me with a beady eye, "a way of thinking quite different from our own. In my view, the Sphinx would in all probability originally have had a lion's head to match its lion's body, and the pharaonic head would have been carved later."[1]

Clearly, the culture that created the Sphinx was prepared to deify an animal on a monolithic scale: a concept quite outside our modern Western anthropocentric philosophical framework. So what imperative led man to immortalize this particular beast on such a grand scale? Could the evolutionary Sterkfontein-type event – when humankind evolved from the hunted to the hunter – represent the beginning and end of the Sphinx riddle? I suspected not.

Looking at the great leonine edifice, I could not forget that it was the real Timbavati lions that had prompted my journey. Here, gazing at humankind's oldest riddle, I kept asking: why a lion? What was so important about lions that generated the production of this 20-meter (66-foot) high, 11.5-meter (38-foot) wide[2] colossus of solid hewn limestone? And why should that lion face due east into the rising sun?

Standing beside the Great Sphinx at sunrise, on the north–south line that linked this precise location on the globe with the land of Timbavati, mulling over the perennial riddle of the Sphinx that has mystified countless generations, I wondered about the mythic connection between the lion and the sun.

The Great Knowledge maintains that the souls of kings assume lion identity and become astral bodies after death. Just as the pharaohs were believed to be embodiments of Horus, the solar lion god, while alive, and returned to the stars when they died, so in the Great African Tradition, the king in death is transformed into the "lion of the ancestor" and his soul ascends to the stars.

It was reasonable to assume that the familiar African traditions of lions as royalty – even that of lions exchanging identity with kings – had their origins in ancient Egyptian mythology, or vice versa. The question is: where does the mythology come from?

The Source

Mutwa tells us that all knowledge in the world is connected and from one great source.

In Egypt, the notion of "the source" is identifiable with "the stars." This is consistent with Mutwa's notion of origins, which pinpoint Sirius, Orion, the Leo constellation, and our sun as the original fountainhead – the source – of this lion–human knowledge on earth. On this Egyptian trip, I followed the astral symbolism of the lion as star beast like a guiding light, for in penetrating to its source, I now felt sure I was encroaching on the central mystery guarded by the secret orders of ancient Egypt.

The high priests of Egypt, those select initiates I believe to have been capable of communication with lions, were adorned in star-spangled lion regalia, while the connection between lion and star – lion as star beast – is celebrated at every turn in the sacred architecture, on wall motifs, and in the Pyramid Texts. Horus in particular is the figure associated with the return to the source (the stars). The ankh that he holds in his hand gives us the key of entry into the soul dimension, which appears to have been viewed as fifth-dimensional reality and associated with the pentacle, or five-pointed star.

Staring out over the desert, into the first rays of the rising sun, I thought of how this great lion monument had been hewn from the bedrock when a dialogue existed between earth and the stars, in a place and time when the star gods were believed to have walked among humans.

Our small group had fallen into intense silence, and I became aware of a tangible sense of the ancient knowledge once custodianed by an enlightened priesthood and invested in this stone enigma. With my great lion-shaman friend in my thoughts, I felt a surging empathy with the "Venerables" in star-spangled lion regalia, the Followers of Horus. There was no longer any doubt in my mind that Mutwa fit into this time-honored shamanic tradition, traceable to the priestly caste of supposedly semi-divine beings, the custodians of the wisdom that is encoded into the earth's greatest leonine monument, and the lion–human mysteries which lie behind our very existence on earth.

What makes the new school of Egyptological work so urgent and compelling, I believe, is that the ancient mysteries convincingly argue that the ancients left encoded messages with specific application for our present times. The argument centers predominantly on the ancient Hermetic dictum, "As above so below," meaning: as it is in the heavens, so it is on Earth. It has been shown that the Giza monuments act as a ground-to-sky map of the heavenly constellations, the chief correspondences being with the constellations of Leo and Orion. As such, the monuments have been used as astronomical instruments to compute earlier epochs, even possibly pinpointing the moment of First Time. They may be used to reflect on our present epoch, believed to be the approach of End Time. In *Keeper of Genesis,* Robert Bauval and Graham Hancock argue that the Orion constellation, which was at its lowest point in the sky over the Nilotic Meridian at the watershed epoch of 10,500 BC, is now approaching its highest point in our time.[3]

Adrian Gilbert's book *Signs in the Sky* revolves around this factor, relating Orion and the Leo constellation to Christ's prophecies of the end of the world.[4] In the Bible, Christ makes the direct correlation between events in heaven and those on Earth, and he specifies that at this prophetic time "the sign that heralds the son of man will appear in the sky."[5]

Osiris – Christlike God

Significantly, the T-cross of Jesus, Christianity's "wounded healer," is taken to be another representation of the ankh. The T-cross of Christ is known as *Tau,* which returns us to the lion-star word *Tsau!*[6] Rather than focusing on the crucifixion aspect of Christ's death, however, I believe this original star-beast word places the emphasis on Christ's resurrection and the return of the soul to the stars.

While the reasons for these striking correspondences were not clear to me yet, it seemed perfectly fitting that Christ, Lion of Judah, should be identified with the very same secret star-beast root word uttered by First Man, the Bushman. While I struggled to put this notion of solar Logos into words, I could feel its powerful vibration in every fiber of my being. Thinking further along these lines, it suddenly struck me that Mutwa's Christian name carried the same connotations. Credo means "I believe" in Latin. It is the first word of an ancient creed.[7] Therefore, Credo is "the Word," the upholder of God's law on Earth.

Thinking of the Christian notion of the second coming, I recalled Mutwa's haunting observation that, for the first time in human history, various world religions are agreed on one thing: the anticipated return of a god, or gods. Synonymous with the wounded healer, the African god that the Zulus called Mvelinqangi (whose leg was bitten off by the monster) resembles the sacrificial god of the Hottentots with the wounded knee, Tsui-goab, who further resembles the white god of the Andes, Viracocha, who sacrificed one leg to a monster in order to facilitate the creation of the earth, and whose return was anticipated by the ancients. It interested me that this wounded healer god, also known as Quetzalcoatl to the Aztecs, should be linked to the Orion constellation.

The Great Hunter: Orion

As our group waited in silence for the sun to rise, I thought over a discussion Gilbert and I had had the previous evening. Trained as a scientist, Gilbert combines an analytical mind with the spirit of a priest. Like scholars before him, he identifies Christ with the sun itself, effectively making Jesus a sun god.

It comes as no surprise, therefore, that along with his sun-god association, Christ is identified with Logos, or a divine principle or "Golden Mean" within man himself, whereby he lives "according to nature."[8] Therefore, Christ is the word of God on Earth and within nature itself. Jesus is the Christian lion king, born as a lion of the tribe of Judah. If Jesus is "the Word," he is also "the Light": the solar Logos, the "word" or vibration of the sun. A sun-god figure, Jesus is the Word, the Truth, the Light.

As an archeoastronomer, Gilbert had been investigating the astronomical factors pertaining to the birth of Christ and relating these directly to the Horus–Osiris mysteries. He identified the moment when the sun conjoins with Regulus, heart star of Leo, as the heavenly moment associated with Christ's birth.[9] This astronomical conjunction was also considered of paramount significance in Egyptian mythology.[10] Mutwa had informed me that the moment when the sun conjoined with Regulus symbolized the birth (or death) of a great king. It was invariably associated with the heart of the lion, Cor Leonis, and in Africa, according to Mutwa, the lion priests looked to Regulus to determine the destiny of kings on earth.

Working from an entirely different premise, Gilbert argues the significance of the moment when the sun passes through Leo's heart star – it is symbolic of the birth of Christ, Lion of Judah and King of Kings.[11]

Sphinx as Equinoctal Marker

The first rays were shining directly into our faces now, breaking into my meditation. John Anthony West was discussing the significance of the Sphinx's placement as an "equinoctial marker."

"At the moment of the equinox," the archeoastronomer was explaining, "and at this moment only – twice yearly when the length of day equals the length of night – the Sphinx is positioned in exact alignment with the rising sun."

West carried a walking stick for the purposes of pointing and dramatic gesture, rather than as a crutch. He was remarkably fit for his age and, like a mountain goat, he sprang onto a huge block of masonry to demonstrate this point. Stretching out his stick toward the east like a sundial casting a shadow, he illustrated how the lion monument's precise positioning served as a beacon for the sun's position in relation to the earth.

"The Sphinx acts as a pointer for the sun on the equinox," he commented, looking pleased with himself, "and can be used as such in measuring the pivotal astronomical notion of precession of the equinoxes."[12] I followed the direction of this walking stick pointing due east, imagining the stately movement of the heavens behind it, a zodiacal band shifting from one of astrological age to another every 2,500 years or so.

Since life on Earth would not be possible without the sun, it is understandable that a civilization would expend such effort to create a megalithic monument to the rising sun, but why should this monument be a lion?

From what I had gleaned from both West and Gilbert, the Sphinx was not only precisely aligned at 90° to the earth's north–south axis, but its square base was locked into the cardinal axis of our planet, that is, in alignment during the four "cardinal moments" of the year (summer solstice, autumn equinox, winter solstice, and spring equinox). Too, the Giza pyramids were precisely aligned on the cardinal points, and the Great Pyramid served as a meridianal (or longitudinal) instrument, something which has been widely acknowledged in astronomical circles.

Using the principles of precession of the equinox, we can determine that over the current couple of decades, the prevailing constellation in the Northern Hemisphere is entering Aquarius. Using the same principles, archeoastronomers (contrary to orthodox Egyptological theory) believe that the Sphinx was built as an equinoctial marker when the prevailing constellation in the Northern Hemisphere was in Leo (10,500 BC). I had little doubt that their conclusion would be met with approval by traditional lion shamans such as Mutwa.

However, there is a critically important point that has not yet been clearly made by the archeoastronomical community. For some reason, the Southern Hemisphere is invariably forgotten in today's raging Giza debates. The point is that, whatever the astrological age in the Northern Hemisphere, the reverse is true for the Southern Hemisphere. Since Leo and Aquarius are polarities in the zodiac, the Age of Aquarius in the Northern Hemisphere is the Age of Leo in the Southern, and vice versa.

By applying the key astronomical notion of precession, I realized now that I had arrived at a neat mirror image: the Sphinx was constructed at the commencement of the Age of Leo in the north while the White Lions appear near the commencement of the Age of Leo in the south. This was an important insight.

The basic idea is that the Sphinx was built in the shape of a lion because it was built in the age of the Lion. On many fronts, this makes a great deal of sense, because it implies that the ancients nurtured a knowledge system that saw connections between the earth and the stars. In some respects, however, this conclusion raises more questions than it provides answers.

West was outlining the argument. "Either the ancients understood the highly advanced astronomical notion of precession, and consequently knew they were living in the Age of Leo, or, as our Egyptological fraternity still maintains, they did not. The question is, if the ancients didn't know they were living in the astrological Age of Leo, how did the formations in the sky (Leo and Orion's Belt) come to correspond so neatly with the man-made creations on the ground in Giza (the Sphinx and the pyramids)?"[13]

He paused for dramatic effect. "This would suggest some kind of dialogue between terrestrial and stellar events way beyond modern man's wildest conjectures."

West's argument leaves one to conclude that, obviously, the ancients must have understood advanced notions such as precession. However, this raises the further question as to why the Leo constellation was called after a lion in the first place. Though it doesn't immediately suggest a lion to the casual observer, when you know how to connect the dots, a lion form becomes obvious.

Mutwa maintains that the Leo constellation has a direct causal connection with lions living on Earth. That led me to ponder the White Lions once more. Following the sun's rising orb, it had gradually begun to dawn on me how the mysterious occurrence of the White Lions of Timbavati in a remote part of Africa was directly related to the Sphinx riddle.

Witnessing the sunrise over Giza bathing the Sphinx in golden desert light, I could picture the Timbavati lions yawning after their nocturnal predations. Since the equinox is that day of the year when night and day are of equal length, it is this time of year, and this time only, when the sun's rays strike the earth at any one longitude at precisely the same time. I could vividly imagine that instant when the sun's rays gilded the manes of Timbavati's lions, just as they radiated from the Sphinx's face – while the rest of the world was either up and about in full daylight, or else shrouded in darkness.

Gradually, it was becoming clear to me that the White Lions' strategic appearance on this longitudinal line might represent living proof of something over and above man-made constructs: that is, nature's law, or the sun's law, the solar Logos.

Here in Northern Africa at a most sacred site, a monolithic lion was hewn from stone, while at a sacred site in Southern Africa, along the same longitudinal line, arose the rarest breed of lions on Earth. The one is a monumental architectural achievement, the other pure flesh-and-blood lion magic.

Akeru: Twin Lion Guardians

John Anthony West was pointing his stick at the engravings on the face of the granite stela between the paws of the Sphinx to reinforce his point. There, carved in relief, is one of the best examples of the recurring double-lion motif, the *akeru*.[14] In the sacred texts and architecture, the *akeru* are usually depicted as double-headed, or back-to-back lions. Since the lion is closely identified with the sun in Egypt, as in other cultures, the back-to-back lion symbol represents the rising and setting sun or, by association, the east–west horizon. Representing the sun's daily course, rising in the east and setting in the west, the paired lion guardians evoke the passage of time along with the birth and death of daylight. Occasionally the double lions are presented one above the other, which then, by association, represents the north–south axis. The *akeru*, in their representation as the north–south-east–west axis, therefore relate to the lion's intrinsic association with the sun itself.

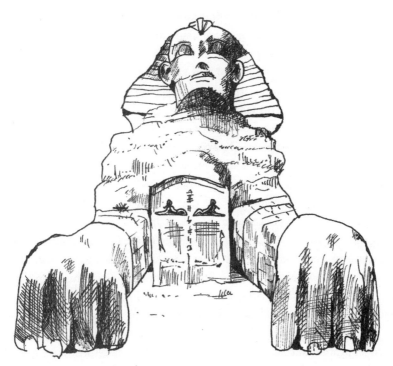

Between the paws of the lion-human Sphinx, the akeru, or back-to-back lions.

In their position between the paws of the east-facing Sphinx, one of these engraved lions faces south while the other faces north, and in this way they define the north–south axis.

I had become accustomed on my Egyptian tour to discovering amazing connections between the Egyptian mysteries and the Great African Tradition. I now saw that the *akeru* symbol so closely resembled the representation of the guarding lion on Mutwa's Talking Stone that it begged comparison. Mutwa had told me that the stone was one of two parts of a lintel, guarding the gateway of the Temple of Prayer of the lion king Shelumi (Solomon).[15] Given that this temple was in all probability on this same Nilotic Meridian,[16] the back-to-back lions of the south would have replicated those of the north. Hoping to find an answer to this piece of hidden knowledge guarded over by the Sphinx-Gryphon, I imprinted the *akeru* symbol on my memory. I was looking forward to sharing a description of it with Mutwa upon my return.

Lion Lady of First Time

Flanked by the sunken Sphinx, with my back to the eternal proto-modernist structures of the pyramids, I began to reflect on the various leonine gods associated with this precise location on the globe.

Since I had been alerted to the importance of the lion-headed goddess Sekhmet, I had gone on to experience what felt like a firsthand encounter with her.

Sekhmet is a very tangible presence in Giza. Her statues are everywhere, and wall reliefs depict her distinctive figure ubiquitously.[17] The previous day, during a visit to her famous statue in the Karnak temple together with Gilbert and West, I had gained an intimate and very powerful sense of this lion goddess's presence. There is nothing meek and mild about Sekhmet. I thought of her in the same spirit as I thought of Maria, Timbavati's Lion Queen. Above all, I associated Sekhmet with Amarava, Mutwa's spirit guide, the fearsome Earth Mother who, unlike Mutwa himself, unashamedly employs fiery primal power. Just as Sekhmet was associated with time before the beginning of time, I recalled Mutwa explaining to me that Amarava was "the mother of the First People on earth, and she will be the mother of the last."

During our visit the archeoastronomers wanted to use Karnak's sanctuary for half an hour's meditation, and I was pleased to participate in the outing. But instead of closing my eyes and meditating along with the others, I found myself focused on the statue of Sekhmet, marveling at the amazing connections that this Egypt trip was revealing. Still musing, I was suddenly startled to see the statue in front of me take on a new light. Half the lion goddess's face, I noticed, was shrouded in a dark shadow and the other half, under a direct beam of sunlight that came from a shaft in the ceiling, was snow white. Of course, my immediate thought was of the White Lions. Sekhmet was staring back at me, an intensity of gaze that is impossible to convey, except to those who have experienced the laser stare of lions in their natural environment. Lions in the wild have an intense fixation in their eye contact quite unlike the desperate blankness of caged animals. Sekhmet's gaze seemed to intensify this. It was unspeakably solemn – as if weeping for humanity. I wasn't hearing voices, but I nevertheless felt as if she were speaking to me. As the snow-whiteness of one side of her face slowly shifted, I found myself mesmerized, watching, until finally the last patch of white was gone. With the beam of sunlight eclipsed, the statue suddenly resumed its overall luster, and became stone again. At this point I shook myself, and the others began to stir.

This first encounter with the Egyptian lion goddess Sekhmet was a moving personal experience – and one that I knew could not easily be shared with anyone, nor readily translated into print.

Sun Gods and Star Beasts

Savoring my last moments beside the Great Sphinx of Giza, one key question kept resounding in my head: why did those followers of Horus, who masterminded these monuments with such ingenuity (the sophistication of which we are only beginning to comprehend), hold onto the notion of sun gods and star beasts?

The answer, simply, was that sun gods and star beasts had a basis in earthly reality. Mythology and ancient symbolism insist on the notions of winged lions and Lions of

God. Should we take them literally? While my rational mind warned against it, I felt flushed at the thought. Why should this conclusion be so inadmissible today? Why should we disbelieve the wealth of ancient knowledge? Why are we so afraid to believe in ascended beings? I smiled at the remembrance of my totem lion's superb debut on the Timbavati runway. Although otherworldly, lions with wings are "angels" of some kind – angelic lion spirits guarding over the affairs of man. The White Lions are angelic beings. There was a time – during the Golden Age of Zep Tepi – when they first came to Earth from the heavens, and there is a reason why they've returned to earth again in our time.

Here on the northern edge of the African continent, I soaked in the atmosphere of antiquity, knowing that a few hours later I would be heading back to the raw bushveld of Southern Africa.

Before leaving the Giza plateau, I took a long, lingering look at the world's greatest lion enigma. Anyone familiar with cats' behavior will recognize that the Sphinx has an intention. It may be basking in the sun, but it is not at ease; nor is it crouched, ready to spring. Stretched out with its head upright, its front paws directly ahead and its hind paws tucked beneath, this cat is in a guarding position. The Sphinx is, and has always been, humankind's guardian: ever alert, guarding the life-giving sun's birthplace on the eastern horizon.

Like Mutwa himself, the Sphinx is a guardian of sacred knowledge, guarding what is routinely referred to by Egyptologists as the "Hall of Records," which is commonly believed to be buried in a chamber beneath the front paws of the giant statue:[18] the hidden subterranean treasure that every Egyptological seeker of fame and fortune is bent on discovering. Over the past two weeks, West had regaled me with amusing anecdotes about the trials and tribulations that had befallen zealous Egyptologists hoping to hit gold. If I understood anything about the Great Knowledge, it had to be that treasure or gold is not a material issue. It is both a physical and metaphysical issue.

If humankind is ever intended to find the "gold" in this secret chamber, I now believed – based on Mutwa's visionary words about the sacred subterranean source of golden wisdom – that this discovery would coincide with a revelatory moment of "enlightenment" in the evolution of the human species.

The group had disbanded, and West was accompanying me down the sloping causeway beside the great stone feline. As if reading my thoughts, he shot me a rueful glance. "Don't give up, my darling. You are going to lose a lot of friends when you go public with this material. They'll think you've gone crazy – while you know that it is they who are crazy and you have only taken the preliminary steps on the long (and perilous) road to sanity!" He gave a rusty chuckle, and I could tell he was reliving his own lifelong gladiatorial battles against rigid orthodoxies.

"That's the problem with the scientifically minded," he quipped, "what they call 'reason' and 'right thinking' is not rational at all; it is simply the rationalization of the spiritually flat earth of their own inner world. Since they experience nothing transcendent or divine, they deduce that there is nothing. And that" – he smiled roguishly – "is just negative credulity, not science! You cannot talk about music to the tone deaf, or moonbeams to the blind, and if you talk about sex to eunuchs, they just get angry."

Encouraged by my amused smile, he went on to deliver his damning closing comment: "I'm afraid it will take a miraculous 'NLE' – near-life experience – before real conversation is possible with such people!" In parting, West gave me a kiss on both cheeks and I wished him a fond farewell. He was the most clued-up and engaging "tour guide" I'd ever met!

When I parted from Adrian Gilbert, the sage researcher gave me his own signed copy of *Hermetica,* the collection of texts written and compiled in ancient Alexandria in the Hellenic era but based on ancient Egyptian wisdom. Gilbert had reissued this seminal text through his own publishing house, Solos Press. Shaking hands, he advised me cautiously, "Whatever you do, don't turn your back on this lion shamanism thing. I've a feeling that you have been picked out to bring this important information to the Western world at this time. You've got work to do, Linda, now go and do it!"

His imperative reminded me of Mutwa's parting words about my being "a bridge" between the African tradition and the traditions of the West, and so, effectively having both "a black and a white face." Well-equipped to continue my bridging work, I felt ready to return to South Africa, in the full expectation of meeting up with Mutwa before long to share my findings with him.

20

NILOTIC MERIDIAN:
SACRED LAND OF THE NORTH,
SACRED LAND OF THE SOUTH

Man must make two connections. He must reconnect with the earth
and he must reconnect with the stars.
– CREDO MUTWA

Although I suspected that none of my findings would be news to Mutwa, I hoped that he would find some gratification in the endorsement I could now offer, in contrast to the scorn and brutal antagonism from which he had suffered for so much of his life. At every turn, my discoveries in Egypt corroborated the Great Knowledge that he had shared with me.

After much investigation, I learned from one of Mutwa's attendants that Cecilia, his wife, was in a critical condition. Moreover, there was the added tragedy that their daughter had now been diagnosed with HIV, after having been raped by an ex-boyfriend. On hearing of his bleak situation, my heart went out to my dear friend, and I thought again of the curse that the great Sanusi believed he had brought upon himself, his children, and his children's children, for speaking of secret knowledge.

Message Behind the Masonry

Endeavoring all the while to keep up with further developments in Mutwa's circumstances, I plowed ahead with research. The Egyptological material had prompted burning questions in respect to the 31°14′ E meridian, and I simply could not let these rest unsolved.

Meanwhile, I continued a lively e-mail exchange with John Anthony West. His informed and unapologetic input after a quarter-century of dedicated research, together with Adrian Gilbert's astute and careful scholarship, continued to provide me with a new understanding of these old constructions. The more I learned about the Giza monuments, the more I understood that nothing was circumstantial, nothing coincidental about these sanctified edifices. Every measurement, every proportion, every dimension carried specific meaning and purpose.[1]

From the pyramids' geometrical proportions to the meticulous stellar alignments of their ground plan, the Giza monuments have symbolic significance. Much has been written about the precision of their latitudinal position, and my own research showed that the same precision applies to their longitude. The architects of these monuments, whose science dictated their faultless alignment to true north, south, east, and west, would have selected their longitudinal placement with the same exactitude displayed in every other geometric and geological consideration. The nicety of the Great Pyramid's internal passageways, running perfectly north–south, and the strategic positioning of the original entrance, exactly homed into the meridian, reinforces this point.[2] The same emphasis on their longitudinal positioning is made by the four "star shafts" within the pyramids themselves, which align with specific stars and targeted along this exact 31°14′ north–south line. Clearly, this is no arbitrary line. So why were the pyramids, Sphinx, and possibly even Nile itself, positioned on this particular longitude?

Man-Made River

Perched on the plateau and located at the apex to the Nile Delta, the Great Pyramid had often been studied as an astonishingly accurate instrument of earth measurement. For example, the pyramid's proportions have been shown to correspond perfectly with the ratio and proportions of the Northern Hemisphere of the earth itself.[3] In respect of the Nilotic Meridian, the Great Pyramid's own meridian has been shown to bisect the Nile Delta precisely, while the pyramid's northeast and northwest diagonals may be extended out to form a triangle that perfectly encompasses the Delta triangle.

More interesting still is the fact that the dimension of the Nile Delta triangle has long been understood by the most serious of scholars to represent a natural instrument of specific and precise measure. The three points of the delta triangle were utilized to define the starting point for longitudinal lines. The three corners of the triangle also provided the ancient Egyptians with the coordinates that determined the proportion and extent of their sacred land of Lower Egypt (Sokar), with the apex of the triangle – the tip of the Nile Delta – delineating the meridianal point. The point itself corresponds with the supremely sacred land in Sokar, called Rostau, believed to be the exact birthplace of the gods.[4]

While the pyramids were masterminded as symbolic geometrical instruments, the principles of sacred geometry used within the Nile Delta itself suggest that the layout of the river mouth is not entirely natural.[5] This supports Mutwa's notion, which had seemed preposterous when he first voiced it, that the course of the Nile was in fact man-made. If, as the sacred symmetry of its Delta suggests, the Nile's outlet was designed by man, not nature, might the same not apply to the course of the entire river?

It was tantalizing to discover that the findings of prominent scholars were leading them to the same conclusion.[6] The question that follows is: if the course of the Nile is an act of art, not nature, what does the art signify?

Time Line

Significantly, the course of the Nile follows a longitudinal line. While latitudinal lines are determined by a fixed factor – specifically the earth's equator – longitudinal lines are arbitrary. That is to say, the line with which we begin measuring longitude might be any longitudinal meridian.

One can take it, therefore, that for the ancients this meridian represented 0° – that is, the line by which they began measuring longitude, at the beginning of time. Rather than the Greenwich Meridian we use today, the ancient Egyptians chose the Nilotic Meridian, the line of the river upon which their entire culture was dependent, and where it was geographically positioned. In a very practical sense, then, time began along this line for the ancients.

Unlike the Greenwich Meridian, the Nilotic Meridian was associated with Zep Tepi – the beginning of time on Earth. It refers to more than mere measurement; it refers to a divine happening, the time when the gods (whom the Egyptians named the *neteru*) visited our planet and mixed with humankind.

Pawprints of the Gods

This notion of star gods remained a deeply compelling one for me on a personal level. Mutwa had informed me that if I continued to trace the tracks of the White Lions I would come to know the answer to the Sphinx riddle.

What bearing might this Zep Tepi time line have on the mystery of the three aligned sacred sites, separated by hemisphere but linked by a common longitudinal thread? If the Giza plateau was a perfect star map on earth, and Timbavati was in perfect alignment with it, what was the significance of the White Lion's birthplace being located precisely here on our globe? On the one hand we were evaluating sacred man-made monuments, on the other we were considering flesh-and-blood lions: could there really be a connection between the two?

Having identified the shared meridian, other correspondences in this geodetic connection became easier to detect. I began to see that Timbavati's location bore uncanny parallels to the land of Sokar, the sacred land of Lower Egypt, defined by the outer corners of the Nile Delta.

Timbavati in the south is virtually a mirror image of the sacred land of Sokar. Of course, one is comparing live lions' territorial ranges with the strategic location of a monumental geodetic marker, yet the two locations demonstrate uncanny geodetic correspondences.

The land of Sokar's southern border lies 24° N while Timbavati's northern border is 24° S.[7] This alone suggests a south-to-north mirror image. To the west, Timbavati's furthermost corner extends out to a point that is in almost perfect alignment to the pyramids at the apex of the Nile Delta: 31°14′ E.[8] I wondered what the designated borders of Timbavati would have been in the days when the early African king, Npepo, declared it a sacred site, and longed, as always, to reach greater clarification through Mutwa. As it was, Timbavati's present-day borders were virtually an inverse image of the sacred land of Sokar, with the equator acting as the centerfold of the African continent.

Why should today's living lion legends align with the lion monument of ancient days? This was the question that kept me awake at night. Why should the birthplace of the White Lions in the south (in our time) correspond, along the same line, with the birthplace of the gods in the north (at First Time)?

Although I hesitated in verbalizing it, I now saw that the answer was staring me in the face. The message was radiantly clear, even if my rational mind could not easily accommodate it: Timbavati's White Lions are living symbols of stars – star beasts walking our earth in our time, just as they had walked among men in the days of old.

Star Beasts on Earth

Significantly, the name of the birthplace of the Egyptian land of the gods, positioned along this line, is Rostau – revealing the hidden suffix *tau,* which identifies it at once with the secret word for both "lion" and "star" in the Great African Tradition.

Recalling Mutwa's allusion to the word *Tsau!,* I saw clearly that his star–beast connection went further than our earthbound Egyptologists' appraisal of the lion and star symbols depicted in the architecture and texts of the ancients. It goes even further than today's archeoastronomers' best-selling observations of the man-made earth map at Giza, mirroring a heavenly star map. As Guardian of Sacred Knowledge, Mutwa's star–beast link goes so far as to draw a causal connection between life on Earth and specific stars in the heavens.

For Mutwa, like the Horus sages of old, Lions of God come from the stars, and return to the stars after death. I was beginning to believe him.

Tsau! – Lions from the Stars

The general consensus among today's archeoastronomers is that the Sphinx is an earthly symbol of the Leo constellation. Along with this clear earth-to-star correspondence, there are other stellar alignments that are now believed to hold the key to the leonine pharaoh's return to the stars. Recently, particular attention has been paid to the so-called "star shafts" within the Great Pyramid. Once believed by archeologists to be mere air vents, these have now been established as strategically positioned shafts of astronomical significance, and are pivotal to the work of today's scholars. In *The Orion Mystery*, Adrian Gilbert and Robert Bauval's argument turns on these shafts, which are directed at specific heavenly bodies – the same heavenly bodies that were identified by Mutwa as vital to the lion message on earth. The first important point is that the shafts

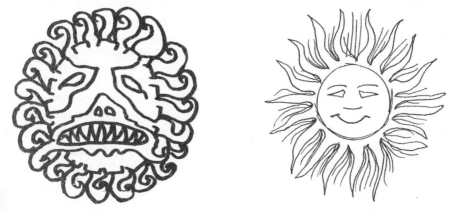

At the mythic level, the sun and the lion are interchangeable symbols. On the left, the Mask of Mithras, a Persian image of the sun.

are directed due south along the Nilotic Meridian. In addition, the shafts are targeted at Sirius and Orion's Belt, respectively.

Mutwa correlates real living lions on Earth not with any star in the heavens, but with specific constellations, and with particular stars within those specific constellations. The stars he identifies are Sirius,[9] the Orion constellation[10] (specifically the central star in the belt),[11] the Leo constellation[12] (specifically Leo's heart star)[13] and, not surprisingly, our nearest star, the sun.

The correlation between the lion and the sun is so obvious as to be virtually a cliché. Any child drawing a lion, with his mane like the rays of a sun, reminds us that a lion is the same symbol as the sun. While the lion–sun association is so familiar across cultures, however, the other stars identified by Mutwa's Great Knowledge are precisely pinpointed by the Giza monuments themselves.

Celestial Meridian

Significantly, a meridian denotes a north–south longitudinal line, not only on Earth, but also in the sky. This line stretches overhead in an arc from the north pole to the south pole. If our line of reference is the Nilotic Meridian on Earth, for instance, then we, like the ancient Egyptians, would need to note the meridian out in space. The Nilotic Meridian corresponds (at certain times of the year) with the Milky Way. In other words, the north–south line of the river Nile is joined at either horizon by the river of stars of the Milky Way.

Following the Hermetic doctrine of the Followers of Horus, "As above, so below," I realized that a mirror image of the connecting thread between Giza and Timbavati could be found in the heavens. The ancient Egyptians called this concept *Duat.*

The ancient Egyptian notion of the Duat goes deeper still, since it appears to represent not only the Nilotic Meridian on earth but also a meridian beneath the earth's crust – a subterranean river of stars. In drawing parallels between the ancient wisdom of the Egyptian lion sages and the living wisdom of Africa's lion shaman, I now believed that the Duat could be identified with Mutwa's notion of the subterranean river, which he called the Lulungwa Mangakatsi.

"Never forget that the story of the White Lions is connected to the stars," Mutwa had told me. When I forgot this connection, the mystery of the White Lions eluded me. When I remembered it, the answers to the White Lion riddle began to fall into place.

Timbavati is consecrated to the lion. Timbavati is also, according to Credo Mutwa, a place of "star" energy. In this bushveld region, star force and lion energy converge. The connection between the White Lions and the stars has to be the critical clue behind the consecration of the Nilotic prime meridian. Timbavati's very name – the place where a "star" came down to earth – speaks of the same mystery that connects the lion pharaohs of Egypt to the notion of the "starry river," or the "eternal river of stars."

Basing their work on ancient Egypt's Funerary and Pyramid Texts, today's archeoastronomers have identified a knowledge system held by generations of high initiates. Their role was to transmit through the ages a body of enlightened wisdom harking back to the time of the gods.[14] The ancient texts not only infuse the men or gods of olden times with leonine characteristics, but, like Mutwa's disclosures about the Abangafi Bapakade – the enlightened ones – they associate them with the word *akhu,* meaning the "Shining Ones," the "Star People," or the "Venerables."[15] Although I was unable to discuss these findings with Africa's venerable lion shaman, my trip to Egypt had encouraged me to conclude that I was now approaching the very essence of the White Lion mysteries. The great conundrum – the so-called Sphinx riddle – leads one around in circles until one simple clear connection is made: the interconnection between the earth and the stars.

Pure Gold

Bearing Mutwa's words in mind, I continued with my quest to understand the White Lion mysteries. Looking back on the amazing journey so far, I felt as if I had been tracking leonine pawprints upon the map of Africa in search of gold. Not gold in terms of mercenary stock-market value, but gold in its highest and purest form: spiritual value.

Throughout world symbolism, gold and lions are closely identified. In Egypt, I had felt this more strongly than ever. Following the moment of First Time, a Golden Age was believed to have existed, during which the star gods walked among humankind. In remembrance of this Golden Age, the lion–gold equation is borne out perpetually in the sacred geometry and proportions of ancient architecture.[16] West and Gilbert had illustrated through example, as we walked about the sites, how the notion of the Golden Mean (sacred ratio and sacred proportion) is the key defining principle behind both the construction and the decoration of the Giza monuments.

The Ancient Egyptian notions of the Golden Mean and Golden Proportion prompted me to remember the gold empire of Zimbabwe and the sacred metal-smelting sites in Timbavati itself. For some reason, gold-smelting sites seemed to cluster around the Nilotic Meridian, reminding me that this strip of the earth's geology appeared to have been the gold-producing center of the ancient world as far back as biblical and ancient Egyptian times (and very possibly further back in prehistory).[17] Zimbabwe's secret word – *zim* – not only had to do with a lion, and the soul of the king, but also with gold. It intrigued me that lions and gold might be associated even at a geographical level, just as they were associated at a symbolic level. As I unraveled the thread through Africa, this would prove vital.

Weighing the Egyptian wisdom together with that of Africa's lion priest helped me to evaluate the central message. Just as the Egyptian sages identify the leonine gods such as Horus and Sekhmet with First Time, so Mutwa associates leonine gods such as Matsieng and Amarava with the creation of humanity. Both the Egyptian and African traditions converge on one conclusion: the Nilotic Meridian is sacred beyond comparison, because it represents the beginning of time when lion gods walked among men. For me, the reappearance on this line of White Lions – the living, breathing, roaring, flesh-and-blood Children of the Sun God – was the physical manifestation of this sacredness. It was no longer of primary concern whether Mutwa's Great Knowledge derived from Egyptian origins or whether the Egyptian priesthood inherited knowledge from an older African tradition. "Which came first" seemed, to me, entirely academic.

At this point in my quest, I suddenly stopped in my tracks. It had become apparent to me that I had to take a stand – either for science or for sacred science.

The former separates fact from faith, and therefore would argue that nothing proves the higher significance of the White Lions. Consequently, while one can analyze the logic and meaning behind the siting and construction of the Sphinx and pyramids, one cannot do the same for the White Lions of Timbavati, since the importance of their arrival at this particular time and place cannot be proved beyond mere coincidence.

By contrast, sacred science argues that faith should not be separated from fact. The design and logic behind the siting and the construction of the Sphinx and pyramids point to divine intention. While the notion of the "Golden Mean" – the sacred ratio and proportion with which these monuments were designed – illustrates a sacred knowledge system encoded into the construction of these monuments, the White Lions are the real-life embodiment of this sacredness. Since the very notion of "sacred" is beyond the bounds of today's scientific method, I now realized it was entirely illogical to expect science to prove the sacredness of the White Lions.

I thought of the weight of academic skepticism. Then I thought of the White Lions. As living symbols, they carried even more weight for me. These radiant creatures, which ancient African tradition tells us have been sent as messengers of God, carry the weight of pure gold enlightenment.

In my mind, I had no trouble visualizing them as modern-day re-embodiments of the ancient star gods of the Golden Age. I now firmly believed what I had been taught by the shamans: that these sacred animals were real-life symbols of a divine purpose: Lions of God, Messengers of God, Children of the Sun God. These genetic rarities gave weight and meaning and physical form to the prophetic intention written into every single aspect of the sacred monuments aligned with this prime meridian.

Now I was presented with an opportunity to put Mutwa's lessons into practice. The first lesson of the lion shaman is to conquer fear. My greatest fear at this time was that my ideas would appear foolish to the academic community.

Golden Balance

Once I made the allowance for faith rather than science, things began to happen. I began to see differently. I began to make connections in a whole new way. Not piecemeal, point by point, but simultaneously. I began to see the African continent not as if I was walking upon it, step by step, but as if I was hovering above it, looking down.

From my new perspective, suspended above the earth, looking down at the vast continent, I began to see the whole picture. My vision was soaring, my thoughts could not keep up, but my heart told me it was seeing true. My logic kept trying to pin the picture down with facts, but it was expanding too fast for rational thought. Clue by clue I had been led to see a sacred geometric pattern presenting itself on Earth in respect of both man-made and geographical structures. Now I saw these clues coming together in one truly amazing hologramatic whole.

For the ancient Egyptians, our north–south polarity was reversed. Their orientation, which was centered on the Nilotic Meridian, meant that the Nile Delta represented a southerly direction, while upstream – heading off in the direction of the land of Timbavati – was construed as north, or "up" on a map. In other words, what is northwards to us was southwards to them; what is southwards was northwards.' The ancients' reversal of the poles along the Nilotic Meridian is highly significant. It relates to the earth's polar reversal. The apparent abnormality of the Nile, as the only great river that runs from south due north, is critically important, as its course along the world's longest prime meridian at the center of the earth's landmasses. The Nile is unique as the only great river that runs from south to north. It originates at the equator, at 0°, which relates directly to the great pyramid as a measuring device of the Northern Hemisphere. At 0°, the source of the Nile is associated with gold, which relates to the notion of the Golden Age. Each of these features is a key to unlocking the mystery of the lion star gods who, I am convinced, walked the earth in the Golden Age following First Time.

What I saw was a bird's-eye perspective – except that I was not in the sky hovering above the earth, but now suspended in outer space like that imaginary eagle in Mutwa's painting. From this perspective, I saw the entire globe beneath me, with the continent of Africa stretched out and encompassed by oceans. Strangely, in my vision, the earth's globe was itself contained within a perfect cube. No doubt the picture was influenced by certain of Mutwa's revelations as well as various sacred texts I had been studying. Ancient symbolism often represents the sacred geometry of the earth as a globe within a perfect square or cube. What John Donne once called "the earth's imagined corners" is a common device, referring to the earth's four cardinal points: north, south, east, and west. Just as other cosmological texts suggested, Mutwa talked about four leonine "brothers" guarding the cardinal points, holding the earth in balance.

These ancient symbols of the earth as a quaternity, or cube, certainly influenced my vision, along with the hard facts and figures with which I had been wrestling in an attempt to analyze the Nilotic Meridian. For once, I did not try to separate symbolism from science, but allowed both levels of meaning to work simultaneously. Then, looking down at the earth in its perfect cube, I saw something I had never noticed before in all the ancient symbolic texts I had studied. I saw a cross within this perfect square around the earth's globe, and the cross was targeted on Africa. One arm of the cross was the north–south Nilotic Meridian, and the other arm was the east–west equator, the epicenter being the very source of the Nile (Lake Victoria) at 0°.

If, as the ancients inform us, this line was identified with First Time on Earth, I now saw how perfectly its positioning was symbolized by a cross, within a sphere, within an imaginary cube. What was taking shape before my very eyes was a Great Master Plan: a star map on Earth unfolding in sublime order and harmony, born out of chaos. From my aerial perspective, the earth itself truly resembled a Golden Cube of perfect sacred symmetry and divine intention, and at the centerpiece, under the overarching wealth of showering stars in the Milky Way, was the golden river running beneath the African continent.

On the question of Zep Tepi, John Anthony West is of the opinion that this notion of First Time refers to a symbolic and cosmological idea, rather than a strictly historical moment in time, "a reference to the inception of time itself, when the absolute first manifested as matter." But he also made it clear to me that "a parallel historical interpretation should not be ruled out either, since myth is capable of expressing many parallel meanings simultaneously." In other words, he combines a symbolic and historically factual interpretation of First Time in one simultaneous notion.

Mutwa had told me that "the First People believe that it was during an equinox that the earth was created, when the Mother Spirit and Father Spirit came together in unity and equality. That was also the time when God the Mother and God the Father created human beings."

In celebration of the moment of First Time, Mutwa had described the marvelous ritual performed by the Bushmen involving the placement of ostrich eggs at the four cardinal points around a shaman dressed as a lion. At this moment of the equinox, the ostrich eggs are able to balance on their sharp points, a seemingly magical feat that Mutwa himself illustrated for me.

Just as I had seen the commonalities between the beliefs of Mutwa's Great Knowledge and the wisdom of the Horus sages, it now seemed to me that this leonine ritual of the First People (celebrating the earth's four cardinal points held in balance) had direct bearing on the ancients' depiction of First Time on this precise time line. If, as today's archeoastronomers tell us, the Great Sphinx, the pyramids, and the Nile itself are part of a sky map on earth mirroring Zep Tepi, it is important that we understand what they are telling us about this moment of First Time. In simple, clear, symbolic terms, the Sphinx indicates the leonine quality of First Time, while the four corners of the pyramids point to the earth's cardinal directions in First Time, and the Nile itself delineates the meridian of First Time.

Earth's Sacred Geometry

What I believed I had identified was a perfect mirror image of the sacred lands of the north – in the Southern Hemisphere. In the cold light of day, however, this notion seemed highly implausible.

The sacred geometry of the monuments of Giza has long since been established. But at first glance, the Southern Hemisphere boasted nothing by way of comparison. So, I returned to the libraries.

If the northernmost border of Timbavati corresponded with the southernmost border of Sokar, the first question that needed to be answered was where exactly the Nile Delta's mirror image fell in the Southern Hemisphere. If I folded a map of Africa in half, and used the equator as the "folding point," I could discern the Delta's Southern Hemisphere geographical equivalent by noting what part of South Africa matched up where the Nile emptied into the Mediterranean. But would the geographical equivalent come close to matching the Nile's spiritual equivalent?

I discovered that the corresponding landmark was a location just southeast of the coastal city of Durban, South Africa, at a point several kilometers into the Indian Ocean. This seemed an unexciting correspondence, to say the least. At 30° North, this precise spot is commemorated by the world's most impressive monuments, while 30° South, the nearest corresponding landmark is the densely populated city of Durban and Zululand's polluted beaches.

Given the sacred geometrical patterns that had emerged in respect of mirror images, I wondered if the sacred underground river, Lulungwa Mangakatsi, believed to run the full length of the continent, might flow into the ocean at this location? This region, once the heart of the Zulu nation, did in fact show many outlets and river mouths near Durban, but no obvious landmark suggested sacredness.

Then I recalled that Mutwa himself had been born precisely here. In fact, there was a group of surviving Bushmen in the region who carried his name: Muthwa. Mutwa had told me of the close association that existed between Bushman shamans and proto-Zulu chiefs in ancient days. He had also spoken about the Valley of a Thousand Hills as a site that housed astrological and astronomical knowledge of the ancients, evident in a system of "standing stones" in Babanango, about 250 kilometers (about 155 miles) north of Durban – known as "the stones of the female" (Nantshe eNsikazi) and the Mcemcemce, the ringing stone high up in the mountains of Zululand, where Mutwa's shaman grandfather had announced the constellations moving into a position of great significance.

These gave some tantalizing suggestions of sacredness, but they could hardly be compared with the Giza monuments and the Nile Delta. If there was truly an ancient delta offshore from Durban, one would have expected an equally impressive demarcation of the territory.

While the idea of some sort of north-to-south mirror image remained too neatly symmetrical for common sense, the vision I had seen of a Great Plan, mapped out in its entirety, kept glimmering in the recesses of my consciousness, resisting all attempts to erase it.

Instead of imposing a preconceived notion of sacred monuments on the Southern Hemisphere, I now attempted to allow the picture to speak for itself. If humankind were seeking evidence of First Time, it struck me that the aforementioned discovery of a colony of coelacanths off the Zululand coast could hardly provide a better symbol. As mysterious examples of the earth's early life-forms, coelacanths are living symbols of time effectively standing still. Believed to have died out in the end-Cretaceous extinction of the dinosaurs some 60 million years ago, these living-fossil fish appear to have survived in a perfectly preserved time warp in the deep sea off Durban. Might the mystery of their sudden reappearance in our day be traced to the outlet of an undiscovered subterranean river in perfect counterpoint to the Nile Delta?

From the mysterious workings of nature itself, it seemed I had been given another clue that I was on the right track. With the coelacanth discovery in mind I returned to the central thread of the mystery I was unraveling. If the Nilotic Meridian was a time line, and if the mysterious river flowing beneath its surface was identifiable with First Time and the "inception of time itself, when the absolute first manifested as matter," what relevance might this have for humankind living today?

It appeared that Zep Tepi was a notion of genesis not only in respect of the advent of time, but to First Matter as well as the appearance of First Man.

Looking down at the form and shape of Africa from above brought to mind a clear memory of Mutwa. I recalled the lion shaman sitting, framed by one of his monumental paintings, unrolling a map of Africa on the table before him. Illustrating his notion of Africa's great underground river, Mutwa had used forefinger and thumb to draw a band down the continent of Africa, with the Nilotic Meridian as its central thread. From my new perspective, I now saw how this band encompassed the Rift Valley stretching out to the east and the Sterkfontein site a little to the west of the meridian defined by the sacred sites. I now realized that this, too, was critically important.

The geodetic alignment of the sacred sites and the notion of the subterranean current implied a relationship with the African continent's most definitive natural landmark: the East African Rift Valley.

Birth Canal of Our Species

Given that the prime meridian on our globe was considered by the ancients to define a place and time on earth when our species was birthed, I saw an immediate association with the great East African Rift Valley, that geographical faultline now understood by modern scientists as "birth canal of the human species."[18]

Africa's geological seam furrows through the earth's crust for some 6,000 kilometers (about 3,728 miles). It is believed to have been formed when two tectonic plates (the African plate to the west and the Somali plate to the east) shifted apart. Its most dramatic section stretches east of the Nilotic Meridian, like a continental corridor from Lebanon to Mozambique (just north of Timbavati). The other fork of the Rift carves through the continent a little to the west of the Nilotic Meridian.

This tectonic margin in the African continent records key archeological evidence relating to man's evolution. The weight and number of these discoveries has led to consensus among the scientific community that Africa was man's birthplace.[19]

Since the Nile runs from the equator due north through most of the African continent, it is contained entirely within the Northern Hemisphere. This is clearly visible on any map of Africa. I recalled, however, how Mutwa's gesture of running his thumb and forefinger in a panel down the map of Africa did not stop at the equator but spanned the whole continent – suggesting the notion of a north–south continental energy belt. I now visualized the same current flowing due south from the equator, down through the continent of Africa, beneath Timbavati and beyond. Only, unlike the Nile in the Northern Hemisphere, this current in the Southern Hemisphere was invisible.[20]

Visualizing Africa in this way, from above, I found questions formulating and reformulating in my mind. The legendary underground river, which Mutwa says "holds the continent of Africa together," is associated with water energy, with a subterranean vein of gold, as well as with a mystifying notion of a shower of stars beneath the earth's crust approximating the "spinal fluid" of the Milky Way in the heavens. Was the Nile redirected into an earth-star alignment with the Milky Way so as to cover an even greater subterranean current, a current so great it was likened to the Duat in the heavens, a sacred river of stars? Could this current be identified with the seismic energies of the continental rift in the geology of Africa? Leading from this, could volcanic activity itself prompt advances in human evolution?

In one of his cosmological tales told one afternoon, Mutwa had described the genesis moment in more detail. Indicating that the creation process was really a re-creation, he had told how "there were stars above and stars in the primordial river. The morning star

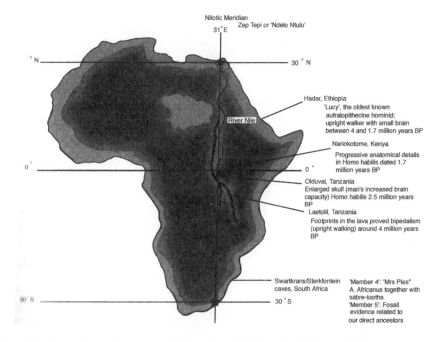

Some of the key evolutionary discoveries establishing Africa's Rift Valley as the "birth canal" of the human species.

signals that creation must begin again. God the Father and God the Mother have to be awakened again."

When he conveyed this genesis myth to me, that is precisely how I understood it – as a myth. I reasoned that the morning star symbolized the sun, and since all life on earth depended on the sun, the dawning sun signaled the creative process. However, the thought of star energy somehow existing beneath the earth's crust sounded like a fairy tale. Now, for the first time, I became aware of profound symbolic implications to these words, and their possible basis in reality. My new aerial perspective had entirely changed my way of looking at things.

Although I did not know the answers yet, from this heightened perspective, the questions at least were becoming clear. Why should our primary hominid fossils have been discovered along this continental power line known as the East African Rift Valley? What is the correlation between the Rift Valley, which scientists view as the birth canal of our species, and the Nilotic Meridian, which the ancients identified with the birthplace of the gods? The answer has to be human evolution.

21

GOLD: SUBTERRANEAN SUN

The lion corresponds principally to gold or the "subterranean sun," and to the sun itself,
and hence it is found as a symbol of sun gods.
– JUAN EDUARDO CIRLOT, *DICTIONARY OF SYMBOLS*

While I missed his company desperately, in Mutwa's absence I continued to make significant connections, not only between the Great African Tradition and the Egyptian mysteries, but connections in an ever-widening web of lion-related discoveries. Sharing some of these with Maria after my return to Timbavati, I was interrogated as to whether I believed this inspired education "came from my mother and father, or from God."

This gave me cause for contemplation. Considering how far my journey into shamanism had removed me from my everyday family inheritance, I admitted to her that this inspiration was certainly not from my father or mother.

In truth, the only way I could describe the knowledge I was receiving was a sense of being "guided" toward the right information. The experience was quite unlike my many years of academic study. I knew for certain that the usual pieces of insight I was being handed were not the product of my own academic endeavors, but rather "gifts" of a guiding will over and above my personal intent. Were the angelic presences of the lion ancestors guiding me? It might sound dramatic to describe receiving information in this spiritual light, but I don't have a better explanation for the synchronistic connections that seemingly began to drop out of the heavens.

Maria appeared to work consciously with her lion spirit ancestors on a daily basis, and at night she received clear messages from them in her dreams. After I inquired more about my own lion guardian, Ingwavuma, Maria disclosed a secret spirit name, which meant "the one who knows and understands all: the Guardian of Knowledge." Receiving her instruction from her own ancestral guides, she informed me that this Timbavati lion "has been incarnating from father to son, father to son, waiting for your return." Moved by this otherworldly explanation, I inquired how Ingwavuma knew who I was. Maria then informed me through her guides that "all the animals in Timbavati know of your return." After I tried to establish what was meant by the word *return*, the ancestral guides offered this answer: "Does it surprise you that you have lived in this land many times before?"

With these words resounding in my head, I lingered in Timbavati, feeling overwhelmingly proud to be alive in one of the last surviving territories under the domain of the king of the beasts. For the first time in this great White Lion mystery, my small part in the grand scheme of things was beginning to fit into place.

While the mystery of the White Lions and their symbolic and geographic link to the Sphinx was partly uncovered, I knew that the riddle went deeper still. The common factor between the ancients' notion of the Nilotic Meridian and our modern understanding of the East African Rift Valley was the story of human evolution. The key difference was that the one took account of the notion of leonine star gods, and the other did not.[1]

Given their perfect alignment with the Nilotic Meridian, I could see that the appearance of White Lions was part of the great star map on Earth. The message encoded in the lion–human Sphinx and the Giza pyramids was directly related to the message carried by the true enlightenment-bearers in the south, the White Lions of Timbavati. The difficulty was how to decode that message.

The Lion and the Sun

On this trip to Timbavati, it seemed I was given a key to unlocking the code. Surprisingly, it became clear that this key had been there all along – I had simply been unable to recognize it before. The key was the lion–sun connection.

On the first night back in Timbavati, I was seated in a circle around the coals, together with Leonard and a group of newly arrived guests from Europe, savoring the harmonious atmosphere of untamed nature. The glowing reeds of the *boma* enclosed the night sky in a ring of fire; the same sky that had once looked down from its river of stars on the snow-White Lions of Timbavati: heavenly presences that still stalked the folklore of this region and, God willing, would grace these lands in physical form once more.

Around the fire we chatted and laughed, while not too far from camp a lion had started up his territorial roars. From the distinctive baritone, Leonard identified my special lion guardian, Ingwavuma, and estimated his position to be a few kilometers to the east, along the Sharalumi riverbed. Ingwavuma had long since become the territory's dominant male, Timbavati's lion king.

Hearing Ingwavuma sounding off in the distance evoked the vivid memory of that fateful night when I was stranded with the group of quivering *Homo sapiens* at the mercy of the Timbavati lions. Then the lions had been mere meters away, whereas now Ingwavuma was a safe distance; yet I could feel the vibration in the soles of my feet. Anyone who has heard the roar of a flesh-and-blood lion will not easily forget it. The sensation is nothing like the lazy wide-openmouthed cinematic growl of the MGM lion. It is unlike anything else. A real lion does not throw his head back and roar to the wind, as in cartoons. He stays level-headed and uses the earth itself as his sounding board. From deep in his bowels, his roar emerges as a full-throated earth-shuddering rumble that shakes one's very soul.

With Ingwavuma rumbling on the horizon, it no longer surprised me that primitive man should have likened the lion not only to the sun, but also to the "subterranean sun," the fiery eruptions boiling at the center of the earth.

The notion of the sun as both a heavenly body and subterranean body (i.e., the earth's molten core) is in accordance with the Duat in ancient Egyptian mythology, visualized as both a celestial and subterranean "river" of stars. And I now believed that this all-important notion had three parallel levels of meaning for the sacred line binding Giza to Timbavati. In the heavens, the Duat is the overarching shower of stars or Milky Way; on earth it is the Nilotic Meridian; and beneath the earth it is the "subterranean river."

As above, so below. The sacred geometry of this notion implies possible interaction between stellar influences and geological factors. As with the other sacred patterns revealing themselves on the face of the African continent, this stellar–earth connection had to be of critical importance.

In fact, today's scientific theory has now linked the earth's molten core to the sun. Modern astrophysics not only identifies a causal linking effect between the sun and the molten core of the earth, but consequently relates seismic activity on earth to the activity of the sun itself.[2] Although astrophysical theory is argued in scientific language, it should not be difficult to see the parallels with shamanic wisdom, which draws the same connection in symbolic language. In his cosmological tales, Mutwa talked about "stars above and stars in the primordial river. The morning star signals that creation must begin again."

Here on the earth's prime time line, with my living sun god sounding forth his primal message, the implications of what I was considering literally shook the earth beneath my feet. The vibration issuing forth from Ingwavuma felt elemental, the decree of the lion king, delivering a divine rule to an earthly kingdom, laying down the law of the sun.

Hidden Gold: Subterranean Sun

One by one, the guests said good night and departed for bed. Ingwavuma had been silent for a while as I mulled over an endless stream of questions, staring up beyond the circle of firelight into the African night. If I watched long enough, I knew I would be rewarded by the flash of a shooting star.

In Timbavati, under the shower of stars, I began to see into the shimmering truth of the White Lion message – as if a smog had lifted to reveal the night sky.

When Ingwavuma resumed his earth rumbles, his roar reverberated upon this sacred meridian. Positioned on the 31° longitude, it issued forth on all four horizons – north, south, east, and west – as if holding the corners of the earth in balance.

Anticipating my lion's next roar, I walked out into the dense Timbavati night and listened. In the darkness, I envisioned him opening his jaw very slightly, and contracting his belly to issue a tremor that resounded over Timbavati's wilderness. His ancestral name meant "he who speaks wise words," and every time he roared, I imagined the wisdom he was sounding forth.

His location had shifted in the intervening period, which meant he was on the move. I could picture him padding proudly through his territory, a living lion and a sacred symbol at one and the same time: king of the beasts, judicious guardian of the land. If, as my sources had informed me, Ingwavuma and his cubs were destined to be the progenitors of Timbavati's future White Lions, then he was at once a symbolic enlightenment-bearer and a flesh-and-blood carrier of the hallowed white gene.

Ingwavuma was also the symbol of gold – the "lion of metals" – along with his fellow lions. Which prompted old questions. Why should lions inextricably be connected with gold? Why should they be connected with the sun itself? On this trip to Timbavati, for the first time I would glimpse the answer.

After my lion's next roar, I hesitated a moment. I assumed the others were fast asleep by now. Even if they weren't, I no longer cared if they heard me. Gathering my courage, on the top of my feeble human voice, I called out the Zulu prayer in honor of the lion, which Mutwa had taught me:

> Lion, symbol of the kings of the Zulus!
> Lion, thunder of the valleys!
> Where your roar is to be heard, there life is found.
> Where your breath is to be smelled, there is no evil.
> And where you are seen, there is no fear!
> Lion, may your footprint never be erased by the passing winds,
> and long may you walk on the plains of this earth.
> To life! *Bayete!*

There was silence. Then Ingwavuma roared again. I heard his message loud and clear this time, and all of a sudden I understood it – in pure, unadulterated solar vibration. I understood the "Word of the Lion"!

The difficulty was how to *translate* it. But even if it took many volumes, reams and reams of written human words inscribed fastidiously, one after the other, even if it was a feeble, inadequate, all-too-human copy of the truth, I made a solemn promise then and there that I was going to do my utmost to make that translation.

The "Word of the Lion" is the solar Logos, the very same vibration as the sun itself, the very essence which first created life on this planet. The sun and the lion are directly linked because they are part of the same sun-god life-force. The lion's association with gold is profound. The sun at the center of our solar system is directly linked with the golden core at the center of the earth. Out of this soul essence, life itself was born.

The White Lions and the Origins of Life

It has long been established that tectonic faultlines are linked with earthquakes and volcanic eruptions. In the case of the Rift Valley, as the earth's crust was wrought apart, so lava was forced to the surface, with the result that numerous volcanoes became a defining geological feature. Given that virtually all our great hominid sites have been found near, or in, this erupting continental seam, the question arises: might the rifting process itself, or rather the seismic energies operative in this faultline, be considered factors prompting genetic mutations – the adaptations that also led to the modern human line?[3]

Today's earth sciences have established a connection between volcanoes and mineral wealth.[4] Is it possible that gold might be connected to the origins of life on Earth?

According to Mutwa, gold is a substance of inestimable value on our planet. He instructed me that gold is not only a metal, but an "entity." He relates gold to a mysterious "X-factor" that controls both the existence and flow of water, and thus of life, on our planet.

As if struck by lightning, I suddenly felt the full magnitude and gravity of the White Lion mystery. Was the myth of the Golden Age a reality? Was gold itself a factor in the moment of creation on Earth?

Barberton, a gold-mining town positioned precisely on the Nilotic Meridian, is important for two reasons. First, it is the prime site where Europeans first discovered gold in South Africa. Second, it is the place where geologists believe life on the planet may have begun.

The antiquity and nature of Barberton's geology has led geoscientists to identify the region as the possible origin of the first organisms on earth to use energy from sunlight to grow. The geology reveals that volcanic activity gave rise to hot springs, the original "primordial slime," which then gave birth to the earth's first life-forms.

Barberton's primordial gold fields would seem to bear witness to the truth of Mutwa's words. "Fly-speck" carbon aggregates have been detected in some of the earliest gold conglomerates, indicating the presence of the earliest advanced life-forms.[5] If this is truly the case, then gold's natural existence in the bowels of our planet is essential to life on earth – clear indication of its metaphysical significance over and above its mercantile value.

Not only First Man, but First Life itself appears to have emerged out of Africa's great birth canal.

Earth's Golden Center

Mutwa had alluded in a guarded fashion to secret practices in the metal-smelting tradition of the Sacred Blacksmiths.

"What we call magic today," he had instructed me, "was the science of the ancient people." From Mutwa's cryptic allusions, I understood that the knowledge of these high priests of African shamanism, "which had to do with herbs and molten matter," drew on the arcane art of combining earth matter with stellar energies. This, Mutwa had told me, enabled the lion shaman élite to "recreate objects which God gave us many centuries ago," relating to "the soul of the earth but also the universe beyond." The belief is that gold not only has a physical dimension but also a *meta*physical dimension, and indeed also an *astro*physical dimension. Significantly, science has now established that the formation of gold is directly related to the birth of the sun itself. In other words, the sun–gold connection in ancient mythology and ancient alchemy is borne-out in current scientific evidence.[6]

Although many of Mutwa's notions had once mystified me, as I stood here now it seemed that I was beginning to catch a glimmer of their truth. In ancient alchemical theory, as in many symbolic texts, gold is the image of solar light and, hence, of divine intelligence, both physical and metaphysical.[7] The sun is also directly identified with the transmutation of prime matter ("earth") into gold.[8]

In alchemy, the lion is often depicted "roaring" the sun, suggesting that the lion's roar issues forth the solar Logos, the Word of the sun. This alchemical image implies that the magma at the earth's core, and the lion's roar itself, are linked by a "common rhythm."[9]

White Lion Message

While I knew these questions would provide a challenge to orthodox Christians and orthodox scientists alike, I no longer feared the consequences. Why should the birthplace of the White Lions in Timbavati align exactly with Africa's most sacred sites, Great Zimbabwe and Giza? Why should the birthplace of the gods in ancient Egyptian times align with the birthplace of the White Lions in our times? Why should that sacred site of Great Zimbabwe – ancient center of gold – be rumored to have once been guarded by White Lions, along with other sites on the Nilotic Meridian? Why should the world's prime meridian, defined by Africa's sacred sites and the Nile itself, run through the continent's gold-mining sites, right down to the mining town of Barberton in the south, where First Gold and First Life were discovered?

The answer has to be that there is inherent meaning and sacred symbolism within the very workings of nature itself. Similarly, there is inherent intention and meaning behind the White Lions' immaculate "choice" of birthplace. These are not chance factors. As the shamans had never tired of telling me: White Lions are Lions of God.

If the White Lions are heavenly messengers bringing the laws of the sun to earth, it is imperative that we understand what message they herald. Their message is related to gold, and it is related to the sun. Our challenge is to understand how and why.

There had been many evenings, as I watched the sun sink into darkness, when I had thought over the lion's symbolic identification with the sun, and how this universal archetype seemed to point to deeper realities, to a truth underlying the myth. Tonight, as the last golden rim of the sun sank below the horizon, and Ingwavuma started his nocturnal rumblings, I went out once more into the twilight to listen. As the father of the future White Lions, Ingwavuma conveyed their message to me in pure lion language. I now believed that I could hear it, clear and true. I could hear it, not as one hears the spoken word, but at a new level of consciousness. A level that told me that I had walked these lands of Timbavati many times before. A level that told me that I was not the possessor of a new consciousness but a very old one, that had been dormant for centuries and was only now beginning to reawaken. A level of consciousness at which the lioness in me and the woman became one. This is my attempt to translate what I heard in Ingwavuma's roar:

It is foolish to demand of God that He prove himself according to the scientific confines which modern man has created for himself. It is foolish to demand the same of the Lions of God. The White Lions will not play the game. Don't demand. Listen. It is then that you might hear the most ancient wisdom which could save your life. And save the world.

22

TENDILE, WHITE LION MOTHER

For the people of Africa, the skies are full of life; yes, even the origin of life may be attributed to the stars! . . . For the African mind, the living animals of the Serengeti plains are reflections of their heavenly cousins. The herds of Eternity are really in the stars; there also is to be found the origin and destiny of humanity.

– CREDO MUTWA

The threat to our earth's ecology is closely linked to its devaluation from a mythical Golden Age. In classical times, the sage-scholar Hesiod described the decline of humankind in terms of four ages: the Ages of Gold, Silver, Bronze, and Iron. Arranged in the reverse order of value, the debasement of metals (from the incorruptible to the corroded, tarnished, and rusty) represented the decline of humanity from Godlike status to base material.[1]

This devaluing process led me to reflect on the White Lions, and how they were ultimately symbols of the highest value: gold. I no longer believed the lion–gold connection to be simply a myth. Behind the myth lies a greater reality, that somehow takes us back to the origins of life on this planet. If lions in mythology are synonymous with gold (the most precious metal), it struck me that the White Lions must equate with gold in its highest essence – its purest, most incorruptible and precious form. The metallic equivalent of the White Lions is pure gold – not the alloy manufactured in our laboratories known as "white gold", but the unique silvery substance created by our earth itself, sometimes referred to as "mononucleonic" gold. Gold in its purest form is a metal associated with the moment of the earth's creation, just as the White Lions are associated with the beginning of time on our planet.[2]

These connections reminded me of veiled allusions of Mutwa's to "gold which is white in color by nature not manufacture" and to the "plants which have concentrated gold within them for millions upon millions of years." Although modern scientists are still gathering related evidence, I believe that in due course they will also come to associate pure gold with the earth's first life-forms.

I also remembered veiled allusions of Mutwa's to the highest goal of the ancient alchemists. As the lion shaman put it: "The Sacred Blacksmiths were not trying to create run-of-the-mill gold – but the gold of immortality." In alchemical terms, this is the pure essence – the highest form of spiritual enlightenment.[3] The goal was not to prolong life on earth; the true elixir, the true gold of immortality, had to do with the eternal life of the soul.

In respect of the possible catastrophic destiny of our planet, Credo Mutwa is considerably more forbidding than the leading scientists of our day. According to his knowledge, derived, as ever, from ancient shamanism rather than modern science, the White Lions are the primary symbol heralding the coming earth changes. I later confirmed with two other *sangomas* – Claude Makhubela and Selby Gumbi – the importance of the White Lions as primary sacred symbols. Gumbi, a Zulu indigenous priest and healer, described to me the White Lions as "the firstborn of creation"; they form "the enlightened priesthood through which we can communicate directly with God" and are part of the "hierarchy of pure light and love . . . next to the throne of God," a symbol of "humankind's soul being."

Mutwa's shamanic warnings square with today's reality. Since the White Lions are the supreme kings of the beasts and guardians of the land, protecting them is the ultimate real-life symbol of preserving our earth. Inversely, their senseless destruction is a primary symptom of how modern humanity is devastating our earth.

Intermittently over this period, I attempted to re-establish contact with Mutwa, hoping he might join Maria and me in Timbavati. I was unable to reach him, and received increasingly bleak secondhand reports on his circumstances. In September 1999, I got through to an attendant, only to be told that Mutwa was out of South Africa, delivering a series of lectures in the United States in the hope of raising money for his wife's medical care. Poignantly, Cecilia, Mutwa's wife of 40 years, died while he was out of the country. Devastated, Mutwa returned and went into retreat and mourning.

Meanwhile, in Timbavati I was informed of an important new development. My ranger friend, Leonard, one of the few people who was aware of the White Lion work I was doing, informed me that a young South African woman had made a pilgrimage to Timbavati. She had told Leonard that Timbavati was a sacred place, that it was on a sacred line on the globe, and that it had age-old connections with Egypt. She also told him that she was a spirit medium, a "channeler," who received her information from spirit guides and stellar sources. Her name was Jackie te Braake.

Knowing I would be interested in meeting her, Leonard had asked for her address, which he now passed on to me. I discovered that she had recently moved to the town called White River, which is also located exactly on the Nilotic Meridian, south of Timbavati. I later learned that her relocation there was no coincidence, but rather a deliberate choice she had made after being told by her spirit guides of the significance of this meridian. The town's name itself – White River – hints at the mysterious connection between the Duat, or "river of stars," and the Milky Way. Just outside White River is a region called Jerusalem, echoing the name of the city addressed as "Ariel," "Lion of God" by the prophet Isaiah.[4] Above this small region in Africa looms a huge mountain called Legogotsi, which is believed to thunder and roar like a lion under certain conditions. According to Mutwa, certain mountains do, in fact, emit roaring sounds. From the town of White River, where this giant volcanic outcrop may be seen, the lion mountain resembles the Great Sphinx itself, only unsculpted by human hands. This was the setting of te Braake's home in White River.

I was sufficiently aware of esoteric activities by now to know that the term "channeling" referred to the ability to "tune in" to information that is usually outside the normal waking state. Along with other pieces of the Timbavati–Giza jigsaw that fell into place one by one, te Braake's arrival signaled more than an everyday coincidence. With a now familiar sense of rising excitement, I made an appointment to see her in October 1999. Not knowing quite what to expect, I took my sister, Serena, along for moral support.

I met te Braake without preconceptions, ready simply to hear what she might have to tell me. I gave her no clues about who I was or what I was doing. But there were many questions that I was curious to have answered. One was the mysterious name that the psychic had passed on to me after my lecture in March 1999. I put the name Count Saint-Germain to her, wondering what might emerge.

Te Braake is an attractive woman so radiantly blonde that she seems to emanate light. She told me that the name Saint-Germain referred to the "ascendant master" responsible for channeling information to do with sacred geometry and human evolutionary development. She also told me that she had been informed through her spirit guide that Saint-Germain's symbol was the winged lion. Given the material with which I had been dealing, the appropriateness of this information was intensely interesting. But that was only the beginning. After she expressed curiosity as to why I should ask this question, I explained that I had been told by an unknown party in a lecture auditorium that I was accompanied by an invisible lion, and that I should take note of this particular name.

"Ah!" she said. "That explains it. I've got a message for you."

I waited expectantly, since these were virtually the same words the psychic himself had used after my lecture.

"There is a White Lion calling to you," she said. "Calling urgently. I heard it very strongly – even before you arrived."

"So, is it that same male lion that I keep seeing in my dreams and who appeared in the flesh in Timbavati?" I asked, ready to explain – for what it was worth – that this lion was, in fact, not white but golden.

"No, it's a little female," she countered.

Again I felt the familiar emotion welling up in me. "You say it's calling to me . . . But from where – Timbavati? As far as I know, the White Lions are extinct in the wild."

"This lion has not been born yet," she said.

"You mean it's a White Lion *spirit* calling me?"

"Yes," she said, "she is waiting to be born – but she needs protection."

I felt the back of my neck tingling. Again, this was precisely the same terminology that the lion spirit, Gegege, had used in the drumming ceremony with Maria and her relatives.

"She is not going to be born in Timbavati. She is saying to me that she will be born in a sacred place of great significance to you."

"Where, I wonder?"

"I'm sorry, that's all I'm getting," te Braake concluded.

After the encounter, as Serena and I prepared to leave, I told te Braake a little about myself and about my work with Mutwa.

"You do know who Credo Mutwa is?" she asked me, after listening patiently.

"How do you mean?" I inquired, not comprehending her question.

"He is the eldest Son of Ra, in his present incarnation."[5]

I stopped dead. I knew that Ra (also known as Re) was the original Egyptian creator sun god.

After a moment's consideration, I inquired, "How did you get that information? Are you channeling now?"

"Yes," she said simply. "That is what I have been told by my spirit guide."

Bizarre and grandiose as these words sounded, they came as no surprise. In what had seemed a highly elevated claim, Maria had described Mutwa as the "son of the sun." Amazingly, the Lion Queen's assertion about Mutwa's higher identity was consistent with that of this unknown spirit medium, although the two women had never met.

Thinking of my great but humble lion-shaman friend, I found the notion was no longer impossible to reconcile. Old Africa, like ancient Egypt, embraces the notion of rebirth. When I considered the date of Mutwa's birth, the place of his birth, as well as the name that he had carried since birth, all pointed to the same truth.

The date of his birth, 21 July, is the cusp of Cancer (the crab) and Leo (the lion). I knew by now that these two animals were, in fact, Credo Mutwa's sacred totems. Ancient astrological theory tells us that Leo is ruled by the sun, while Cancer is ruled by the moon. Mutwa's date of birth, therefore, implies a reconciliation between solar (male) and lunar (female) principles, while in reality I had witnessed the inner struggle within Mutwa between the great lion shaman and the original Creator Goddess Amarava.

His very name, Credo, is the belief in God's law, "the Word," just as, in Egypt, the sun god Ra is identified with the Word or solar Logos: "I am Ra . . . I am that which created the Word . . . I am the Word."[6]

Finally, his birthplace counterpoints the birthplace of the Sons of Ra in Egypt. Like those other Children of the Sun God, Timbavati's White Lions, Mutwa was born on the Nilotic Meridian. Only, in his case, the positioning of his birthplace in the south, just outside Durban in Zululand, corresponds (both longitudinally *and* latitudinally) with the birthplace of the gods in the north: Giza. If the Son of Ra were to reincarnate in our present day, he could hardly choose a more appropriate site.

Birth of a Sun Goddess

On returning to my sister's home, I found the idea of the White Lioness calling for my protection gave rise to a keen sense of foreboding. While echoing the spirit ancestor's message and the urgency of some of Mutwa's imperatives, the notion of my being able to protect the White Lions remained so unlikely that I had no idea what I was meant to do about this task. Once more, I decided to return to Timbavati to share my worries with Maria.

Watching Maria throw the bones again, I saw the smaller of the two lion bones fall outside the rectangular borders of the grass mat. Thanks to Maria, my bones-reading technique had advanced to a point where I had no trouble interpreting this: it indicated, as Maria duly went on to explain, that the lion cub was outside the Lion Queen's territorial domain of Timbavati. Although te Braake had said as much, this came as a great surprise to me. No White Lion had been born in Timbavati since 1991, the year of my near-death encounter. Yet each season that followed increased my longing for their return. Now that I had been told of Ingwavuma's role in their continuance, I hoped in time that I would see him sire white cubs. If there was one sacred place for the White Lions to make their appearance, it had to be Timbavati. After further divination with the bones, I was surprised when Maria reported that the White Lioness was already alive: newborn and safe. She reassured me that I had no immediate need to worry; in time I would meet my special lioness.

A couple of days later, I was filled with amazement and sheer exhilaration when I was contacted unexpectedly by lion-man Gareth Patterson with the message that a white female lion cub had been born in the vicinity of Sterkfontein.

Sterkfontein! The land abutting the famous hominid caves had been bought and made into a reserve by a retired stockbroker, Ed Hern. Along with a menagerie of African and exotic felines and other animals, he had a pride of tawny lions (originally of Timbavati stock) that turned out to be carriers of the white gene. From the two gene-bearing parents, a white cub had been conceived and born. A tourist driving through the lion enclosure had spotted a lone bit of snow-white fluff moving on the opposite embankment and reported it to the game warden, imagining it to be a white hare. Abandoned by its mother and left to die, possibly because of the confines of their enclosure, the baby lioness, her eyes not yet opened, was discovered and rescued.[7]

Her birth in this place and time seemed profoundly meaningful. Immediately after receiving the news of her birth, I remember walking out into the Timbavati night and staring up into the brilliant sky above, overcome by a sense of the miraculous workings of nature. Assessing the direct association that spirit mediums had established between me and this special White Lioness, I felt deeply "connected" – that's the best word I can find. I felt the connection between the spirit world and the physical world; between humans and the animal world; between nature and the civilized world; between the past and the present worlds. Ultimately, in the magic of this human–feline moment, I began to feel a connection between the stars and our earthly world.

After Maria had conveyed the message from the lion ancestors that my title was "Keeper of the White Lions," I had come to understand that with this highest of honors, came the weight of responsibility that would change my life forever.

Ed Hern named the White Lioness Tendile. Within weeks of her birth, the cold-hearted merchants for trophy hunters were in discussion with Ed Hern about a price for her. To my profound relief, Hern remained unswayed, although, I suspect, the temptations of financial gain must have been substantial.

Tendile was my first direct physical contact with a White Lion. A bundle of white fleece, she was a lioness in lamb's clothing. According to Hern, the name meant "something special" and I could not have agreed more. She was special beyond anything I had ever encountered in my life before. On the question of how I might protect her, Maria instructed me that, as long as I honored the White Lioness, and never forgot her (not even for one single day), she would be "protected." And consequently she would grow proud and immensely strong. Maria recited a prayer for Tendile, and sent offerings for the White Lioness – crystals from the Timbavati riverbeds and grains of sand scooped up from beneath the pawprints of Timbavati lions – that I duly presented to the little cub on meeting her. Hern was hand-rearing her in his home, with the intention of later moving her into an enclosed area where she could be viewed by tourists. He was a warm and personable individual, who allowed me access to the White Lioness whenever I requested it.

Amazingly for a lion, Tendile had the gentlest of natures. Yet, on first meeting me, while she was still a little cub, she showed uncharacteristic anger. After I asked Maria why this should be, she told me the sacred lioness was irritated that I had taken so long to "wake up" to who I really was. She also told me that a mother–daughter bond existed between this lioness and me, and compelled me to look after Tendile as if she were my own child, for once I had been *her* "cub."

I had long since stopped rationalizing Maria's words. At a deeper level than the everyday, they made absolute sense. I could understand why the little lioness was angry. Looking back, it seemed as if I had been living my entire life in a dream state, and only now had I begun to wake up to the truth.

At six weeks, Tendile was about the size of a domestic cat, but much more weighty of build – an irrepressible powerhouse of energy. Romping with this small lion creature was an indescribably electrifying experience – as if I were playing with fire and lightning. In return for all her fiery warmth, I was overcome by an overwhelming tenderness and affection. It was so tempting to cuddle and baby her, yet I could never forget where the true power lay. She would use her mesmerizing blue eyes to freeze me to the spot – then pounce. By the age of four months, she had the power to knock me over and club me playfully with furry paws, while – amazingly – never allowing her sharp claws to emerge.

Together with Hern, I followed Tendile's progress very closely, and was delighted to watch how she grew into a sublime specimen of White Lionhood. She had a tawny lion as a playmate, but she soon outgrew this male companion and started bullying him mercilessly because of her advantage of superior strength and size. Commenting on what a fine specimen she was, Hern told me that he had acquired the tawny male from a zoo, so he assumed that a degree of inbreeding had taken place there. By contrast, the sacred white gene in Tendile was radiantly undamaged.

Tendile was living proof that the suppositions of many geneticists are incorrect: the White Lions are by no means a weaker species. On the contrary, I believe that they represent a genetic upgrade on the tawny species. I believe that, in due course, this will be identified by geneticists.

Unlike albinos, White Lions show no indication of abnormality or weakness. Whereas albinos suffer from a genetic malfunction, namely that the pigment is entirely missing from their eyes, the eyes of the White Lions are not watery and pink; they are the same pulverizing gold that characterizes the razor-sharp stare of Africa's tawny lions. Sometimes, as in the case of little Tendile, they are the deepest, gentlest aquamarine. In terms of bearing and physical make-up, the White Lions are always reported to be the finest of specimens.

In his study, Chris McBride recorded how the young white cubs proved more tenacious and courageous than their siblings, darting in to steal meat from the kill and scampering off before they could be punished by the dominant males. Their primary challenge remained their lack of camouflage. In the tawny bushveld, a snowy-white cub is constantly at risk. I thought of Tendile, a little ball of white fluff in the midst of the burned grasslands, vulnerable as a lamb. In Timbavati, she could have been picked out by birds of prey or loitering hyenas.

Studies have shown there is 80 percent mortality rate of lion cubs to adulthood in the wild. It isn't natural predators, but humans who pose the greatest threat to the White Lions' survival in the wild. I spent several months interviewing eye-witnesses, who confirmed that despite their unique coloring, the White Lions were very capable hunters in the wild, well adapted to their natural environment and on occasions even making kills for their tawny prides. After many removals from the wild, however, their survival was increasingly threatened.

If the White Lions are identified with the star gods at First Time, what does their reappearance mean for *our* age? In terms of the White Lion message, I recalled the words of Mutwa's moving speech at the zoo on our last day spent together: "These animals are said to herald coming changes on this earth."

What coming changes on earth might the White Lions herald? What is meant by the sun's ominous "disappearance"? While my own opinion of Mutwa had long since moved from skepticism to admiration, te Braake's allusion to his hidden identity as the Son of Ra placed an entirely new weight and authority upon his humble shoulders. It gave the lion shaman's words the highest prophetic dimension.

Mutwa points out that lions "show every evidence of being snow animals originally", citing the thick mane and paw formations as features appropriate for glacial conditions.

I now began to wonder whether these might be the approaching earth changes of which the White Lions are here to forewarn us. Are we in danger of moving headlong into the next Ice Age?

The obvious fact is that a tawny landscape is not an appropriate environment for a snow-White Lion. Only under freak conditions would mutations such as the White Lions be favored with an ecological niche where they could survive and reproduce. If we ask what ecological circumstances would be favorable, the answer can only be: Ice Age conditions.

For some time now, scientists have been warning us of the possible catastrophic onset of the next Ice Age. The Cambridge astrophysicist John Gribbin, for instance, points out that Northern Hemisphere summer sunshine, the key indicator of approaching glaciation, "has declined steadily since 11,000 years ago to the point where, other things being equal, there is a real risk of a sudden spread of snow and ice cover, a 'snow blitz' heralding the start of the next Ice Age."[8]

Despite substantial scientific support for an impending Ice Age, the idea that a unique white gene might make an appearance *in anticipation of a radical climatic change* has, to my knowledge, no scientific basis as yet. But in respect of Mutwa's view of the White Lions as prophetic messengers, this makes absolute sense.

As Chris McBride wrote soon after experiencing what he believed to be the "discovery" of the White Lions: "As far as lions are concerned . . . I can see no set of circumstances that would ever make it advantageous for them to be white, so I really don't see this white strain developing unless man steps in and does a certain amount of stage managing."[9]

McBride talks about "stage managing" with the best possible intentions, meaning that we clever humans should "direct operations" and "step in" to guide in the natural processes when it comes to protecting the unique white genes. I believe, however, that he has seriously missed the point. The White Lions don't require any "stage managing" of natural forces to survive. They *are* natural force personified. Lion shamanism helped me understand that the spirit should not be separated from the physical form. The White Lions are *spirit made flesh*, radiant light-beings in White Lion form. They will survive the forces of nature, for they embody the law of nature, the law of the sun, the solar Logos. It is humankind, rather, that has become unnatural, dissociating itself from natural forces to such a degree that its own survival is threatened.

Blueprints for White Lions

Symbolically (if not yet scientifically), the White Lions are identifiable with pure gold and with the first life-forms on earth. Applying genetic theory to the ancient Hermetic teachings left me in no doubt that the White Lions could be identified with the Abangafi Bapakade, the shining lion gods known as the *akeru* by Egyptians, the star beasts who walked among humans in the Golden Age following First Time. The golden question is:

why have these *akeru* returned to Earth in our time? If, as Mutwa indicated, they herald earth changes (very possibly of a catastrophic glacial nature), then it would appear these symbols of First Time may have returned to forewarn us of End Time.

Despite the present-day environmental conditions being stacked against them, the truth is that these genetic rarities have proved they are able to survive in their natural (and spiritual) homeland of Timbavati. It appalled me, therefore, to learn that it was humans themselves who were attempting to wipe the sacred White Lions off the map.

23

TROPHY HUNTING

What kind of man would breed her kind
For the gun?
What kind of man would separate a mother
From her young?
And what kind of man would shoot her dead
In front of those young eyes?
She died, dying to be free.
– GARETH PATTERSON'S IMPASSIONED PLEA,
WRITTEN AFTER VIEWING A "CANNED" LION HUNT
IN WHICH A LACTATING LIONESS WAS SHOT AS A TROPHY
IN AN ENCLOSURE IN FRONT OF HER CUBS

In the light of messages that had been directed to me through shamans and ancestral spirit guides about my role as a guardian of the White Lions, I could no longer stand by as an academic or detached outsider and watch while Africa's most precious living resource came under threat by humanity

Essentially, two views exist on the White Lions today. Both of these are, in their own way, seriously misguided. The first sees the White Lions as misfits, unusual animals that have arrived at the wrong place at the wrong time. As such, no particular consequence is attached to their survival, since White Lions in a tawny environment have no "conservation value." The endpoint of this view would be to argue that if the uncamouflaged White Lions cannot fend for themselves under present circumstances they should be left to die out.

By contrast, the second view sees that the White Lions are worth preserving – but as phenomenally precious money spinners. In wildlife circles, one commonly hears the motto "If it pays, it stays." The rationale is that its existence is justified in material gain. It is only viable if it pays its way. Only if nature is financially self-supporting will it be maintained by humanity; alternatively, the land and all it sustains will be taken over by humankind's immediate needs.

Given the White Lions' rarity, it is not surprising that they equate with high revenue. By the same token, it is not altogether surprising that White Lions attract, as custodians, people of power and material influence, money men such as Las Vegas showmen or retired stockbrokers. Significantly, the world's premier evolutionary site in the Sterkfontein Valley, where Tendile was born, abuts the old gold-mining town of Krugersdorp. A large percentage of land in the region is owned jointly by the corporate giants First National Bank of South Africa and Anglo American, based in London. AngloGold, the premier mining house that uses a lion as its corporate logo, opened its listing on the New York Stock Exchange in 1998 by parading a live lion across the selling floor. Underlining the implicit lion–gold association, the mining house sponsored a $1.1 million new enclosure for the White Lions at the Johannesburg Zoo. Johannesburg, housing the only zoo in South Africa where White Lions have been bred successfully, is known as the "city of gold." The name of the province in which it is situated, "Gauteng," derives from the Tswana term meaning "place of gold." In Timbavati itself, those few landowners who remember sightings of the White Lions speak in terms of "hitting gold."

Such gilt-edged associations add weight to the connection between White Lions and money. But the association goes deeper than the obvious material level. In sacred texts throughout world mythology, a direct association is made between lions and gold: gold is the "lion of metals" and the lion is the "guardian of gold."

Most important, in real terms, the White Lions' manifestation on the geological vein of gold that runs the course of the African continent – that very meridian that the ancient Egyptians associated with the Golden Age – forces us to consider a profound truth underlying the lion–gold association in world mythology: while money is associated with White Lions, the White Lions are, by the same token, manifestly associated with gold sites.

White Gold

Along with every other aspect of the White Lion story, the association between the White Lion and gold sites is an illustration of nature's immaculate logic. The symbolism is so fitting, it would seem illogical to view the equation of pure-gold White Lions in any other way. Yet, unfortunately, that is precisely what we humans have done: we have turned real value upside down. Following the White Lion story in real life today reveals just how corrupted the notion of pure gold has become. Sterkfontein, for instance, a world heritage site of unparalleled evolutionary significance for humankind – and the site where White Lions are once again beginning to appear – has recently been proposed as a prime location for a high-end casino project. The same dangerous contradiction exists in Las Vegas, the sanctuary for our rare White Lions, which is not only the world's premier gambling Mecca, but also where international hunting conventions take place. The test for us is to identify the real value in these equations.

Lions are hunted in South Africa, including in Timbavati. This method of bringing in high revenue is generally disguised as "sustainable utilization," and consequently is not frowned upon, even in conservationist circles. The danger lies in the assumption that nature reserves must be profitable to justify their right to exist. The hidden questions that should be asked are: *Who* exactly profits? And what exactly *is* profit? Is profit the material benefit for a few exploitative individuals, or is it the long-term profit for humanity and our earth itself? The objectives behind conservation depend on how we define value. Is paper money real value? Or is value the survival of our earth and its true riches?

The argument that the earth is here for human utilization is, of course, an easy one for humans to defend (since it is in our immediate interests), and until fairly recently, it is one that I bought into without questioning. I went along with the idea that nature is here primarily for humankind's enjoyment and enrichment. But "sustainable utilization" – sustaining the earth so that it may be utilized by humans – holds good only if it does not rely on short-term monetary incentives at the expense of ethics and devaluing the earth. Clearly, we need to entirely re-evaluate the management of our earth's resources, and wildlife areas. For a start, we need to shift from concepts of ownership and cost to those of responsible custodianship and long-term investment, in which we humans give back as much as we take.

Lions in the Can

The most cynical and ruthless of man's mercenary hunting attitudes toward nature is that of the "canned" lion trophy industry. The term *canned* refers to the practice of breeding lions in captivity to be shot on demand. It is a practice that continues in South Africa and is legitimized despite public outcry. Gareth Patterson has exposed the systematic breeding and hunting of lions in his books and on film. He shows how organizations neighboring Timbavati are not only happy to offer lions to professional hunters to shoot for exorbitant sums, but also how these lions are housed in enclosed areas and drugged on request to make the hunter's task all the easier.[1] This takes the "if it pays, it stays" argument to its inevitable conclusion, with the individuals involved treating Africa's White Lions as nothing other than a high-income-yielding commodity. The attitude of those who breed White Lions for trophy hunters to kill is simple and brutal: the closer the White Lions remain to the verge of extinction, the higher their value on the international trophy market. Just as merchants control a commodity's price by artificially holding back distribution, so canned trophy hunting outfits handle Africa's most sacred animal.

With the scale of money involved, Mafia-like secrecy surrounds trophy-hunting operations in Timbavati and other game areas throughout South Africa. Patterson, who so courageously exposed the activities of these game hunters, lives in constant fear of his life. Others who have attempted to reintroduce the white gene back into South Africa (by importing white-gene-bearing lions from Timbavati that had found their way into zoos overseas) have received serious death threats. Some of these lions have also been killed under mysterious circumstances. Since White Lion trophies command high rewards, competition means loss of revenue.

The fact is: the only White Lions in the vicinity of Timbavati today are being bred for shooting, in captive breeding programs. A web of hunting operations exists in a stranglehold around Timbavati's borders. The Timbavati fences are being lifted, and white-gene-bearing lions are being lured out and abducted by neighboring owners for canned hunting purposes. While hunting is legal, poaching neighbors' lions is not. Yet, for unaccountable reasons, this practice continues, despite incidents of offenders being caught red-handed.[2] South African trophy hunting draws big, "brave" hunting clients from prosperous first-world countries, including Britain, the United States, and Germany. Local canned lion farmers justify their operations by saying they are simply meeting an international demand.

In our modern day, the notion of "man, the hunter" is a myth. Today this is no more than a virtual reality, which does not exist in the real world of Africa. I have spoken to some of the rangers responsible for taking hunters by four-wheel-drive vehicle to dispatch their trophy. Some describe how, despite being armed to the teeth with heavy weapons, these supposed great hunters are so nervous, ill-prepared, and clearly out of their league that they often misfire and wound the animal. The ranger himself is often forced to do the dirty work and kill the badly wounded lion. These unromanticized descriptions led me to reflect on the nature of a man who gets pleasure out of murdering a magnificent, endangered animal – and then pays for that pleasure. What kind of inflated ego or inferiority complex results in a person deriving fun out of killing the king of beasts? The most miserable of men, making a sport of playing God.

The hunting industry is controlled by tight syndicates. To protect vested interests, unauthorized persons are not allowed access to breeding premises. Nevertheless, footage does occasionally get out, some of which reveals reprehensible conditions for the White Lions in captivity. Some lions appear to be suffering from the effects of inbreeding, including bone defects, and are filmed dragging their hind quarters; others have no tail tufts. One lion captured on film has an open wound in his forehead that resembles a bullet hole.

Most distressingly for me, White Lion cubs have also been admitted to Onderstepoort Veterinary Hospital for open-heart surgery. At a physical level, this is a clear indication of genetic damage. When one considers the symbolic level, the implications are even more grave. Newborn cubs with their hearts already failing signals something beyond simple genetic malfunction. In world mythology, the lion is man's guardian, the symbol of the heart in man. In the Bible, for instance, Daniel's dream involves the winged lion descending to earth and giving its heart to man. The lion is connected with humanity's heart in world symbolism, and lion shamans, at least, have never forgotten this. The last surviving Bushman hunter-gatherers honor humanity's heart as the Heart of the Hunter, the Heart of a Star: braveheart, trueheart, lionheart (*Tsau!*). They were truly lionhearted. We need to ask: what happened to our hearts?

24

WHITE LIONS: PROPHETS OF THE FUTURE

What is the trophy price for a sun god? What is the cost to our earth?

– LINDA TUCKER

Though sorely missing my mentor's tutelage, I found my special connection with the lions of Timbavati continued to grow. While ten years before I had had little conception of what "psychic" meant, and I had imagined it to be concerned with processes and phenomena that appeared outside physical or natural laws,[1] I now understood psychic processes to be part of natural law. Given that the word *psyche* refers to the soul, I suspect that apparently psychic or telepathic connections between different species may represent communication at a soul level – with far-reaching implications in restoring the ancient bond between humankind and lions.

An event in Timbavati at around this time reminded me of this soul bond.

Mozambican Floods

In February and March of 2000, thousands lost their lives in the devastating floods that ravaged Mozambique. Large areas of Timbavati and the Kruger Park (which borders on Mozambique) were badly damaged. Leonard's camp was fortunately unscathed, but the heavy rains fell unabated for more than two months. The earth was so sodden that even rangers in all-terrain vehicles stopped venturing out onto the roads for fear of getting trapped in the mud.

My sister, Serena, and the elder of her two daughters, Faith, had decided to pay me a visit in Timbavati. With them was Richard Wicksteed, a documentary filmmaker I had met during my shamanic journey who by now had become a close friend. After spending the first few days in the reeded huts listening to the relentless pummeling of rain on the thatch, we decided to risk a game drive. After the information I had been receiving from psychic sources about my affiliation with the White Lions, I longed to see my special "winged lion," Ingwavuma, again. I had visited Timbavati many times since his debut appearance on the runway. Although he regularly found his way into my dreams, and although I had heard his roars on many occasions, I had not seen him again in the flesh.

The newspapers informed us that many thousands of people had drowned and many more had been left homeless. They made no mention of the animals that had similarly suffered. I was concerned that Ingwavuma might have been harmed in the flood but had no way of determining his whereabouts. Since his appearance on the runway, he had become the dominant male of the area, Timbavati's lion king. But he had last been spotted in this region before the flooding began, more than two months before, and this worried me. Working with Maria and her bones of divination during the past rainy days, I was relieved when she informed me that Ingwavuma was alive and well. Furthermore, she instructed me that, if the skies cleared, my lion would come out to greet me. She explained that it was a matter of calling him "in my mind."

That night we decided to weather the storm, and head out for a game drive regardless. Restless after several days of being cooped up in *rondavels*, we pulled on hooded rain jackets and set out into the drenched evening. Despite having four-wheel-drive, we took care not to leave the dirt roads so as to avoid getting stuck axle-deep in the mud. As a consequence, we saw no game whatsoever.

At my request the ranger, Rexon, drove us to the runway. Once there, we stopped the Land Rover. After shining his spotlight into the darkness as a standard safety precaution, Rexon allowed us to disembark. The rain had let up momentarily, and I sat with Faith, who was five at the time, on the wet tar. Remembering Maria's words, I conveyed to Faith that she and I were going to call Ingwavuma "in our minds." We both closed our eyes, and I found I could see him clearly, just as he appeared to me in my dreams: a regal face, with an intense expression of wisdom and power.

A moment later, a lion started to roar nearby. Rexon, whose many years of tracking experience in the bush had taught him extreme caution, ordered us to climb back into the Land Rover immediately. We obeyed. That familiar primal excitement welled up in me as we drove in the direction of the roaring lion. We could not leave the dirt road, but it did not matter. We had no need to track the lion: the lion came to greet us.

Like a flash of gold in our spotlight, a living example of those beaten gilt masks of sun gods from ancient mythology, the lion stared straight at me with that fierce, all-knowing expression that I knew so well from my dreams. Rexon identified him immediately: Ingwavuma.

I was amazed and humbled. Of all animals, at that very moment, at that symbolic site in the midst of the Timbavati wilderness, under these weather conditions – *my* special lion declaring himself was a supreme occasion, recorded on film by Richard Wicksteed, who was sitting beside me at the time. Our group returned to camp in a state of mild euphoria. I was thrilled at the sight of my lion, and relieved that he was safe. Above all, I felt an almost umbilical sense of "connectedness" – the same sense that had overcome me at the birth of the White Lioness Tendile. The possibility that Faith and I had somehow called Ingwavuma in our minds was an idea that gave me a newfound sense of personal meaning in my life.

This was one of several signals that I had been given that, one day, I would be capable of crossing from my world into his, and back again. Shamans know that every living creature on this planet has a spirit or soul. The art of the shaman is to cross barriers, and among the most challenging of these is the apparent divide between the physical world and the spirit world. In the tradition of the shaman, I no longer feared dealing with the ancestral spirit realms. For some time now, my greatest inspiration had come from messages delivered through spirit sources, who seemed to guide my every step.

Just as on the occasion of my surreal journey through the zoo with Mutwa in his Sanusi regalia, my experience with spirit mediums felt like I was living a fairy tale. Only, the mythic realm was more real than everyday reality. Although deeply mysterious, it made profound sense of life.

Jackie te Braake was one spirit medium with whom I worked closely, but there were others. What impressed me was the consistency of information that came through different sources. I was surprised to discover that there were specific spirit entities who chose various channels by which to communicate their messages. According to mediums, the enlightened beings we call angels do exist – and can intermittently take on physical form, although they generally abide in an other-dimensional reality. After following the lead that the psychic had given me in respect of two specific names, I learned that a group of "ascended beings" (once human, now in the angelic realms, sometimes referred to as the "ascendant masters")[2] presided over the activities of humankind from the spirit realm. I tended to reconcile this view with Mutwa's notion of beings of semi-divine origin, the Abangafi Bapakade, and the ancient Egyptian notion of leonine star-beings. The name Count Saint-Germain turned out to be a leonine master spirit who addressed information to me through a number of different spirit mediums. His characteristics coincided closely with the fabled King Solomon of the Old Testament, not only in the identification with the lion symbol, but also in the teachings of gold as wealth in both material terms and alchemical terms – the path toward the highest soul essence. According to Mutwa, King Solomon, "the Alchemist," was renowned not only for his wisdom but also for his magic. His sword was used in the manner of a wand rather than as a weapon of bloodshed. Drawing from an entirely different source of knowledge, Adrian Gilbert had discussed with me how Solomon's Temple was astronomically aligned with the Leo constellation in the sky, thereby underwriting the notion of the lion as star beast.[3]

The other name the psychic had conveyed to me was Serapis Bey, who turned out to be the ascendant master spirit identified with pure white light, and therefore closely akin to the symbolism behind the White Lions. Whether understood as angels, ascendant masters, spirit guides, or leonine star gods, I discovered that these intelligences from the ancestral realm transmitted messages of astonishing guidance and wisdom.

While for me it was a new experience, I gathered there was a long precedent for the notion of receiving wisdom from other-dimensional realms. The "readings" by Edgar Cayce (while in a hypnotic state) on the significance of the Sphinx and pyramids, for instance, are now widely quoted by scholars and archeoastronomers. Our biblical texts speak of sages who conveyed wisdom from apparently angelic realms. Religious meditation through the ages has depended on creating a direct line or "channel" between the initiate and God or the gods, thereby receiving higher wisdom.[4]

Today, this technique has been labeled "channeling" and is in danger of being dismissed as a New Age fad, without reference to its possible ancient shamanic origins. Whether such mediums or "channelers" are tapping into a "higher self" within themselves, whether they have the ability to read their subject's deepest psyche telepathically, or whether there are, in fact, outside spirit sources or angelic guides speaking through them was not of immediate concern to me. The information being channeled was always entirely relevant to my quest for the meaning behind the White Lion mysteries. A thread ran through all my discourses with these spirits, a thread of continuity that acted as an invaluable lifeline to the mysteries I was unraveling.

Fragile Balance

When I next returned to Ingwavuma's territory, the catastrophic floods had abated.

In the wake of this natural disaster, I became acutely aware of the fragility of our earth. Timbavati's bushveld wilderness exists in a tenuous balance of natural forces presided over, on the one hand, by a consortium of wealthy landowners and, on the other, by the natural guardians of the land, the lion prides. For the first time, I began to appreciate how far removed the people's laws and objectives are from the solar Logos, the sun's law on Earth.

My journey into African shamanism had taught me an entirely new way of seeing the idea of ownership. Simply because an individual has the means to buy a piece of land does not give him the right to destroy the natural resources on that land for personal gain. Simply because an individual has the money to buy an animal does not give him the right to abuse that animal. In old Africa, the idea of ownership was a highly sophisticated one, in which the king's or the chief's role was one of custodianship over the land, rather than ownership.

Through his shamanic advisors, the king worked in accordance with the ancestral forces, who were understood to be God's agents guarding over the land. This understanding of the natural order of things has now all but disintegrated.

Even in the few years since I first embarked on my quest for understanding the true meaning behind the White Lions, irreparable changes had undermined the natural order. Structures that had held good for millennia were breaking down. The lion–human tradition of First Man, which had lasted for countless seasons of time – long before the remote hominid–sabertooth events that took place in the Sterkfontein Valley caves – had sadly come to an end. Today, the oldest fabrics of life on earth are unraveling with devastating rapidity. Along with the loss of rain forests and rare species, our oldest indigenous cultures – the Bushmen, the Aborigines, the Native Americans, and the other examples of what is known as the original 12 tribes of humankind, and whose primordial wisdom is so sorely needed in these times of change – have all but died out. If the world's oldest peoples, who survived the millennia intact, are departing this earth, what does it signify about the times in which we live? It is not difficult to appreciate that we may be rapidly heading toward global mass self-destruction.

Convergence of Lion Force

Facing up to the breakdown of natural order is an intensely sobering exercise. It is easy to lose courage and believe one is incapable of making any positive difference. If a plan had not been taking shape in me, if a feeling of light-force had not been building up in me, I might have felt despair. Instead, back in Timbavati, I tried to gather strength, listening to the most ancient wisdom in the sounds of the wild and searching the earth for signs. I spent the afternoons on foot with Rexon and Foreman, the trackers, tracing animal spoor through the intricate web of diverse living kingdoms, each dependent on the other, returning to camp as dusk set in. In the mornings, I lay outside my hut, in a hammock under a mopane tree in the heat, watching the translucent geckos curve into the bark, listening to the sweet song of the paradise flycatcher – *chira-weeet-tzweet-tzweeet* – and wondering how long these precious last stages of natural equilibrium would hold out.

For some reason, lions have recently started migrating to Timbavati in large numbers, creating one of the highest-density lion populations in the world.[5] I wondered why this should be. According to the law of the lion shaman, and the laws of nature, everything has a purpose and higher meaning. What might the lions converging on Lion Holy Land signify?

Considering this, I closed my eyes as I swung to and fro in the hammock. I tried not to demand an easy explanation; I simply tried to listen. Due north, I could picture the inimitable Sphinx in its position facing the sun and beneath its paws the back-to-back lion symbol of the *akeru*, defining the Nilotic Meridian. I remembered now how Adrian Gilbert had discussed with me his argument that this prime meridian represented the gateway to return to the Duat region, the "river of stars."[6] Was this significant?

The Egyptian Funerary Texts tell of the ascension of the pharaoh's soul to the overarching shower of stars along this meridian, while the Great Pyramid's four star shafts are believed to provide a channel through which the soul of the pharaoh may make its ascent through the "star gate."[7] The Sphinx itself symbolizes the Leo constellation, while the Great Pyramid's star shafts are targeted at Orion's Belt and Sirius – the specific luminaries that Mutwa had identified with the lion gods of First Time. Given that these star shafts are directed due south along this meridian, I now suddenly recalled Mutwa's hint that not only was Timbavati the location where star gods once appeared in the form of White Lions, but it was equally the location where an ascension back to the stars may take place.

While it seemed a far-fetched idea, I could not dismiss the possibility that the lions were congregating on this time line, like the pharaohs of old, in preparation for their souls' departure back to the stars. If lions are star beasts, and they are converging on this sacred meridian, the question we should look at is: why?[8]

Gold Enlightenment

Through my knowledge of lions and all that they symbolize for us humans, I had begun to see metaphysical meaning behind physical events on Earth. Information from the spirit world (whether derived from ancestral sources speaking through lion shamans or messages through channeled sources) had helped me identify deeper causes to natural catastrophes taking place in our day.

Shamanism teaches that beneath physical events is clear metaphysical logic. Devastating volcanic eruptions, floods, and tsunamis are in direct accord with the prophetic warnings of global divinity texts, which speak of our world ending in earthquakes and cataclysm. The Mayan notion of the Four Ages (or "Suns") forecasts that our Age (or "Sun") will culminate in earthquakes, because humans are imperfect. The world is eternally threatened as both the direct and indirect result of fallen humanity's mismanagement of its responsibilities. It strikes me that the logic behind these sacred texts is sound. Can we really begin to know the repercussions, for instance, of detonating nuclear bombs beneath the earth's crust, as different countries around the globe still persist in doing?[9] Is it any surprise that our earth convulses?

The information that has been conveyed to me, both of a scientific and shamanic nature, has led me to conclude that natural disasters are the consequence of the destructive human attitudes and practices at this time, which threaten our very survival on this planet. The solution lies within the earth itself, and our reconnection with it as modern scientists are, at last, starting to view our earth as a living organism.[10]

We tend to think of evolution as simply a physiological event. But if the shamans and lion ancestral spirits are anything to go by, humankind's challenge at this time appears to be in the nature of spiritual evolution: raising our consciousness. In its present course, our mass mind-set can only lead to disaster.

Return of the White Lion

Since I had first embarked on this quest for knowledge, I had found myself increasingly privileged with an abundant wealth of information through different spirit sources. Gradually, I was given reasons for why I was honored in this way.

Over the years, my awareness had been challenged by the information that was handed over to me. The lion ancestors, speaking through Maria, had told me that I had lived in Timbavati over many many lifetimes, which was consistent with Mutwa's teaching that

I was "a bridge" with a long ancestral history in Africa, an interface between black and white. I was instructed, "Remember who you are," as if my true identity was not fully understood, even by myself. Now I was told an extraordinary story by a channeled spirit:

> Many, many years ago, you came to earth in service to humankind, as a being of pure light and truth. A Sirian light-being. The form that you took was the shape and guise of a White Lion. You were a White Lioness and you were accompanied by your twin-flame, who was a great White Lion. You were beasts of truth and you carried the knowledge with you. And the place where you roamed is that place of which you now speak as Timbavati. Then came the hunters who wanted to take the power of the White Lions for themselves. They forgot that it is impossible to take the power of light by force. It is forever beyond their reach. One hunter pretended that he was giving offerings to these magnificent creatures, but it was only a means by which to gain access to their sacred lands and attempt to steal their light force. And then it was that you were killed, Beloved One, you and your lion-mate. But you did not die – for you were immortal Sirian beings. Instead, your spirits leapt into the bodies of human beings. You may call it transmigration – perhaps you know the term? And so it was that you transmigrated and took on human form and body to be of service to humankind – but you retained the soul of the White Lion.

My journey into lion shamanism had left me with no option but to treat the information from the spirit world with the greatest respect, and the most intense curiosity. Honoring Maria's imperative never to forget that there were Lions of God who walked beside me every step of the way helped me to feel strong, supported, and protected, despite the doubts that often plagued me. Sometimes my discoveries seemed so otherworldly that I wondered how I would ever find the words to express them. Yet, in my mind, I was beyond questioning the existence of these lion guides – their presence was manifest in too many subtle ways, over too many years. With every step that I took through the Timbavati wilderness, the same thoughts imprinted themselves in my consciousness. When will the White Lions walk this wilderness once more? And when they do so, will we humans be fit to welcome them back to earth?

How we humans understand the White Lions, and how we treat them and honor them – just as how we understand, treat, and honor all forms of nature – will ultimately determine whether we as a species have a future. To me, it was deeply satisfying to find that channeled sources corroborated Mutwa's words: the White Lions *will* survive, they will be the last beasts at the end of this age, and the new age will bring the White Lions to "reign once again upon this planet." It is our own survival, rather, that we urgently need to re-evaluate at this time.

The Hunter and the Hunted

Illuminated with this new information from spirit sources, I returned to the real world of trophy hunters and White Lions in captivity.

If part of the divine intention behind the White Lions is to highlight the question of value – monetary value as opposed to higher spiritual value – then it is not just the material values of those individuals responsible for "farming" the White Lions and shooting them that are being tested. Rather, it is humankind's value system at large that is in the spotlight.

If the mysterious notion of White Lions as guardians of our souls is difficult for our rational minds to comprehend, might the simple answer be that we have forgotten we have souls?

Wounded Healers

Shamans believe that, for every lion killed, a human associated with this atrocity will lose his or her soul. What exactly is a human without a soul? It's hard to imagine, but whatever it may be, a human soul for a lion's life suggests a profoundly grim correlation. Whenever I returned to Timbavati, my route took me past the road sign indicating the hunting camps and, with nausea in my heart, I was compelled to read and reread the crass euphemism: WHITE LION BREEDING PROJECT.

In the publicity brochure for this farm, the owner brazenly advertises himself as a "professional hunter," followed by the title "breeder of white lions." One does not even need to read between the lines.

It continued to bewilder me why the Creator should allow the White Lions to be mowed down as trophies. If they are indeed Children of the Sun God, why should they allow themselves to be so maltreated?

Of course, the same argument may be applied to Credo Mutwa. Why doesn't the Son of Ra stand up and defend himself against wounding ridicule and savage physical attacks? In terms of his own health, why doesn't the great shaman simply cure himself? Maria had explained that one of the oldest laws of the Sanusis is that a healer may not heal himself. When I inquired of Maria why such a great man as Mutwa, who knows the most secret arts of healing, should have to endure such personal suffering, and along with it, such personal ill health, she responded that there was no shaman "higher than Mutwa – only God. Only God can heal him."

It is not difficult to identify parallels with the idea of Christ, the ultimate wounded healer, dying for humanity's sins. Why did God allow his beloved son to be harmed? The answer must surely be: in the hope of creating spiritual awareness in humankind. The White Lions are an archetypal symbol of the wounded healer, the injured God, whose life or death is seemingly in the hands of humankind. Humankind has free will to choose the outcome. What will it be?

Modern Western man's consciousness seems only to be able to extend as far back as the beginning of the last astrological age, 2,000 years ago (the Age of Pisces, the fish) when Christ was born. For this reason, Christians identify Christ as the one and only Son of God. If we could extend our consciousness farther back, as shamans are able to do, we would know that there have been many such "children" of God, sent to our earth in the hope of creating spiritual awareness in humankind.

Quetzalcoatl, Osiris, Mithras, Mvelinqangi – if we go deeply into the mythology behind these figures, we will see that they stand for the same divine consciousness, the same self-sacrifice for flawed humanity, for which Christ himself lived and died. Behind all these radiant, altruistic figures exists what one might term "Christ consciousness."

Like Quetzalcoatl, the feathered feline god of ancient America; like Horus, the falcon-headed lion god of the Egyptians; like Mithras, the lion shaman king of Mesopotamia, I now saw how the winged White Lions could be identified with our own solar lion god, or Christ, with his crown of thorns – suffering not for their own sins, but ours. As Lions of God, the White Lions are heavenly symbols reminding us that human evolution is not only a physical or genetic issue, but ultimately a spiritual or soul issue. Our first challenge is to be aware of ourselves as ethical and spiritual beings made flesh, not simply as physical human beings.

Death of a Lion King

The Timbavati landowners have a policy of raising money through trophy hunting lions. To my dismay, I was informed by one of the Timbavati lodge owners that the prize lion they had earmarked was Ingwavuma. My first thought was: of all the lions in Timbavati, why my lion? *Why any lion?*

Sickened, I retreated to my thatched *rondavel*. Feeling desperate and powerless, I thought over what, if any, practical steps were still open to me. The majority of Timbavati's management are intelligent, moneyed people but, with few exceptions, they view controlled hunting as a perfectly reasonable practice: a means of bringing income into the region. And even an anti-hunting chief warden still has the unenviable task of implementing the landowners' wishes when they are legally supported by the government.

I might have tried to make a special case for Ingwavuma on the grounds that I believed he was carrying the white gene. But there is no way of telling whether a tawny lion is a gene carrier until he actually produces white offspring. Citing Maria as my source would have carried little weight for an upper-income group of predominantly European landowners, who have little regard for, or even knowledge of, traditional *sangoma* wisdom.

Rangers Pierre Gallagher and Grant Furniss had compiled an identikit of prime territorial males, including Ingwavuma, with the purpose of protecting them. Ironically, this identikit was used by the hunter to identify his quarry. This was not some common stereotyped criminal, but a lion king who had ruled over his territory with dignity, wisdom, courage, and pride. They were hunting a living example of the divine laws of rulership that we humans might do well to follow.

A landowner told me that Ingwavuma was selected to be killed over and above other lions in the larger vicinity, since his cubs were said not to be surviving. But if Ingwavuma's genes were not of the strongest, he would have been ousted long ago – by natural law. Dominant lions commanding a territory come under fierce pressure from younger males, who sometimes form a coalition of up to five members or more in their bid for takeover. In his time, Ingwavuma had survived many overthrow attempts. By lion standards, his rulership had been long and particularly impressive for its solo nature. There could be no better indication of the strength of his genes.

After receiving the news of my lion's imminent death, I could not prevent the vision of his magnificent, proud face stuffed into a fake snarl by a taxidermist, with marbles in his eye sockets. Ingwavuma's golden eyes, which so closely resembled the "sacred eye" of the Egyptians (with three tear ducts symbolizing the rays of God) would be gouged out and replaced by manufactured glass eyes from a factory in Germany.

I now visualized his pelt gruesomely spread out on a wall, in a mockery of a five-pointed star. These power-points, which Mutwa had indicated were the symbol and source of star power, would be rendered powerless and lifeless and meaningless. I saw his four paws staked into a wall, like a crucifix – and the figure of Christ rose up in my mind. I recalled reading in the New Testament how "the earth did quake" at the moment of Christ's death on the cross.[11] If the lion is our guardian, holding the four corners of the earth in balance, as our sacred texts compel us to remember, what does it mean to kill a lion? Why do we destabilize the balance on our precious earth? It was all too sickeningly real for me, knowing there was no one I could appeal to.

Retreating, exhausted, to my *rondavel,* I spent a desperately troubled night. I woke intermittently, realizing I had been dreaming of Mutwa's sacred weaponry of the spirit: the bow with the three arrows symbolizing the rays and powers of God. More than ever I felt desperate to discover Mutwa's whereabouts. I thought of the prayer of protection he had placed over Ngwazi a lion-generation ago, and how that great lion had been saved from the hunter's bullet. His words were resounding in my head: "I am history, ma'am, you are the future. Sharpen your sword and *assegaai* of the spirit . . . Sharpen the gifts which God gave you!" And Maria Khosa's injunction advised that I never forget the umbilical cord that connected me to Tendile – that, if I were ever killed, this matriarchal White Lioness' fury would be unleashed upon her keepers. Now I felt the inverse impulse – if Ingwavuma were shot, I knew that I would take up arms, and Mutwa's spiritual weapons, and fight ceaselessly until my term on earth was up. In my desperate half-dream state, I knew that this was a cause for which I was prepared to die.

When I awoke before first light, it suddenly struck me that I knew exactly what to do. I immediately told Maria the news of the impending hunt. She listened intently and soberly. Then she responded: "No one will touch that lion. Go and rest."

That day passed. Then another, and another. It was weeks later that I finally determined that my prayers had been answered. Timbavati reported that the trophy hunters had had the greatest difficulty and inconvenience trying to locate Ingwavuma. The mysterious fact was that he literally seemed to have disappeared from the territory, as if instinctively sensing danger. The hunters finally gave up the search.

The final result was that some other great lion, alas, ended up as a trophy on some hunter's wall, but at least my lion king was spared. But for how long?

25

ICE AGES AND SNOW LIONS

Kingship came from the skies. There is a Zulu saying which asks leaders to link their minds to the gods in the skies, because that is where kingship and law came from.
— CREDO MUTWA

It felt as if my ancestral lion was forever following me, even guarding me while I slept. There were times in my daily life when his presence was almost tangible. Now, after his narrow escape from the hunter's bullet, the connection between us felt all the more intense.

If, as Maria had revealed, a "soul bond" existed between me and this particular lion (my ancestral spirit guide, my lion brother), then I was beginning to appreciate what this might mean on a real, everyday level. I was fortified by his invisible presence, even in a city context. While my dreams were still emblazoned with Ingwavuma's proud face, he was no longer roaring as if trying to make himself heard. In general, his appearances had become peaceful. In one dream, I saw him padding beside me through the Timbavati bushveld. On looking down, I discovered that my own feet were lion's paws, as were my hands. I took this as symbolic of how one day I would learn to cross into his world, just as he made an occasional appearance in mine.

I traveled to London to follow up on some of channeled information I had received, in an attempt to corroborate it with scientific material. I am particularly familiar with the streets of London, but this visit felt different. The lion guardian spirit was protecting me.

Earth in the Balance

Having just entered the crowded hysteria of Trafalgar Square, where the sculpture of Nelson stood on his column with Landseer's famous lions placed precisely between the four cardinal points beneath him, I paused and considered for a moment. I had passed this symbol, unwittingly, hundreds of times on my way to my former advertising job. But now I stopped to read the meaning behind the monument for the first time.

Just as the lion symbol guards the earth, so it guards the earth's axis. Ancient mythologies show the earth held in balance by four leonine animal figures. While Mutwa identifies four great lion brothers as guardians of the earth's cardinal axis, here, in one of the world's most civilized of cities – where flesh-and-blood lions have not roamed for many centuries – the lion symbol lives on.

The equinox and, leading on from it, the notion of the "precession of the equinoxes," remains one of the most important notions in astronomy, both ancient and modern.

But the astronomical principles behind the equinox are only part of the story. As the astronomer-priests of old Africa, such as Mutwa, knew, there is meaning behind cosmic events. Therefore, one should look equally at the astrological principles behind the equinox; in other words, the causal connection at this time between events on Earth and heavenly events.[1]

In astronomical terms, the equinox is that moment of paramount significance in the yearly cycle when the earth comes into a special relationship of balance with the sun – night and day being equal. It is also that moment in the year when the sun's rays strike the earth along the length of each line of longitude *at precisely the same time*. In respect of the Nilotic Meridian of the First Time, for example, the equinox is that day of the year when the Sphinx and the lions in Timbavati meet the sunrise *simultaneously*.

The equinox and the precession of the equinoxes were notions that I needed to keep constantly in mind when working with the messages that had been delivered to me from the ancestral spirit world.

Since lions link with the sun symbol, the lion "brothers" at each of the cardinal points indicate our globe's rotation on its axis, with the sun rising in its present position (due east) at the equinox, and setting due west. Our earth is held in the most fragile of balances. Should this balance be destabilized, the condition of the earth would approximate hell on earth in a furnace of cataclysms, earthquakes, fire, plague, flooding, and darkness.

Suddenly the cacophony of human voices and the odors of automobiles belching black smoke into my nostrils dragged me out of my reverie, and back into the London streets. I continued my walk to the public libraries to investigate the information I had received from spiritual sources regarding the White Lions and Ice Age theory.

Ice Lions

One of the most significant fragments of information channeled from the spirit ancestors was an implied connection between Ice Ages and astrological ages of Leo – a correspondence that ultimately has far-reaching implications for the White Lions' appearance in our present age.

These were the words of the spirit guide:

> When man destroys the agents of light in his world, he freezes conscious-
> ness, through fear. Unfortunately, this appears to be a recurring phenom-
> enon upon your planet because mankind destroys the bringers of light, such
> as the quintessential light-beings, the White Lions. Each time consciousness
> becomes frozen from fear, it suffers an Ice Age. Only when it experiences a
> change of heart, and the lion heart warms the earth again during a Lion Age,
> do you experience the great meltdown.[2]

Couched in highly esoteric language, this message had taken some concentrated effort to interpret. The notion of "consciousness" affecting climatic conditions at first appeared an entirely new one.

It soon became clear that the message made sense of two conclusions that I had recently reached. The one was that the sudden recurrence of the white gene represented a forerunner to the impending Ice Age. The other was that the White Lions had significance in terms of the forthcoming Age of Leo.

Since Mutwa linked real lions with the Leo constellation in the heavens, I had used this premise as a basis for understanding the astrological principles underlying African cosmology. I had also used it as background to Western archeoastronomers' conclusions that the Great Sphinx of Giza was built at the beginning of the last Age of Leo (the period during which the constellation of Leo resided behind the sun on the vernal equinox). It makes sense that a civilization should build a great lion monument to celebrate the prevailing constellation in the sky. Significantly, this last Leo Age coincided with the end of the last Ice Age, the great meltdown approximately 11,500 years ago, which ushered in the warm interglacial period known as the "recent period." According to modern evolutionary theory, the recent period spans the entire development of human civilization, at the tail end of which we modern humans are living.

If the Sphinx was built at the end of the last Ice Age cycle, it means that the lions at the time would in all likelihood have been white. A white coat would naturally provide a selective advantage in glacial environs. The thought that the Sphinx was modeled after a White Lion – and hence on the original source breed of today's tawny lions – provides a tantalizing correlation between White Lions as Ice Age animals in the Age of Leo.

More immediately, it continues to raise the question of why the White Lions should have reappeared in our own age. The channeled information about "humankind freezing consciousness through fear" sheds a whole new light on the question of the White Lions as genetic precursors to glacial conditions. It seems to suggest that the White Lions are here as an early warning signal, alerting us to the danger that humankind's mental attitude of tyranny over our earth is threatening to plunge us into the next Ice Age.

Lion of Learning

Determined not to let this spirit message about White Lions and Ice Ages fall on deaf ears, despite my not understanding it fully, I used my time in England to visit my old academic haunts, where I secured entry passes into the science libraries. Still not knowing quite what I was looking for, but only too familiar with the grind of academic endeavor, I was surprised when the perfect references seemed to drop into my lap. It was almost as if my sage lion was there with me in the library stretching up on his hind legs, pulling books and manuscripts and journals off the shelf with his paws, and presenting them to me at precisely the moment when I needed them.

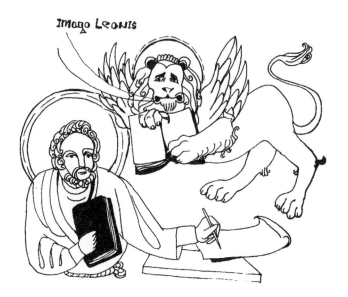

Imago Leonis

One after one, the pieces of the Ice Age puzzle fell into place. In no time at all, I seemed to have been given precisely what I needed to validate the Ice Age/Leo Age correlation. It was a radiantly illuminating exercise, the likes of which I had never experienced before. I almost felt as if I was doing no work at all, only listening and concentrating intensely on what was being said to me.

According to the laws of precession, we are on the brink of the Age of Aquarius in the Northern Hemisphere, while in the Southern Hemisphere we are on the brink of the Age of Leo. Modern science has also now determined that Ice Age cycles are related to precessional cycles and, in turn, that human evolution is related to these Ice Age cycles. The correlation between Ice Ages and precession of the equinoxes was first determined by a Yugoslavian astronomer, Milutin Milankovitch, almost a century ago. Milankovitch's precessionary models of Ice Ages was recently corroborated by more recent independent scientific advancements with the analysis of microscopic sediment cores from deep ocean beds.

Many evolutionary scientists have now identified a direct correlation between Ice Age cycles and human evolution. That is to say, human evolution is contingent upon Ice Ages. Furthermore, the evolutionary events correspond with prehistoric lion–human interaction. Bob Brain's research in the Sterkfontein caves supports these scientific models for evolution.

Further information was handed down from the shelves, adding weight to this theory. My ultimate conclusion was that the White Lions were precursors to an impending Ice Age, in the approaching Leo/Aquarius Age.

My primary objective now was to get my book out without further delay, in the hope that it might make a little difference to the present circumstances on our earth, and the ecological and psychological crisis in which we find ourselves.

Shamans, who see the fast-approaching future, believe our earth is on the brink of catastrophe because the actions of its human inhabitants have brought about critical instability. I concur with this thinking. There are causes, reasons, and consequences, the patterns of which are identifiable – if we simply open our eyes and our consciousness.

To speak of lions "forewarning" implies that they bear a "consciousness." I believe this to be so. Yet, rather than the ego-consciousness so familiar to humankind, I believe that they carry the consciousness of the Original Source, the Creator identifiable with the solar Logos. Like the shamans of Africa, I accept that the White Lions are agents of light: Lions of God.

In this way, the words of the spirit master gradually became clear to me: "When man destroys the agents of light in his world, he freezes consciousness." Humankind's mismanagement of its planet, and the consequences of this mismanagement, have instilled fear on earth, and for good reason.

The thought of an Ice Age of imminent apocalypse and global catastrophe is frightening in the extreme, yet the White Lions' message to us is not to succumb to our fear. They are here as the symbol we might draw upon to overcome this fear – and change the consciousness that is heading us into devastation. As the symbol of the heart of humankind, they are here to teach us the power of being brave and truly lionhearted. We as a species can evolve – not only physically, but ultimately also spiritually. We can overcome fear by summoning principles of courage, faith, and love. Love, in shamanic understanding, is faith in a divine presence. It is the knowledge that we are not alone, that we are all connected, we are all One.

Caught in the treadmill of our consumer societies, we might feel impotent against the ongoing destruction of our earth. This is not so. I do not believe that we are helpless. We become intensely powerful and effective once we start believing in the light within us, and allow this inner light to guide us toward the right action.

There are many ways to reconnect. We might not choose the White Lion as our symbol. Our totem might be the doves that we feed at Trafalgar Square, or the stray cat that we rescue along the road, or the vegetables that we plant in our garden, or even the crystal that we cherish as a light-radiating stone in our house. There are many ways to reinvest in our earth and its riches. There are many ways to give something back for what we have received. The important thing is to start making the connections, and the interconnections.

The truth is that we *can* make a difference.

The very first step is to confront, and overcome, our own fears. Fear can hold us back from believing in our own inner radiance. The lion symbol is not a lifeless statue in bronze or marble guarding the entrances of our state buildings. It is alive. It lives in the courage and truth and light of every one of us. Like Christ himself, and all the other avatars of light who walked this planet in physical form, the White Lions are here on earth as a beacon to guide us to reclaim that light within us.

The White Lion mysteries take us back in time to the evolutionary beginnings of our species, but they also take us forward to our future. I believe that we are being offered the rarest opportunity to experience the principles of the Golden Age once more, in accordance with divine symmetries being revealed within our earth – on the brink of our potentially catastrophic Leo–Aquarius Age.

Whether or not there is a future for human life on this planet, I believe, is dependent at this evolutionary moment upon humankind's consciousness-raising powers as a species. As guardians of the soul essence of humankind, the White Lions offer us entrance into other dimensions. In particular, into what is known in spirit sources as the fifth dimension of the spiritual evolution of the soul.[3] It might sound esoteric, but from my own limited experience of other-dimensional realities, I believe that what seems paranormal to us now will, in time, become perfectly normal – if we are brave enough to take the path of spiritual evolution of the human soul.

Star Beast Returns to the Stars

On 22 August 2000, Ingwavuma was hunted as a trophy. I was still in London at the time the tragedy occurred. I remember a night full of distressing dreams, after which I knew I had to return to Timbavati. I arrived at Ingwavuma's territory to pick up the pieces of what had happened in my absence.

Following the search and failure to find him, the annual Timbavati trophy quota had been used up on an unknown nomadic male. But the previous year's quota remained. After an extended period of roaming in the wilderness, Ingwavuma had returned to his kingdom, where he was shot. The picture I received was of him walking right up to the trophy hunters, proudly and defiantly, offering humankind a choice. And they paid $35,000 for the pleasure of killing him.

My feelings on this matter are not easily describable. It was as if the light went out. My important family member had been shot, execution-style. And with his death on

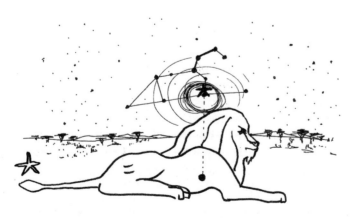

On the day Ingwavuma was shot, there was a rare alignment of the sun with Regulus, heart star of Leo.

this auspicious day, everything I had been researching in theory now became all-too-real. He died in the late afternoon as the sun set over Timbavati, on the last day of the month of Leo at the turn of the millennium. The shot was fired shortly before 6 P.M. The timing is profoundly poignant. From my studies in ancient astrology, I could now determine that on this day, and this day only, at this very time, the setting sun was in perfect alignment with Regulus, the heart star of the Leo constellation.[4] Regulus is the star that Credo Mutwa tells us is the heart of the great sky lion. Regulus is the star that Adrian Gilbert identifies with Christ. Both Mutwa and Gilbert pinpoint the unique moment when the sun passes through Regulus as symbolizing the birth, or death, of a lion king. And, consequently, with the birth or death of a kingdom on earth.

This was confirmation of the sacredness of my great lion of Timbavati. I only wept that he should suffer such devastatingly real circumstances on earth in order for me to see his status in the sky. Ingwavuma's relevance as star beast was written across the heavens. As for me, I had lost my guardian angel, the golden lion with invisible wings who was meant to father the future Star Lions of Timbavati.

26

LION OF JUDAH

Our deepest fear is not that we are inadequate. Our deepest fear is that we are powerful beyond measure. It is our light, not our darkness, that most frightens us.
– NELSON MANDELA (FROM HIS INAUGURAL SPEECH)

In my state of mourning, I turned to Gareth Patterson for consolation. Over the past couple of years, he and I had spent much time exchanging ideas. In his courageous fight for the protection of lions' rights, Gareth had always drawn on his firsthand physical experience with lions. After our intimate discussions, he was now brave enough to go public for the first time with his spiritual experiences with lions.

In commiserating with me over Ingwavuma's death, Gareth attempted to provide comfort with the kind words, "All I can say is that your lion will remain with you as a guide."

Message from Ingwavuma

What made my grief all the more intense was that I had truly believed Ingwavuma was protected. Distraught and confused, I tried to contact Jackie te Braake for a reading. Unfortunately, she was away at the time, so I had to approach a spirit medium in Cape Town whom I had never been to before. I heard from several sources that she was good at her work and, as usual, I followed the procedure of offering no background information. On arrival, I simply explained that a relative of mine had recently died and I wanted to know whether he had a message for me. I told her his name was Ingwavuma.

After a short meditation, she began to describe my relative. She said that she saw a regal and very wise man standing on a high promontory, surveying his lands. She said that he looked like a great chief, or king, and he carried a staff of some kind in one hand. She then went on to describe his proud face, which she said was covered with "a great deal of tawny facial hair" – at which point, despite my sadness, I couldn't help laughing and interjecting that she was, in fact, talking about a lion. She laughed, too. She had naturally imagined that I had meant a human relative.

Then the reading became serious again. Now that she knew it was a lion she was viewing, the picture was clearer. She saw Ingwavuma making his way through the bushveld, padding straight up to the hunting party, with a low growl, as if to say: "All right. I am ready. Do your damnedest."

This detail moved me deeply. It implied that, at some level, he had anticipated his own death, and was reconciled to the outcome. It suddenly reminded me of Mutwa's words about camouflage being a product of the soul. The implication is that once an animal becomes visible to its prey, the animal's soul has chosen its destiny. Hard as it was for me to accept this version of the truth, I now understood that, at a soul level, Ingwavuma had allowed himself to being sacrificed for the higher good of humankind.

My lion did, indeed, have a message for me. It was this: "Do not mourn me, beloved one. You have work to do, Worker of Light. I am forever with you."

I still mourn Ingwavuma every day, but I continue the work that I do in the belief that I can make a difference. In respect to my lion's death, I remember the profoundly disturbing information that was conveyed to me, by shamanic sources, on the lion-hunting issue. "For every lion shot, a human soul will be lost."

There is something eternally damning about this statement. This is not the rough justice of the human variety: a tooth for a tooth, a life for a life. The correlation is *a soul for a life*: a human soul for a lion's life. This balance of scales has the ring of divine justice about it.

Because shamans can cross the threshold between this world and the spirit world, death itself is not the issue. Nature, after all, is a never-ending cycle of birth, procreation, and death. Death, therefore, is a natural part of life, and rebirth. If we do not acknowledge death in our lives, this is yet another index of how we have cut ourselves off from reality. We will all die sooner or later. The question is: what happens to our souls? Shamans know that everything in the real world has a soul, therefore nothing ultimately dies. I know that Ingwavuma has not died. He still exists. He still guides me from the spirit world. The tragedy is that a human soul has died in killing him.

Our oldest morality tales tell us that if we sell our souls, we are lost souls. If we sell ourselves to darkness, not enlightenment, we will exist in eternal darkness. If we kill the sun god, we kill the sun in our lives, and our souls will die with the dying sun.

As to the future, I know that several of the cubs sired by Ingwavuma live on in Timbavati. Some of them are surprisingly light in color. There are a couple that have green eyes. I believe this signifies that they bear the white gene. I believe the White Lions will one day return to their rightful kingdom of Timbavati. However, I do not believe they will show themselves again until human consciousness is ready to be uplifted, and we human animals are prepared to open our hearts to the true meaning that the White Lions bring us.

Lion and the Lamb of Judah

In the months following Ingwavuma's death, I made a pilgrimage to Legogotsi, the lion mountain overlooking White River, beside the region called Jerusalem. Legend (from Swazi elders)[1] has it that Legogotsi is associated with the crucifixion of Christ. Situated on top of the volcanic leonine mountain, among ancient Bushman rock paintings, I found a Christian mission training school. There I met a man named Dr Johannes Malherbe, the principal of the ministry, whom I discovered to be a very knowledgeable and enlightened person.

I had always associated Jesus with the idea of the lamb. While the symbol of the lamb (as well as the shepherd) is regularly drawn upon as an easy and gentle image for us to accommodate, the origins of Christ are, in fact, quite plainly leonine. This point is made many times in the Bible.

Malherbe pointed me to the biblical references equating Christ with the lion. The Bible tells us that Christ is of the tribe of Judah. In Genesis, it is explained that the tribe of Judah are the lion people. Jacob says of his beloved son: "Judah is a lion's whelp: from the prey, my son, thou art gone up: he stooped down, he crouched as a lion, and as an old lion; who shall rouse him up? The sceptre shall not depart from Judah . . ."[2] Jacob was the father of Judah, from whose line was born King David, who in turn begat King Solomon. Further in the same lineage, Joseph was born, "the husband of Mary, of whom was born Jesus, who is called Christ."[3] This genealogy of Jesus from the Judaic lion tribe of David is specified over and over in the Bible.

So the question is: if we do not take Jesus Christ, Son of God, Lion of Judah, King of Kings, *literally* as the Son of God on earth, then how do we understand him? As a mere mortal?

The Bible makes it plain that Christ is both human and God. The four evangelists raise this issue four times – and resolve it four times. Each from a different angle, Matthew, Mark, Luke, and John pose the same question: if Jesus was the son of David, of the leonine Judaic line, how could he also be the Son of God?

Each and every one of the four evangelists arrives at the same answer: Jesus is both son of God and son of man.[4]

In the Book of Revelation, Christ himself is quoted as saying, "I, Jesus . . . am the root and offspring of David, and the bright Morning Star."[5]

Star Gods

Meaningful symbols are all around us in nature. The trouble is that most of us no longer know how to interpret them; or worse, don't even see them. Significantly, children's stories from all over the globe have drawn inspiration from the White Lion symbol as a guiding light for our future generations. We adults may choose to dismiss these as fairy tales, or we may choose to recognize truth in them, subtly disguised as stories that children (unindoctrinated, as yet, by our artificial world) still believe in.

C.S. Lewis' famous children's story *The Lion, the Witch, and the Wardrobe,* for instance, delivers a profound message to our children, which we adults seem to have forgotten. In Lewis's story, the lion, Aslan, has Christlike associations. The lion is symbolic of light and the witch is symbolic of darkness, while the wardrobe may be understood as the agent of change (or evolution): the shamanic "fifth dimension," through which humankind must travel to reach the path of the soul.

Appropriately, the lion in *The Wizard of Oz* needs a heart to animate him with life-force. In the early German fairy tale *The True Bride,* a radiant White Lion appears as an angelic guardian figure when the trials and tribulations of life threaten to overwhelm the heroine. Again, in another children's book called *The Butterfly Lion,* it is infinitely appropriate that a real White Lion becomes a spirit guardian.[6]

It is not enough for adults to classify this recurring symbol in human consciousness as an "archetype," and leave the matter there. Only in finding satisfactory answers to why this archetype should be embedded in our memories and where this archetype first originated will we reach the truth. The lion as sun god, or star beast, is imprinted in our collective unconscious and manifests in every corner of our globe, because it carries meaning and validity. It simply will not go away.

Although I had been slow to wake up, Ingwavuma's death had shaken me out of unconsciousness. There, upon the lion mountain of Legogotsi, I made a silent promise that I would never again overlook a message that nature sent to me.

The presence of the original Creator God is manifest in all of original creation: nature. God lives in every living, wild, and wondrous creature on this planet. God lives in the White Lions, and manifests His divine presence through them.

It is important to remember that, unlike many of us who have dissociated ourselves from the natural world, Jesus is directly connected with wildlife and the laws of nature. When Jesus spent 40 days in the desert, the Son of God was with "the wild animals, and the angels attended him."[7] Christ was one with nature. In fact, the word *Logos* (God's law on earth, the rule of nature) is used as Christ's very title.[8]

We are all familiar with Christ's description as the sacrificial "Lamb of God, who takes away the sin of the world." Yet, while the lamb is the meek and mild image of Christ with which we are comfortable, it should not blind us to his true godlike leonine powers. Johannes Malherbe was of the opinion that only the most committed of Christians can deal with the notion of Christ as the lion. In William Blake's poem *The Tyger,* he wrestles with the idea that the same God who made the lamb created the feline's "fearful symmetry." Both lamb and lion are symbols of light, but Christ as Lion God may be terrifying to some – because it implies the power to destroy. Yet the truth we should face up to is that there are many occasions in the Bible when God's judgment is likened to a lion's attack.[9]

In Revelation, the last book of the Christian Bible, we are instructed: "Do not weep! See, the Lion of the tribe of Judah, the Root of David, has triumphed. He is able to open the scroll and the seven seals."[10]

This corresponds directly with the first book of Genesis where Jacob describes his son Judah as a lion's whelp and predicts: "The sceptre shall not depart from Judah."[11] Rather than a lion, however, it is in fact a sacrificial lamb that opens the seven seals. Upon prophesying the seals' opening, John says, "Then I saw a lamb, looking as if it had been slain, standing in the center of the throne, encircled by four living creatures and the elders."[12]

This lamb is of course Christ, Lion of Judah, who ultimately reconciles lion and lamb, predator and prey, since in him all are One.

In the Bible it is prophesied that at the end of the world, the lamb of God looks "as if it has been slain." Yet I knew only too well that in our day it is not simply the lamb but equally the Lion of God, the sacred White Lion of Timbavati, who is sacrificed to humanity's greed.

Jesus describes the end of the world to his disciples, sitting on the Mount of Olives. His words are reported four times, in the four gospels of the evangelists. When asked by his disciples how they will recognize his "second coming," he explains that there will be "many pretenders and many false prophets." He talks about nation rising against nation, and kingdom against kingdom, and earthquakes and famines. He also makes reference to the prophet Daniel's apocalyptic dreams.[13]

White Lion Saviors

At the end of days, Christ says, "The sun will be darkened and the moon will not give its light, the stars will fall from the sky and the heavenly bodies will be shaken."[14] At this prophetic time, events on Earth will be quite clearly manifest in the heavens. Christ tells us that, "At that time, the sign of the son of man will appear in the sky."[15]

For me, the death of Ingwavuma signaled the death of a kingdom on Earth, with ominous resonances of Christ's prophetic words about the signs in the sky preceding the end of the world. Earth tremors and tsunamis are early warning signals that, although we might believe otherwise, we are not lords of the planet. We might believe we can control the power of the king of the beasts in man-made confines. We might believe we can breed the sun god's hallowed children as stuffed trophies. We might believe we can mess with genetics. In these beliefs, we are profoundly misguided. We cannot master nature; nature is one with God the Master.

Sometimes I wonder about the trophy hunter who killed Ingwavuma, and what led him to commit this atrocity. His decision was obviously a conscious one, but yet without consciousness. Whether he knows it or not, he carries the blood of my lion on his soul.

There are times when I feel personal anguish and outrage at the treatment of this great king and his royal lineage, but then I am suddenly reminded of Ingwavuma's message to me not to mope and mourn, but to get back on track and assist the Light Workers with what I now believe to be a Great Plan on earth. As a Lioness of God, I realize that it is not for me to cast judgment. I humbly leave that in higher hands.

When asked what God's greatest commandment was, Christ replied:

> The Lord is One. Love the Lord your God with all your heart and all your soul and all your mind and all your strength. The second is this:

"Love your neighbor as yourself." There is no greater commandment than these.[16]

We humans forget that our "neighbor" is not simply the member of the species of *Homo sapiens* living next door to us over the picket fence. Our "neighbor" is each and every wondrous creation – plant, animal, and mineral – which is intended, according to nature's law and God's will, to share this planet with us. In the great circle of life, we are all connected, we are all One.

It is about time we started remembering. In accordance with the oldest principles of Christ consciousness, the symbolic message behind the White Lions is pure and simple, and delivered out of sheer love. The White Lion message is the same as ever: Save the world.

Christ, Lion of Bethlehem

Shortly after my time at the ministry on Legogotsi, I received extraordinary news. I learnt that a White Lion male (from original Timbavati stock) had been born in a canned hunting camp in a town called Bethlehem, in the "Free State" province of South Africa.[17] After my promise not to overlook any further clue from nature, the sacred symbolism of a lion born in Bethlehem was not lost on me.

From this moment on, all my studies about the mythic and legendary aspects of the White Lions shifted from mere theory to living practice.

The Second Coming

From Sterkfontein to Bethlehem; from the cradle of human origins to the namesake of Christ's birthplace – this lion's arrival struck me as a truly miraculous real-life story, with suggestions of the coming of the new Messiah. It was a declaration that the fabled enlightenment-bearers of the ancient scriptures were not a myth, but a very urgent reality.

The town of Bethlehem in the Free State is in the foothills of the Drakensberg Mountains. At this high altitude, Bethlehem is often the coldest town in South Africa. It has been known to snow in the height of summer, at Christmas time. The thought of a White Lion in the snow at Christmas, during the peak of summer in the Southern Hemisphere, was so unlikely, yet somehow appropriate, given changes in global climate patterns. It confirmed my belief that the White Lions are, in fact, snow animals *ahead* of their time, precursors to a coming ice age, angelic messengers returned to earth at a time of ecological and psychological fragility – to assist humankind through the coming challenges. In perfect attunement with the gilded symbolism of the White Lions, the Bethlehem area is known as the Golden Gate, and is one of the richest treasure houses of Bushman paintings in the country. The mountains are studded with shamanic feline messages. In true therianthrophic spirit, almost as if prophesying the lion–human event that would unfold here. Bushman paintings in the surrounding mountains show felines superimposed on human figures and, inversely, human figures superimposed on felines.[18] In fact, some of South Africa's most important lion shaman paintings – those of Coerland and Clocolan – are to be found in the mountains cradling Bethlehem.[19]

Yet all that is gold does not glitter. The truth is that Bethlehem in South Africa's Free State province is the black heart of the canned hunting industry.

In mockery of its name, the so-called Free State is a land of imprisonment for all things wild and wonderful, where lions are not born free, nor are they permitted to die free. They are locked in enclosures, "canned," and trophy hunted. This trophy hunting operation in Bethlehem was reputed to be one of the worst: golden lion cubs were removed from their mothers at birth using lawnmowers to separate them, bottle fed, hand-reared in the family household, then sold to be shot in enclosures. The thought of such a magnificent lion being killed for fun and money, was like switching off the sun.

I do not believe that the Creator allowed his lions to be born in God-forsaken lion-trophy country because humans decided to breed them there. He sent his Lions of God to Bethlehem in order to bring us light.

When I informed Maria of this White Lion held captive in the canned hunting camp in Bethlehem, she reminded me that despite humans' worst efforts to destroy sacredness in nature, God's "Enlightenment-Bearers" would continue to manifest. I remember clearly how we were seated on her ceremonial mat at the time and, as was customary, she gathered up her bones of divination in her hands, and cast these out onto the mat. The lion bone rolled off the mat to me. Scrutinizing the complex symbolic picture laid out on the mat, as if it confirmed what she already knew, she went on to indicate something of immense gravitas to me. She said that a lioness was about to be born in a place of great sacred significance to humanity. She said that I was due to take over Maria's own mantel as the "Keeper of the White Lions" and, furthermore, that it was my life's task to guard over this lioness.

A couple of months later, at the end of the first year of the new millennium, I made a pilgrimage to Bethlehem to meet the King of the King of the Beasts, held captive there. I arrived the day after Christmas, to discover an event that I knew would change my life forever.

Bethlehem Baby

A second White Lion had been born in the trophy hunting farm in Bethlehem: on Christmas Day, 2000. I was utterly overwhelmed. When I held this little lion-lamb in my arms, I felt an overwhelming joy and pain simultaneously: the indescribable joy that a mother feels in clasping her newborn to her breast, and the heart-rending pain of knowing that this baby had been wrenched from her own mother, in a 'factory-farming' facility where lions are bred as trophies . . . At that moment, I made a solemn pact with this baby lioness: I vowed I would not rest until I had freed her from the canned hunting camp and returned her to the land that was her birthright: Timbavati.

I will never forget Credo Mutwa's words, when I informed him of this cub's arrival. He said, "Ah! She has come. The One the African elders have been waiting for: Marah, Mother of Ra, the sun god."

At the time of this book first going to press in 2001, the situation in respect to predator farming and hunting in South Africa was bleak, and the treatment of the earth's most precious animals was nothing less than reprehensible. By 2010, the time of this book's republication, the situation is somewhat better – and somewhat worse. After more than a decade of campaigning, together with other animal rights groups and conservationists, I was relieved when the South African government finally prohibited canned lion hunting in 2009. But by this time, approximately 4,000 lions had been bred for killing, and their fate is yet to be determined. If we take the shamanic view that for every lion killed, a human soul will be lost – we are left with the picture of a soul-less consumer society.

However, over this past decade many more thousands of people have committed to an enlightened and responsible way of living in love and respect for Mother Earth, and they are actively following their soul's path.

The White Lion message – nature's message – is unfolding at this very moment. It is radiant. It is magnificent. And it is not too late.

We all know what is needed. We need to protect the White Lions, just as we need to protect all forms of life on our planet. We need to stop damaging our planet. We need to start seeing the signs being shown to us in each and every aspect of our natural world. We need to start taking responsibility for the state of our earth. We need to stop walking blindly into our self-created doom. We need to stand still for a moment – and start *waking up*.

Our route toward spiritual evolution is radiantly clear. We all have our own unique individual journey to walk toward enlightenment. Living on the brink of evolutionary change means that new ground is being broken and new consciousness is being raised. Truth is of the essence – we have no dogma, no set formula, no prescribed rules, no false standards to follow. All we have is the truth within our souls. I believe most of us want to follow the light, the path of healing and not destroying our earth, but we don't have the courage, the lion heart, to follow our individual truth toward enlightenment. Giving in to our fears, we bury our "gold" beneath the false value systems of our societies, and we attempt to comfort ourselves with the notion that we have no power or responsibility for what is happening to our world.

The reality is that, potentially, we all have the power of light – the White Lion – within us. The very first step is to overcome our fears. Thereafter, our hearts will lead the way.

Until we realign ourselves with the forces of light, of sunlight, of light energy that breathes the very word *life* to each and every life form on this planet, we are aligning ourselves with darkness. Until we reinstate, within our own lives, the sacred geometry and divine principles of balance and harmony in accordance with the natural laws of the sun we are inevitably plunging ourselves into appalling upheaval and chaos. The cosmic laws of our universe are meaningful and profoundly logical; it is we humans, rather, who have lost our divine logic.

In the dark and challenging days that lie ahead, there are two truths we should never forget in our quest for golden enlightenment. The lion is the symbol of the soul essence of humankind. And the soul is eternal.

POSTSCRIPT

And the sun god said: "You are no longer alive, Mbube, but your soul shall remain up here amongst the stars until the end of time. You will be one with the stars, and guide the fate of many people on earth."
– CREDO MUTWA, ON THE CREATION OF THE LEO CONSTELLATION IN THE HEAVENS

Early in the new millennium, Credo Mutwa and I re-established contact. Increasingly, people are making pilgrimages from all over the world to see Mutwa. When I questioned him about what I had heard, in channeled information, concerning his identity as "the eldest Son of Ra," he chuckled and replied, "Would the Son of Ra really have his bottom beaten by his nasty stepmother?"

Despite obstacles, he is attempting to commit further oral material to print. His health is frail, but stable.

On 22 April 2001, on the eve of this book's South African publication, Maria of Timbavati passed away. its, I found this devastatingly sad timing. It seems she was not due to receive the recognition she so dearly deserved in her lifetime. I have come to believe, however, as Maria herself did, that lions and lionesses of God are able to work even more powerfully for good from the ancestral realms.

PUBLISHER'S UPDATE: MARAH'S STORY

In 2002, Linda Tucker founded the **Global White Lion Protection Trust** to protect both the White Lions, which remained under threat by the trophy-hunting industry, and the indigenous knowledge which holds these animals sacred.

In 2003, Linda teamed up with lion ecologist Jason Turner and together with their advisors from the **Global White Lion Protection Trust,** they managed to secure the freedom of Marah from the canned hunting camp, against formidable odds. For a period after her rescue, Marah had to be housed in a zoo, and this institution was, in turn, reluctant to release her, because she was identified as a prime genetic specimen for breeding. Once again, Linda Tucker and her trusted team had to secure Marah's freedom.

While a battle took place over the guardianship of Marah, the beautiful lioness gave birth to her first litter of snow-white cubs, in a concrete cell. They were named Regeus, Letaba, and Zihra by the ancestral elders, their names meaning "first ray of sunlight" in three different root languages, although they would not see the sun for the next nine months.

Through legal action, the White Lion Trust ensured that Marah was allowed to raise her cubs herself, without human handling or imprinting, because this was vital for their rewilding process. It was now no longer a campaign simply for Marah's freedom but also for the freedom of her three precious cubs. They were Marah's lineage, and Linda could not abandon them to a lifetime of captivity. Finally, the White Lion Trust won the long battle, and mother and all three cubs were flown from the zoo to a safe haven in the Karoo mountain lands. This was made possible because of the extraordinary love and patronage of Mireille Vince, one of the White Lion Trust's first patrons, who was prepared to put up the funding for all four lions.

However, the safe haven was simply the next step in Marah's long walk to freedom. Since Timbavati is the only endemic birthplace of the White Lions, Linda was committed to returning them to their natural range.

The next monumental step was the acquisition of strategic tracts of land in the Timbavati region identified by African elders as the Sacred Heartland of the White Lions, where the Marah and her cubs' reintroduction could safely take place.

Many institutions housing the White Lions in captivity maintain that these genetic rarities could never survive in the wild. Marah proved them wrong when she learned to hunt and provide for her cubs only weeks after her release into her wild habitat.

Today, Linda Tucker lives in this White Lion protected area, together with her two prides, free-roaming in their natural habitat. Marah's two sons now form part of an integrated pride having bonded with two golden lionesses from that region; while Marah's daughter, Zihra, has her own pride of three snow-white cubs, their father a magnificent male of another genetic bloodline.

The day after Marah and her cubs were released in 2005, natural occurrences of White Lion births started being recorded in the greater Timbavati region.

Linda is working with the indigenous Tsonga people to have a White Lion heritage site declared, and she continues to campaign for the White Lions' protection. In 2009, the South African government finally agreed to prohibit the notorious canned hunting industry. However, the White Lions remain unprotected by law – regionally, nationally, or internationally – and tragically, even today, these rare animals may be legally hunted in the wilds of Timbavati.

In her role as "Keeper of the White Lions," Linda continues Maria Khosa's work as a lion shaman. She has established a school of Sacred Warriorship together with Andrew Harvey and The Institute of Sacred Activism, which applies the ancient universal laws of lion shamanism in redressing the all-encompassing crisis of our day. It will have its first sessions on White Lion territories in March 2011 (see **www.whitelions.org** and **www .instituteofsacredactivism.org**).

ACKNOWLEDGMENTS

My heartfelt thanks to the many lionhearted people who have made this book, and the consequent White Lion conservation work, possible. First and foremost, Jason Turner, my partner, a lion ecologist who dedicated his life and expertise to protecting the White Lions through scientific research and by ensuring this rare animal's reintroduction into its endemic habitat. Jen and Pat Turner for their unconditional support at all times. My sister Mae and my family for their unwavering enthusiasm and support for my cause throughout the years.

Sheryl Leach and Mireille Vince, my godmother, for supporting the foundation of the White Lion sanctuary and Heritage Lands, while also providing the "ransom money" to free the most sacred animals on earth. Ray and Liz Vince for assisting me in building on these foundations. Ileen Maisel, Jane McGregor, Andrew Harvey, and Jill Angelo for seeing the importance of this book and dedicating their expertise to the next steps in getting its message to a greater audience. Organisations and individuals such as Howard Rosenfield, Martin Bornman, Brad Laughlin, Lesley-Temple Thurston, Ruth Underwood, Jen Gardy, Mike Booth (Aurasoma), Gillian Keane (Dandelion Trust), Vance Martin (Wild Foundation), Stephen Pomeroy (Remarkable Group), Stephen Leigh (Leigh Group), Paul Saayman – leading lights among the many who have supported this book and its principles in establishing a safe haven for the White Lions in their natural and spiritual homelands.

There are many people who have selflessly assisted my conservation and community upliftment work. Amongst them, my particular thanks goes to the advisors of the **Global White Lion Protection Trust**, Dr Ian Player, Don MacRobert, Harold Posnik, Marianne van Wyk, Coenraad Jonker, Adv. Nkosi Pathekile Holomisa, M.P. Mninwa Mahlangu, Hosi Solly Sekhororo, and other traditional leaders in South Africa. Among the many indigenous elders from other continents who have given their approval to the content of these pages, I would like to acknowledge, with eternal gratitude Dr Apela Colerado (Oneida People, Hawaii), Retired High Chief Francois Paulette (Dene People, Canada), Dr E. Richard Atleo (Nuu-chah-nul People, Canada), Mother Moon (Chippewa People, Ojibwa Nation, America), Jan Si Ku (Ku Koi San People, southern Africa), Angaangaq Lyberth (Inuit People, Greenland), and Ilarion lmerculieff (Aleut People, Alaska). My eternal thank-you to the many shamans, primarily Maria Khosa, Credo Vusamazula Mutwa, Baba Mathaba, Selby Gumbi, Mathabi Nyedi, and Wilberforce Maringa, who have lent an authentic voice to the protection of the White

Lions as a sacred animal of global importance. Wynter Worsthorne, Anna Breytenbach, Amelia Kinkade, Jackie Freemantle, and others who have supported this project and its principles by upholding and practising responsible and loving animal communication techniques on White Lion territories. Wendy Strauss, Karen-Jane Dudley, Connie Neubold, Berit Brusletto, Philippa Hankinson, Alison Effting, Jane Bell, Steffie Betts, Wendy Hardie, Linda Hall, Kathy Pierce, Mary Selby, Lianne Cox, Sharon Brett, Michelle Stewart, and the extended pride of dedicated lionesses who selflessly support this project from different corners of the globe. Nelson Mathebula, Nelias and Winnah Ntete, Xolani Ngewu, Amon Mashile and Patrick Mkansi, the security officers, and our whole team and staff who serve the protection of the White Lions on the ground. Rob Thompson, Chris Job, Lindie Serrurier, Leander Gaum, and the many dedicated enviro-lawyers who have generously given their time and expertise to the White Lion cause. A battle-weary thank-you to the many individuals and organizations who have united over many years in campaigning for the abolishment of canned hunting, amongst them Gareth Patterson, Karen Trendler, Paul Hart, Greg McKewen, and Mike Cadman.

Finally, my gratitude to Michelle Pilley, Patty Gift, and all the other people at my publisher, **Hay House,** for seeing the true value of the White Lions; and for taking my message, as the White Lions' protector and representative, to the world.

ENDNOTES

For more information about the topics discussed in *Mystery of the White Lions,* please see page 307 for a list of the appendices that are available online.

Chapter 1: Timbavati

1. Sirius is the star that follows the constellation of Orion. It has central importance for many ancient cultures, including those of Africa.

Chapter 2: Maria, Lion Queen of Timbavati

1. Traditional snuff powder, such as *buchu,* or even commercial snuff, is sniffed by African shamans as a means of clearing the route to the ancestral realm.
2. Such a belief, so foreign to my own Western background, seemed to account for the ritualized ingestion of lion parts, such as the heart or spleen, by primitive tribes seeking to take on the identity of the beast.

Chapter 3: Lions of God: People of Lion Identity

1. See the works of David Lewis-Williams, Thomas Dowson, and Peter Garlake, which are now matched by similar theories in respect of the prehistoric paintings in Europe, such as those of Lascaux, France.
2. In considering the subject of shamanism, Ken Wilber employs the term *typhonic* for any hybrid human–animal figure, the same term he employs to describe the mode of consciousness that characterized Paleolithic times. See *Up from Eden.* I choose the more commonly used *therianthropic* to describe the same notion.
3. Frazer reports the same phenomenon, observing that "The prevailing belief amongst African tribes . . . is that their ruling chiefs live on as lions." *The Golden Bough,* vol. 2, p.287.
4. For a comparative discussion of the hierarchical relationship between lion chief, lion shaman, and Lion Ancestral Spirit in the Mashona tribes around Great Zimbabwe, see Bourdillon's *The Shona Peoples:* "The territorial proprietorship of the lion spirits of a chiefdom . . . concern the land and its fertility rather than the care of individual persons" (p.255). He says that, as always, lion and ruler are interchangeable: "The lion spirits exercise their control over their territory by appointing and maintaining the chief of the country."
5. There is also a Tibetan lion-headed goddess called Senge-dong-ma and the Egyptian lion-headed goddess Sekhmet, as well as the feline-riding Hindu earth goddess Doorgah.

6. Laurens van der Post, "The Other Side of Silence," lecture delivered at the World Wilderness Congress, published under the title *Voices of the Wilderness*, p.9.

7. *Song of the Stars*, p.59. *Abangafi* means "they who do not die," and *Bapakade* means "they of all eternity." According to Mutwa, this term is incorrectly given as *Abangafi Bakafi* in *Song of the Stars*.

8. Alan Oken, *Complete Astrology*, rev. ed., p.94.

9. Sometimes spelled Nrisimha. See Nicholas Campion and Steve Eddy, *The New Astrology*, p.52.

10. Most dictionaries give a similar explanation, e.g., *Oxford English Dictionary, Advanced Learners,* 4th ed.

11. In Gareth Patterson's book *With My Soul Amongst Lions,* he gives a few accounts of intimate experiences that suggest communication with the lion spirit realm. See his account of Batian, his beloved hand-reared lion, killed by humans, whose collar reappeared on the second anniversary of his death, pp.152–153.

12. See Evan Hadingham, *Lines to the Mountain Gods: Nazca and the Mysteries of Peru*, section headed "When Men Turn into Jaguars," p.270.

13. Various practices, such as murder for body parts (known as "muti-killing"), continues today, and is given ghoulish prominence in the press.

14. See, for instance, the Assyrian cylinder in the British Museum. That these lion goddesses have the star as their symbol is of central import.

Chapter 4: Lion Priest of Africa

1. Watson, *Return of the Moon: Versions from the /Xam*. All Bushman quotes in epigraphs are from this work.

2. Note that the Freemasons' secret handshake is described in similar terms: "the Lion's Paw or the Eagle's Claw grip, which is given by taking a firm hold on the sinews of the wrist of the right hand with the points of the fingers." Knight and Lomas, *The Hiram Key*, p.16.

3. In the context of South Africa's sensitive race relations, Mutwa's beliefs (derived from his oral knowledge) have contributed to his notoriety.

4. The Bushmen experience the psychic power of trance, *Kia*, as invisible arrows that are being shot into their bodies from the spirit world. Invisible "arrows of potency" were believed to activate shamanic powers. See Katz, *Boiling Energy*, and Garlake, *The Hunter's Vision: Prehistoric Art of Zimbabwe*, p.144.

5. Mutwa recounts the story of Mageba in detail in his published animal tales, entitled *Isilwane, the Animal: Tales and Fables of Africa*, pp.152–153.

Chapter 5: Credo: The Word of Africa

1. Mutwa, *Song of the Stars*, p.57.

2. As De Santillana puts it, "a shaman is elected by the spirits, meaning that he cannot choose his profession." *Hamlet's Mill*, p.122.

3. Mutwa, *op. cit.*, p.59.

4. Great healers responsible for Mutwa's training and initiation, according to Mutwa, include

Myna Mkhaliphi, Telaphakathi Zwane, Mankanyezi Jabane, Chikerema, Chiringa Mwesi, and Simbasultani Mutsoni.

5. See his dedication in *Song of the Stars.*
6. Mutwa, *Indaba, My Children*, Introduction (Kahn & Averill ed.).
7. Ibid., Introduction, ix.
8. Ibid., xiii.
9. *Song of the Stars*, p.61.
10. *Drum* Magazine, vol. 310, 13 August 1998, p.43.
11. Ibid.
12. *Song of the Stars*, p.44.
13. Ibid.
14. Ibid., p.65.
15. Ibid.
16. The term is borrowed from Jung and refers to an archetype of the shaman who heals others through his own suffering. This takes on particular relevance in respect of the White Lions, and the comparison might be made with Christ himself, the great healer who suffered for humankind's sins.
17. Mutwa, *Song of the Stars*, p.83.
18. *Twak* also means snuff or tobacco, a common ingredient in preparations used by shamans to cross into the spirit world.
19. On the Bushmen as the first true humans, see H.J. Deacon and Janette Deacon, *Human Beginnings in South Africa: Uncovering the Secrets of the Stone Age*, in particular the chapter entitled "The First True Humans." The ancestors of today's surviving Bushmen, known to paleoanthropologists as "proto-Khoisan," have been shown by genetic, linguistic, and archeological evidence to have been the first true *Homo sapiens* to walk this earth, appearing in Southern Africa from about 140,000 years ago.
20. For shocking documentation, photographs, and archive records of the systematic destruction of the Bushmen communities, see Skotnes, *Miscast: Negotiating the Presence of the Bushmen, passim.*
21. The antbear or pangolin is considered a sacred animal, symbolic of the *sangoma.*
22. It would be incorrect to call the traditional guardians of tribal history a "brotherhood," because in the Great African Tradition, a matriarchal system of inherited knowledge applies equally.
23. Mutwa, *Indaba, My Children*, viii (Kahn & Averill ed.).
24. Van der Post, *The Lost World of the Kalahari*, p.224.

Chapter 6: Hunter or Hunted?

1. It may be of interest to note that leopards and baboons still share the same caves in many parts of Southern Africa, and their relationship is one of relentless animosity – leopards kill baboons; baboons gang up against leopards. See Eugène Marais's *The Soul of the Ape* and Lawrence Green's *Karoo.*
2. Chatwin, *The Songlines*, p.284.
3. Ibid., p.283.
4. Ibid., p.284.

5. In Africa, *Homo erectus* has recently been classified as *Homo ergaster*; however, for the purposes of discussion of bipedalism, I prefer to use the term *erectus*.

6. Leakey, *The Making of Mankind*, p.58.

7. Ibid., p.61.

8. Brain, *The Hunters or the Hunted?*, p.273. While espousing the notion of the predatory origins of our species, the picture at the Sterkfontein site has since become more complicated, with Member 5 revealing several different layers.

9. Ibid.

10. See the conclusions to C.K. Brain's lecture entitled "Do We Owe Our Intelligence to a Predatory Past?", presented to the James Arthur series on the evolution of the human brain, New York, 2000.

11. Mutwa, *Song of the Stars*, p.81.

12. Ibid., p.82.

13. Ibid.

14. Ibid., p.83.

15. Brain, *op. cit.*, p.273.

16. Ibid., p.3.

17. In the story, a jackal (the traditional trickster figure) plays a key role in stealing the fire tools and giving them to man.

18. Mutwa, *op. cit.*, p90.

19. Ibid., p.94.

Chapter 7: Great Hunters and Mighty Predators

1. Mutwa, *Isilwane, the Animal*, p.35.

2. For more on the symbolism of the cat in world culture, see Saunders, *Animal Spirits*, pp.70–71.

3. Mutwa explored the quarry site together with Adrian Boshier, anthropologist (and subject of Lyall Watson's book *Lightning Bird*). Known as "wonder stone" for its heat-resistant properties, the pyropheline rock was quarried and utilized by the former South African Defence Force in rockets (as a buffer against metal melting) and in the lining of high-temperature kilns. In the course of quarrying, possibly as many as 200 golf-sized balls were discovered embedded in the pyrophelite. One of these balls is still in the possession of the Klerksdorp Museum. Further indication that this is an important site is demonstrated by the fact that the quarry mound was formerly decorated by ancient Bushman engravings – some of which are also preserved in the Klerksdorp Museum.

4. This theoretical assertion has its counterpart in the revolutionary scientific research of Giorgio de Santillana, the respected historian and anthropologist who risked his academic reputation by publishing a highly controversial work, together with his student, Hertha von Dechend, entitled *Hamlet's Mill: An Essay on Myth and the Frame of Time*. The complexity of the subject matter and originality of the approach made it inaccessible to a larger readership. Only today, since popularizers such as Graham Hancock have taken up his theories, is the true value of Santillana's research beginning to be recognized. Santillana spent his life probing archeological sites for the origins of scientific thought, and concluded that these

could be traced back to a lost Neolithic civilization which displayed prodigious feats of intellect and technological sophistication: a race of "Newtons and Einsteins long forgotten." More controversially still, Santillana views shamans (initiates into ancient wisdom and arcane practices) as an offshoot of this ancient civilization.

5. Frazer, *The Golden Bough*, pp.221–223. Also see Frazer on how the contents of the stomach of the Bushman hunter influenced the chase, p.495.

6. In the film *The Great Dance*, Craig Foster plants a couple of seeds of the future film on lion shamanism which we intend making with Richard Wicksteed.

7. Liebenberg, *The Art of Tracking*, Introduction, p.ix. In later discussions with Liebenberg, he explained his belief that endurance hunting (tracking and stalking a particular prey continually for days at a time) eventually induces a trance state. Understandably, at this point of physical exhaustion, with the sustained concentrated focus on the prey, the hunter feels virtually inextricable from the animal he has hunted.

8. Garlake, *The Hunter's Vision*, p.145.

9. Mutwa, *My People*, p.121.

10. Compare this and the other tusked lion paintings such as those at Coerland and Cloclolan.

11. See, for instance, tomb of Rameses VI, where lions are depicted in guarding positions at the queen's feet.

12. See the sequence in the northern frieze of the Temple of Hatshepsut.

13. Balandier and Macquet, *Dictionary of Black African Civilization*, p.215.

Chapter 8: The White Lions According to the Great Knowledge

1. Mutwa, *Isilwane*, p.16.

2. Ibid.

3. Ibid., pp.15–16.

4. There are limited records of the hunting and poaching that took place. For some background, see the article "Timbavati's Heritage Triumphs over Poaching," *(Toronto) Star*, 26 June 1991.

5. For one of many articles on the coelacanth discovery, see *Mail & Guardian* (Johannesburg), 9–15 February 2001, p.5.

6. Mutwa, *Indaba, My Children*, p.vii (Kahn & Averill ed.). For mention of the "High Curse" that befalls those who change the oral knowledge, see viii. Bear in mind, however, that the English translation makes certain adaptations.

7. The snow-white eland with a single horn evokes the mythical creature we know as the unicorn. Mutwa later told me its name in the Great Tradition is Mbuti Yanebange. This legendary animal is depicted in Bushman paintings – see Knox-Shaw, "Unicorns on Rocks: The Expressionism of Olive Schreiner," *English Studies in Africa* 40, no. 2 (1997): 13–32.

8. Mutwa later identified the date of 1906, after the Zulu rebellion, in which Dinizulu had suffered great personal injuries under the British. Dinizulu was given the white *kaross* by Bapedi traders as compensation for his beatings.

9. It is possible that the knowledge rather than the stones themselves were carried from Zimbabwe to Timbavati. When I posed this question to Mutwa, he allowed that this might have been the case.

10. Interestingly, the wolf is not an African animal, unlike the hyena or jackal.

Chapter 9: White Lion Genetics

1. McBride, *The White Lions of Timbavati*, p.113.
2. The spot where McBride first discovered the White Lions, roughly speaking in the middle of the Timbavati region, is a location known today as Vlakgesigt, approximately 24°S 22'; 31°E 20´.
3. McBride, *op. cit.*, p.54.
4. Ibid., p.56.
5. Ibid., p.114.
6. Ibid.
7. Ibid., p.112.
8. For more on cometary debris prompting genetic mutations, see Robert Ardrey and others who proposed links between meteorite activity and genetic leaps in human evolution. In his book *African Genesis*, Ardrey relates the so-called brain explosion to a meteorite or small asteroid that exploded over the Indian Ocean around 700,000 years ago.

Chapter 10: Great Zimbabwe: Resting Place of the Lion

1. See, for instance, an article in the London *Times* of 5 March 1951: "The natives who lived in that dark corner of Africa were no more capable of working as skilfully in stone as the forgotten architects of Zimbabwe than they were of constructing a Cape to Cairo railway."
2. President Robert Mugabe, for instance, claims to be directly descended from the original dynasty that built Great Zimbabwe.
3. There may be parallels with the mysterious bearded travelers who brought wisdom to the world, according to ancient legends in many cultures.
4. Mutwa compared the style of this sword to a Bushman painting in the Brandburg Mountains, the famous "White Lady," which he maintains holds clues to the Zimbabwe story.
5. Some scholars translate *Monomotapa* as meaning "Lord of the Mines" – see Hall and Neal, *The Ancient Ruins of Rhodesia*, xiii; Keane, in *The Gold of Ophir*, writes that *tapa* means to dig or excavate – therefore mine. According to Mutwa, this is incorrect. The original word, he says, derives from *Mwene Mutaba*, "King of the Whole World."
6. For more detail, see *Indaba, My Children*. In it, Mutwa refers to Zimbabwe in distasteful and shameful terms, describing it as "a place we must forget." According to his knowledge, "Bad, immoral things were done in this place," the original name of which he identifies as Luvijiti, a cursed title. In echoes of the Atlantis story, Mutwa described how, prior to its total destruction, the great civilization of Zima-Mbje declined into decadence, slavery, and bestiality. By way of example, Mutwa cites cross-species breeding attempts to mate the finest maidens together with lions, with a view to producing a super-race which combined leonine courage and ferocity with human intelligence. Such genetic engineering practices between the royal bloodline and the king of the beasts seriously debases the nobler message inherent in the lion shamanism (*Indaba, My Children*, Kahn & Averill ed., p.70). While these practices might seem remote from our modern context, they may have relevance for the dangers of genetic engineering and notions of breeding a super-race that have surfaced in our day.
7. The National Monuments Commission of Rhodesia published their findings in an *Occa-*

sional Paper of National Museums in 1961. C.K. Cooke, director of the Historical Monuments Commission, represents the orthodox view still held today: "From the scientific excavation in 1906 until the present day nothing has been found that proves anything but of African origin for the whole complex of ruins."

8. See, for instance, the London *Times*, 5 March 1951: Zimbabwe is referred to as "a cluster of glorified kraals erected only at a comparatively recent date."

9. See Keane, *The Gold of Ophir, passim.*

10. See Hall and Neal, and Johnson, *passim.*

11. See, for example, Genesis 10.

12. See Keane, x, for commentary on Zimbabwe's possible link with King Solomon and the Queen of Sheba.

13. Mutwa later informed me that the Land of Punt is in present-day Botswana.

14. See Keane, also Peters and his speculations on the statuette of Thotmes III (nephew of Queen Hatshepsut) in the London *Times,* 20 August 1901.

15. Keane, *The Gold of Ophir*, p.33.

16. Cooke, *The Ancient Ruins of Rhodesia* (reprint ed.), Foreword.

17. In their comprehensive investigation of the smelting sites, Hall and Neal conclude that the ancient goldsmith's craft was pre-eminently more sophisticated than in the more recent period – see *The Ancient Ruins of Rhodesia*, Chapter VII.

18. For a detailed account of the controversy surrounding the Golden Rhino of Mapungubwe, see the South African Broadcasting Corporation's documentary *Mapungubwe: Secret of the Sacred Hill*, 1999, produced by Katerina Weineck and Lance Gewer.

19. See, for instance, the London *Times*, 5 March 1951.

20. Much of De Barros's original text is translated by Keane in *The Gold of Ophir.*

21. De Barros in Keane, *The Gold of Ophir*, pp.3–6.

22. Mutwa, *Isilwane*, fable entitled "How the Cat Came to Live with Human Beings," p.35.

Chapter 11: Zimba: Golden Lion Shrine

1. See, for instance, Marsh, *Unsolved Mysteries of Southern Africa*, p.74.

2. The roots of this word appear in Sanskrit: *simha* meaning "lion." See Vishnu's incarnation as man-lion Narasimhu in Saunders, *Animal Spirits*, p.29.

3. The historical relationship between Mapungubwe and Zimbabwe is well established. They are believed to be sites of the same culture, which shifted its capital.

4. Summers, in *Ancient Mining in Rhodesia*, argues that gold mining probably started there in the AD 8th century and continued into the 17th century. This contradicts the notion that the Egyptians and King Solomon obtained their gold from Zimbabwe.

5. Unfortunately, Mutwa's book on the Lembas is one of many of his works that remain unpublished.

6. Tudor Parfitt took genetic samples from the Lemba, which, after testing by biologists in London, revealed that the Lembas' genealogy was directly related to that of the Hadramaut Yemeni Jews. Saunders, "Invisible races," p.90.

7. For more details, see Gareth Patterson's *exposé, Dying to be Free: The Canned Lion Scandal.*

8. Parfitt, *Journey to the Vanished Land*, p.180.

9. Ibid., p.107.
10. Ibid., pp.158–159.

Chapter 12: Lion Priests and Eagle Shamans

1. Mutwa here alludes to Hamlet's words to the rationalist Horatio.
2. See this practice described in *Isilwane*, p.21.
3. See Campion and Eddy, *The New Astrology*, p.52.
4. The wild lioness symbol is widely associated with the Earth Mother, the *magna mater.* See Cirlot, *Dictionary of Symbols*, p.182.
5. For more on Horus as the solar lion-hawk god, see Wallis Budge, *Gods of the Egyptians*, *passim.*
6. Mutwa pointed out a number of goddesses in the Egyptian pantheon who are undeniably African in appearance. Others, such as John Anthony West, have pointed out the negroid features of the Sphinx itself.
7. Professor Barry Fell (of the International Epigraphic Society of California, known for his work in deciphering the Easter Island inscriptions), who was shown this artefact by Mutwa, confirmed its authenticity, but was unable to decipher the texts comprehensively. Fell believed the message might be related to the ten commandments.
8. For the significance of dolphins and whales as "record keepers" in the Great African Tradition, see Mutwa's article, "Born under African skies," *Drum* 203 (November 1996): 24.
9. The temple, says Mutwa, was located in Venda (also on the Giza–Timbavati meridian).
10. See, for instance, Summers, *Ancient Mining in Rhodesia.* Using evidence based on isotope testing of samples from the site, he concludes: "It is impossible for any scientist or archaeologist to accept theories giving dates of thousands of years ago to any phase of the Zimbabwe building, and for the same reason they reject the idea of a link with the Queen of Sheba or Solomon." Also, the London *Times* article, 5 March 1951.
11. Epigraphy is the study and classification of ancient inscriptions.
12. See article on Mutwa's "sacred tablet" in *Epigraphic Society Occasional Publication* 12, no. 284 (1984). The "Talking Stone" is also referred to as *Twe ya bula bula.*
13. According to Mutwa, these are the people who call themselves the Balubetu or Bashapa.
14. According to Hermetic doctrine, it appears that there are two Sirian star seeds, the whale/dolphin people and the lion people. The whale and dolphin people are the symbol of the first four "ages" of man. The lion is the symbol of the Fifth Race in the Fifth Age – as well as the races of past and future ages. See the lion–star connection in "Solomon's seal" or "Solomon's shield" in medieval Jewish mysticism, Liungman, *Dictionary of Symbols*, p.298. For more on the importance of the lion in Solomon's temple, see Gilbert, *Signs in the Sky.*
15. See Bell, *Somewhere over the Rainbow*, p.198. Describing the Venda area, the author refers to *sangoma* and traditional healer Mashudu Dima, who describes a White Lion that protects the Thathe Vondo forest, explaining that "You can hear him roar at midnight, but you cannot see him." Bell recounts: "The story goes that a chief called Nethathe had been a magician with the power to transform himself into animals to watch his people. Since lions were feared more than any other creature, his spirit naturally assumed this form to guard his burial place."

Chapter 13: Underground River of Gold

1. The Shilluk people, a tribe in southern Sudan, also have a myth of their great king, Reth, being born of a river goddess and the sky god Nyikang. He fights a battle with the sun, and divides the waters of the White Nile – thus the dual interface between river and sky is evoked. These North African people also lived alongside the Nile itself, albeit thousands of kilometers from Giza.

2. Bauval and Gilbert, *The Orion Mystery*, p.124.

3. See, for instance, Cirlot, *Dictionary of Symbols*, p.190. Also on the lion symbol linked with gold and with water, see Bailey, *The Caves of the Sun*, pp.139–143.

4. See, for instance, mining engineer Telford Edwards's "Gold Production in Matabeleland," *Bulawayo Chronicle*, 26 June 1897, and Keane, *The Gold of Ophir*. Also, Hall and Neal, *The Ancient Ruins of Rhodesia,* which argued that the goldfields of Monomotapa were the centre of gold production and export to civilizations such as Egypt and Arabia. Scholars early in the last century, citing numerous extracts from the Old Testament, concluded: "One thing which appeared to be established beyond doubt was that [Zimbabwe was,] one thousand years before the Christian Era, a gold-producing country of a large extent, and colonised by the early Semitic races round the Red Sea, viz., the Jews, Phoenicians and Western Arabians." Hall and Neal, p.32. The precise dating of gold production, however, remains contentious to this day.

5. For detailed descriptions of ancient gold-smelting apparatus in the Zimbabwe area, see Hall and Neal, *The Ancient Ruins of Rhodesia.*

6. *Minerals Yearbook*, Area Reports, International United States Government Printing Office, 1999, p.SS2.

7. Translated by Keane, *The Gold of Ophir*, pp.3–4.

8. Quoted by Keane, *The Gold of Ophir*, p.15.

9. See the breakdown of gold production in the years 1943–1947 in William van Royen, *Mineral Resources of the World*, pp.125–127. In 1970, South Africa produced 68 percent of the world's gold; see *Minerals Yearbook*.

Chapter 14: Winged Lion of Timbavati

1. In some versions of the Bible the word *heart* is replaced by *mind*.

2. I would later discover that Count Saint-Germain and Serapis Bey are titles given to spirit entities (known as ascendant masters) believed to be guiding events in the physical world from the ancestral spirit world.

Chapter 15: Playing God with the Sun God's Children

1. Daniel 6:23.

2. Siegfried and Roy embarked on the white tiger project two decades ago when they met the Maharajah of Rewa, the dignitary responsible for the preservation of Indian Wildlife. Typically, the Maharajah's royal ancestry was associated with felines. Rather than lions, the royal coat of arms traditionally depicted sacred tigers. Interestingly, the tigers were snow white.

Note that European heraldry also shows White Lions, e.g., the White Lion of Mortimer bearing a Yorkist badge – the white rose *"en soleil."* The lion is depicted holding a shield which is "emblazoned with another Yorkist badge, the white *rose en soleil,"* and is shown against a sun, the badge of the king. Like the Timbavati lions, the mythical white tiger was a phantom species believed to be the reincarnation of the gods, and had been the subject of legend and myth long before its sudden appearance. Upon discovering a white tiger cub in the forests of Rewa in 1951, the Maharajah took it home to his 120-room palace and gardens, which became the royal tigers' breeding grounds. His son, the present Maharajah, approached Siegfried and Roy in the 1970s with the idea of a joint breeding project.

A further contribution of the joint breeding project is that analysis of the hereditary patterns of both the Las Vegas and Johannesburg cubs can be systematically undertaken: a process of genetically fingerprinting every lion born, which may assist in unraveling genetic questions and, more pressingly, in offering ways of aiding the white strain's survival. The White Tigers of Rewa represent a corresponding genetic phenomenon to the White Lions of Timbavati: both are the product of an unexplained mutant pigmentation. Like the tawny lions of Timbavati, certain of the golden tigers in Rewa are "heterozygous" – which means that they are white-gene-bearers.

Chapter 16: White Lions and Magic Men

1. Siegfried and Roy's Secret Garden is one of several playgrounds available to the lions, well designed with caves and outcrops, ponds and water fountains, rockeries, palm trees, and rolling lawns. The Jungle Palace is Siegfried and Roy's private home, a spectacular jungle gym of a mansion. Little Bavaria is a sprawling wonderland of natural habitation in which the lions are regularly exercised and let free to roam. The holding facilities, four square kilometers (about one and a half square miles) of pristine animal accommodations are meticulously well planned and organized. These and other factors led Dr Condy to conclude that although Siegfried and Roy are not qualified conservationists in the conventional sense, their husbandry of predators is excellent.

2. Siegfried and Roy (with Annette Tapert), *Mastering the Impossible*, p.15.

3. Ibid.

4. Ibid.

5. "This would not be the first time, nor would it be the last, that I should be thankful to one of my animals for my safety," Roy writes. See the early example of Hexe, his dog, *Mastering the Impossible*, pp.4–5.

6. Ibid.

7. See figures gained on Serengeti lions in David MacDonald, *The Velvet Claw*, p.68.

8. Blythe was discovered in 1932 by ex-U.S. Army pilot George Palmer on a private excursion. Human figures are depicted alongside figures of huge felines, some over 35 meters (about 38 yards) long. These desert drawings, like the famous Nazca plain of southern Peru, were created by scraping off the top surface of gravel so as to reveal the lighter color beneath. They may have existed here for many centuries. It was only in the 20th century, when aviation was invented, that the Blythe site and other similar earth canvases came to light.

9. In a chapter entitled "When Men Turn into Jaguars," Evan Hadington maintains that these

four-legged creatures in the Blythe desert are mountain lions or jaguars, reminding us that "These beasts were among the most important supernatural beings that Mojave healers, or shamans, traditionally attempted to contact through their dreams." Hadingham, *Lines to the Mountain Gods: Nazca and the Mysteries of Peru*, p.270.

Chapter 17: Lion, Star Beast

1. See, for instance, Hadingham, *Lines to the Mountain Gods*, p.272; also discussions of Quetzalcoatl as feathered god of feline origins, Willis, *World Mythology*, p.239.
2. Note the Chinese use of the term *Sza/Tzse!* for the Leo constellation; Campion and Eddy, *The New Astrology*, p.51.
3. Van der Post, *The Heart of the Hunter*, p.46.
4. Regulus is the star at the center of the Leo constellation, also known as *Cor Leonis* – the Lion's Heart; see Campion and Eddy, *The New Astrology*, p.52. Mutwa called this red heart star of Leo "Mthalhinkosi" or "Winsinkosi."
5. This song was made famous by Miriam Makeba and released by Gallo Records around the world. For more on the story see *The Sunday Times*, 4 June 2000, p.5.
6. Mutwa speaks of the zodiac or *Mulu-Mulu* in *Song of the Stars* and in his article "Born under African Skies", *Drum* 203 (November 1996): 22–24, 104–105, 107–109.
7. Hermetic doctrine: "As above, so below." In the great African tradition there are not 12 constellations, but 13. The 13th (Umkhomo, the Whale) is associated with shamanism and other-dimensional reality, termed Indidamadoda, meaning "the puzzler of men." See Mutwa's story of the Wounded Healer Ngoza born under this 13th sign of the zodiac, in *African Signs of the Zodiac*, pp.78–79.
8. Mutwa also associates him with Sozabile, the great hunter and healer of the Sagittarius constellation. For more on Sozabile, see "Born under African Skies."
9. Sirius is known as the "dog star." The Leo constellation is Orion's "friend lion."
10. Sirius is also linked with Valisango, the dog, protector of the *Mulu-Mulu*, or Closer of the Gate, and thus possibly compared with the Sothic Cycle or "dog days" of ancient Egypt. See Credo Mutwa's essay, "Born under African Skies," p.24. Sirius is also referred to as Inja Ebomvu.
11. It also had a reptilian quality. See Icke, *The World's Biggest Secret*. It is important to note that in certain matters of critical importance, Mutwa's disclosures have been misrepresented in Icke's work.
12. In the Great African Tradition, a skull is a sacred object, and not potentially evil as Westerners believe (e.g., the skull and crossbones flag). For recent Western research into this phenomenon, see Morton and Thomas, *The Mystery of the Crystal Skulls*.
13. In 1996, the British Museum of Mankind consulted Credo Mutwa as the authority on more than 5,000 South African artifacts in their possession. Among these are artifacts relating to astronomical knowledge, including an important beaded piece in colored diamond sections used by African astronomer-priests for measuring the months of the year. See reference to this in an article by Benison Makele, "African Soul Still Held Captive in Europe," *City Press*, 22 December 1996.
14. The mythology of the Dogon people in respect of the binary star Sirius was widely publicized by Robert Temple in his best-selling book *The Sirius Mystery*. Also, Griaule, *Conver-*

sations with Ogotemelli. The Dogons' mythology detailed a knowledge of Sirius's invisible companion "dwarf star" (known to astronomers as Sirius B) before it was discovered by Western astronomers.

15. Mutwa spoke to me about certain "star races" in Africa who carry star knowledge – these include the Bushmen, Ndebele, Mashona, Zulu and Dogon.

16. The Zulus say they descended to earth through space. To travel in space is *ukuzulu,* says Mutwa.

17. In the lead-up to the speech, Mutwa had made a comparison between the ravens in England, "the very ugly birds at the Tower of London . . . which have been preserved by the English monarchy for several hundred years. It is said that if these ravens were to perish, then England and her people would cease to exist."

18. According to Mutwa, the notion of reincarnation is a founding belief in old Africa.

Chapter 18: Birthplace of the Gods

1. Quoted in Chatwin, *The Songlines,* p.208.
2. Berendt, *Nada Brahma: The World Is Sound.*
3. See, for instance, the work on stone emission frequencies, e.g., Elkington, *In the Name of the Gods.*
4. West discusses the "Word" in *Serpent in the Sky,* p.69.
5. *Logos* does not just mean "word," it means something more like "law" or "decree," the truth behind natural law; see Gilbert's discussion of this notion in his introduction to *Hermetica: The Writings Attributed to Hermes Trismegistus,* edited and translated by Walter Scott, p.9.
6. See *The Illustrated Bible Dictionary,* p.908.
7. Laurens van der Post, *The Heart of the Hunter,* p.46.
8. Gilbert's investigations into the sacred teachings of the Mesoamericans (*The Mayan Prophecies*) and the ancient Egyptians (*The Orion Mystery*), as well as the unknown origins of more familiar Christian teachings (*Magi* and *The Holy Kingdom*), make him well placed to detect parallels across continents. He relates Mesoamerican cosmology to the Sphinx question, as well as to Christian and ancient Mesopotamian mysteries.
9. See, for instance, the wall relief on Dendera's stairwell, depicting a procession of priests in lion masks in honor of the goddess Sekhmet.
10. Balandier and Macquet, *Dictionary of Black African Civilization,* p.215. For more on priestly lions in temple of Heliopolis, see Spence, *Myths and Legends of Ancient Egypt.*
11. Rundle Clark, *Myth and Symbol in Ancient Egypt,* p.146.
12. For a discussion of Horus, Bast, and Hathor as leonine entities, see West, *The Traveller's Key to Ancient Egypt,* p.394. For the lion symbol in ancient Egypt, associated with Bast and Hathor, the lioness symbol of the Sphinx known as "the Destroyer," see Wallis Budge, *Egyptian Language,* p.61.
13. Rundle Clark, *Myth and Symbol in Ancient Egypt,* p.160.
14. See Bauval and Hancock, *Keeper of Genesis,* pp.71–73. This belief is held by other archeoastronomers such as John Anthony West, Adrian Gilbert, and David Elkington.
15. Bauval and Hancock, *Keeper of Genesis,* pp.230–233; Gilbert, *Magi* and *Signs in the Sky, passim.*

16. For a different angle on the shamanic route of evolution reconciled with the heroic route (Osiris versus Horus), see West's discussion of the two roads of the return to the Source, *Serpent in the Sky*, p.83. For the identification of Osiris and Christ, see Gilbert, *Signs in the Sky*, and Elkington, *In the Name of the Gods, passim*.

17. See Bauval and Hancock's discussion of *Zep Tepi* in *Keeper of Genesis*, p.219.

18. See discussion of hieroglyph *Rwty* and lion deities associated with lion guardians, *Keeper of Genesis*, p.165.

19. See discussion of Atum by Swiss Egyptologist Edouard Naville, as quoted in *Keeper of Genesis*, p.164; also see p.166. The leonine overtones of the key Egyptian luminaries, including the Creator God himself, should be compared with the Mesoamerican pantheons, which are founded on precisely the same feline basis.

20. Wallis Budge, *Egyptian Language*, p.61

21. See, for instance, Gilbert and Bauval's discussion of *Zep Tepi* in *The Orion Mystery*, p.189; also Bauval and Hancock's various discussions in *Keeper of Genesis*, in particular, Chapter 17, and Hassan, *Excavations at Giza*, p.265.

22. For some scientific advancements in the notion of stellar influences on events on earth, see the work of Gribbin and Plagemann, *The Jupiter Effect*, in which possible causal interaction is identified between "the earth, the sun and the Planets." See also the work of Greenwich astronomer Percy Seymour, *Astrology: The Evidence of Science*. For statistical analysis of astrology, see the work of Michel Gauquelin, *Planetary Heredity* and *Cosmic Influences on Human Behavior*. For a defense of astrology see West, *The Case for Astrology*.

Chapter 19: Lion of the Desert; Lions of the Bushveld

1. From the proportions of the Sphinx, West deduces that the present edifice represents a renovation of an original lion sculpture; see *Traveller's Key to Ancient Egypt*.

2. In the metric system, it amounts to 20m high and 11.5m wide.

3. Bauval and Hancock, *Keeper of Genesis*, p.74.

4. Matthew 24:29.

5. Matthew 24:30.

6. See Fontana on the T-cross as *Tau*, *The Secret Language of Symbols*, p.57.

7. See, for instance, *The Shorter Oxford English Dictionary on Historical Principles*, p.453.

8. See *The Illustrated Bible Dictionary*, p.908.

9. See Gilbert, *Signs in the Sky*, Appendix 3, "Lion of God," p.307. Also *Magi*, pp.222–227.

10. Plutarch observed, for instance, that the Egyptians "hold the lion in honor," and they adorn the doorways of their shrines with gaping lion's heads, because the Nile overflows "when for the first time the sun comes into conjunction with Leo."

11. For his reasons behind coming to this conclusion, see Gilbert, *op. cit.*

12. The astronomical-astrological notion of precession remains a key notion in today's astronomy. The astrological "ages" are defined by the period during which a particular constellation – in this case the constellation of Leo – forms the starry backdrop behind the sun at the all-important date of the vernal equinox. Precession (i.e., "precession of the equinoxes") is the apparent movement of the stellar band surrounding the earth, so that the constellations

in this band appear to change approximately every 2,200 years, from one zodiacal constellation to another.

13. Archeoastronomers like Adrian Gilbert, Robert Bauval, and Graham Hancock argue the case for the Giza monuments representing a star map on earth, laid down to specify a critically significant moment in time; see Gilbert's *The Orion Mystery* and *Signs in the Sky*, and Hancock's *Fingerprints of the Gods* and *Heaven's Mirror*.

14. While the stela itself long postdates the Sphinx, the dual lion motif is recognized as one of the oldest archetypes in this region. See, for instance, the research of Egyptian scholar Bassam el Shammaa, Lecture at the Annual Quest for Knowledge Conference, March 1998.

15. On the question of the temple of Solomon in the Southern Hemisphere, Gilbert was particularly helpful. In his book *Signs in the Sky*, he points out that David and his son, Solomon, were the lion kings of the tribe of Judah. Solomon built the first temple in around 900 BC and housed the Ark containing the tablets of Moses bearing the Ten Commandments. (See *Signs in the Sky*, pp.157–158.) Even today, the drapes protecting the Torah show the twin lion symbol, while the six-pointed star of David recalls the six-pointed star of Sirius. See this illustrated in *Signs in the Sky*, opposite p.239. The lion–pentacle connection remains, with the pentagram called Solomon's Seal or Solomon's Shield in medieval Jewish mysticism. See Liungman, *Dictionary of Symbols*, p.298. Based on potsherds in Palestine, this symbol can be dated back to 4000 BC, and it appears as a sign on the official seal of the city of Jerusalem during the period 300–150 BC.

16. Venda, where Mutwa said this temple was located, is located around the Nilotic Meridian.

17. "Sekhmet, in ancient Egypt," West writes, "was portrayed as a female figure with the head of a lioness. In the mythology, it was Sekhmet who meted out Divine vengeance when errant humanity neglected to worship the Gods and took matters into its own unknowing hands. Her destructive rampages were designed to restore rightful order, she was the Goddess who heals . . . but by fire." West, "Sekhmet Speaks," in *Quest for Knowledge* magazine. On legends associating lion-headed gods with the Sphinx, see Hunt-Williamson, *Secret Places of the Lion*, p.21: "The Pyramid was the place of the 'second birth,' the 'womb of the mysteries.' Tradition says that somewhere in its depths resided an unknown being called 'The Dweller.' He was a lion-faced master that few men ever saw."

18. See, for instance, Lawton and Ogilvie-Herald, *Giza: The Truth*, and Bauval, *The Secret Chamber*.

Chapter 20: Nilotic Meridian: Sacred Land of the North; Sacred Land of the South

1. For a concise summary of some of the precision measurements of the Sphinx and pyramids, see Bauval and Hancock, *Keeper of Genesis*, pp.40–44; Hancock, *Fingerprints of the Gods*, Chapter 48; LeMesurier, *Decoding the Great Pyramid, passim*.

2. See LeMesurier, *Decoding the Great Pyramid*, p.12.

3. Ibid., or Hancock and Faiia, *Heaven's Mirror*, p.54.

4. See this laid out schematically in Alford, *When the Gods Came Down*, p.146.

5. Tompkins, *Secrets of the Great Pyramid*, p.46.

6. Geologically speaking, the Nile carved its bed and formed its Delta relatively recently – that is, only during the Quaternary period. Deposits left on the riverbanks testify to the fact that

in the previous geological epoch – the so-called Tertiary – the Mediterranean engulfed the Nile Valley, flowing in as far as Aswan, Egypt, like a narrow fjord. See Schwaller de Lubicz, *Sacred Science*, p.945. Schwaller de Lubicz alerts us to significant geological aberrations in respect of the Nile. He speaks of the "unbroken tradition" concerning the alluvial origin of the Delta and the existence of a maritime gulf before the ushering in of the earth by the Nile, which finally submerged the Sphinx in silt. Mutwa's "Great Knowledge" may be part of this unbroken oral tradition.

7. More precisely, Sokar's southern border is 24°N (and 6′) while Timbavati's northern border is 24°S (and approximately 11′). Therefore, Timbavati's northern border correlates with the latitudinal location of Mapungubwe (30°E, 24°S).

8. Most poignantly, the canned trophy project on Timbavati's borders where the White Lions are being bred and trophy-hunted is located on exactly the 31°14′ E. This reprehensible practice of breeding lions for killing is discussed in more detail in Chapter 24.

9. Much has been made in recent times of the fact that one of the two southern "star shafts" of the Great Pyramid is targeted on Sirius. See Bauval and Gilbert, *The Orion Mystery*, and Hancock and Bauval, *Keeper of Genesis*. Sirius is the bright star on which the Egyptian calendrical system is based, the so-called Sothic calendar. According to Mutwa, life on earth originated from the Sirius planetary system.

10. Orion is associated with the creative deity Matsieng, who also brought lions to earth. Mutwa told me that there were certain "star tribes" in Africa who carried star knowledge. While the Ndebele people carry the knowledge of the Mbube star of Orion (*Umhabi* – "the far-walking constellation"), the Dogons in Sudan, among others, carry the Sirian story.

11. The second of the two southern star shafts of the Great Pyramid is directed on Orion's Belt. Archeoastronomers argue that these star shafts represent the ascension of the pharaoh's soul to the stellar source: Sirius and Orion. Mutwa ascribes the source of life on earth to the central star of the Belt, in particular Al Nilam (the star the Nbebeles called Mbube – meaning "lion of the dark").

12. The Leo constellation is identified by virtually all today's archaeoastronomers – Gilbert, West, Bauval, and Hancock among them – as the stellar formation that the leonine Sphinx exactly mirrors. Mutwa maintains that in the African zodiac (the *Mulu-Mulu*), the constellation of Leo (Mbube Edingile) has direct bearing on the genesis of the lion species on Earth.

13. While the Sphinx itself symbolizes the Leo constellation, the conjoining of the sun with Leo's heart star is believed by scholars such as Gilbert to symbolize the moment of the lion–human identity embodied by the Sphinx. Similarly, Mutwa maintains the sun–Regulus conjunction is a moment of critical importance in the Great African Tradition, symbolizing both the birth and the death of a great epoch.

14. See, for instance, Bauval and Hancock, *Keeper of Genesis*, p.205.

15. See Bauval and Hancock's discussions on this, *Keeper of Genesis*, p.219.

16. For examples of the lion connected with the Golden Mean, see wall reliefs of lions in the Tomb of Mere-Ruka, Saqqara, and in Karnak Temple.

17. Recent investigations into the quality of gold ornaments in ancient African burial sites in the Kruger/Timbavati area have revealed that the gold was mined and not surface gold – further indication of the sophistication of the ancient culture that existed at this time. For more research on the gold finds, and the sophisticated community which must have pro-

duced them, see the South African Broadcasting Corporation's documentary *Mapungubwe: Secrets of the Sacred Hill*, 1999, produced by Katerina Weinek and Lance Gewer.

18. Christopher Wills, in his book on the evolution of the human species, *The Runaway Brain: The Evolution of Human Uniqueness*, entitles his chapter on the Rift Valley "The Birth Canal of Our Species."

19. *Past Worlds: The Times Atlas of Archaeology*, p.54.

20. On the question of subterranean watercourses, we do know that a subterranean river, carrying as much water as the Nile, is today being tapped in Libya, Egypt's neighbor. Colonel Gaddaffi commissioned a team of South Korean engineers to access the water source in the Great Man-Made River project, the largest irrigation endeavor in the world.

Chapter 21: Gold: Subterranean Sun

1. In their book of symbols, the French scholars of ancient symbolism Chevalier and Gheerbront write that the zodiacal lion (Leo) represents the principle of evolution, or "metamorphosis" (*Dictionnaire des Symboles*, p.577). On the number symbolism of the numeral 5, they explain that it describes both the "biological and spiritual evolution" of humankind (pp.254–255).

2. Recent findings of leading astrophysicists reveal that volcanic activity from the earth's molten core is directly related to the sun's activity. In 1977, leading Cambridge astrophysicists John Gribbin and Stephen Plagermann identified "a causal effect linking the activity of the sun . . . and geomagnetic disturbances of the earth's ionosphere by high energy particles emitted from the sun." This led them to conclude that "the overall seismicity of the earth is related to the solar activity." *The Jupiter Effect*, p.93.

3. There is some research to suggest that this may be the case. See, for example, Robert Ardrey, *African Genesis*.

4. BBC *Earth Story* series, program entitled "Ring of Fire."

5. See Society for Geology Applied Mineral Deposits, *Ore Genesis: The State of the Art*, special publication no. 2 (Berlin: Springer-Verlag, 1982), p.38.

6. It is generally understood in geology, chemistry, and planetary physics that most elements, in particular gold, are produced in the life cycles of stars as well as the process by which those stars evolve solar systems. Our sun, the star at the center of our solar systems, is the nuclear energy behind the molecular makeup of gold. See, for example, the work of Stephan Rosswog of Leicester University on the alchemy of gold and stellar energy.

7. Cirlot, *Dictionary of Symbols*, p.114.

8. Ibid., p.304.

9. Schneider, *El origen musical de los animales-simbolos en la mitologia y la escultura antiguas*; Cirlot, introduction.

Chapter 22: Tendile: White Lion Mother

1. See Hesiod's *Works and Days*, described in Bruce Chatwin's *The Songlines*, p.226.

2. Mutwa himself identifies this gold as "mononucleonic gold," although its existence is in question by geologists with whom I have spoken.

3. Wasserman, *The Art and Symbols of the Occult*, pp.91–93.
4. See Gilbert, *Signs in the Sky*, p.307.
5. The notion of rebirth is central to ancient belief systems, both Egyptian and African.
6. This extract from the world's oldest written text, the *Egyptian Book of the Dead*. For a discussion of Ra as "the Word," see West, *Serpent in the Sky*, p.69.
7. Conservationists explain that the behavior of abandoning newborn cubs is directly related to lions' territorial ranges.
8. Gribbin and Cherfas, *The Monkey Puzzle*, p.207.
9. McBride, *op. cit.*, p.112.

Chapter 23: Trophy Hunting

1. In collaboration with the ITN investigative documentary program *The Cook Report* and video footage handed to him, Patterson captured canned lion hunting on film. For more details, see Gareth Patterson's *exposé*, *Dying to be Free: The Canned Lion Scandal*.
2. See the trial of Mfuwa Malatjie reported in *(Toronto) Mail & Guardian*, 20–27 April 2000, p.3.

Chapter 24: White Lions: Prophets of the Future

1. See dictionary definitions of *psychic*, e.g., *Oxford English Dictionary*: "relating to or denoting faculties or phenomena that are apparently inexplicable by natural laws, especially involving telepathy or clairvoyance . . . of or relating to the soul or mind."
2. For a comprehensive documentation on this phenomenon through hypnosis of patients, see the work of the psychiatrist Dr Brain Weiss, *Many Lives, Many Masters*. Also the work of Magdel Shackleton, PhD, Physics and Medicine (UCT), who has spent the latter part of her life working with channeled information from the masters: *Georgina and her Guardian Angels*. Probably the first recorded contact with the ascendant masters are the accounts of 19th-century clairvoyant Helena Blavatsky. See her works, *The Secret Doctrines* and *Isis Unveiled*.
3. Gilbert, *Signs in the Sky*, pp.167–170.
4. Carl Jung's theories on the collective unconscious, as well as his notion of "synchronicity" ("an acausal connecting principle" operating over and above the scientific method of cause and effect) go some way to explaining the workings of phenomena that defy common reason. To Jung, the supernatural was largely the product of archetypes emanating from an original source, or a higher reality. Channeling of information, therefore, may represent the ability of certain individuals, knowingly or unknowingly, to tap into this "super-realm" of superior wisdom. See also Carlos Castaneda on the "tonal" (everyday reality) and the "nagual" (spirit reality) in *Tales of Power*.
5. The Timbavati authorities have brought in master's student Jason Turner to investigate.
6. See Gilbert's discussion of this in *The Orion Mystery*, p.123, and his later findings in *Signs in the Sky*. His focus is on Rostau (Giza).
7. See the writings of the Egyptologist-astronomers Prof. Alexander Badawy and Dr Virginia Trimble on the ventilation shafts as astronomical instruments, and the subsequent theories of Gilbert, Hancock, and Bauval.

8. The lions in the neighboring Kruger Park are infected with tuberculosis and a leonine form of HIV, which are ultimately man-made problems. Even game "sanctuaries" are no longer safe havens.
9. In January 2001, tens of thousands of people died in an earthquake in India. Atomic bombs had been detonated in the region shortly before this "natural" disaster.
10. See BBC documentary series entitled *Earth Story*.
11. Matthew 27:15.

Chapter 25: Ice Ages and Snow Lions

1. The name that Mutwa was given during initiation as a Sanusi has to do with the observation of the stars.
2. Azti, channeled by Jackie te Braake.
3. Fifth-dimensional reality combines time (one dimension) with space (three dimensions) into a space-time coalescence. Symbolically, it is represented as a five-pointed star, or as the center of the cross
4. On the day of Ingwavuma's death, the sun and Regulus were at precisely 20°50′ in the constellation of Leo. Plutarch identified the importance of this moment for the Egyptians, who "hold the lion in honor . . . because the Nile overflows when for the first time the sun comes into conjunction with Leo."

Chapter 26: Lion of Judah

1. This view is held by the Chief Masoyi and Swazi elder Solomon Mabuza.
2. Genesis 49:9–10.
3. Matthew 1:16.
4. See Matthew 1:1–17; Mark 12:35; Luke 21:44; John 7:41.
5. Revelation 22:16.
6. Michael Morpurgo, *The Butterfly Lion* (New York: HarperCollins, 1996). See also *The Roi Leo*, a children's television cartoon screened in Canada with father-and-son White Lions as the central characters.
7. Mark 1:12.
8. The *Illustrated Bible Dictionary*, part 2, p.908. For a detailed discussion of the Christ as Logos, see Freke and Gandy, *The Jesus Mysteries*, pp.82–85.
9. See Isaiah 38:13; Lamentations 3:10; Hosea 5:14, 13:8.
10. Revelation 4:5.
11. Genesis 49:10.
12. Revelation 4:6.
13. Matthew 24:15; Mark 13:14.
14. Matthew 24:29.
15. Matthew 24:30.
16. Mark 12:29–31.

17. It should be noted that the east–west passage of the Great Pyramid is angled in such a manner as to pass directly through the Jewish town of Bethlehem; see LeMesurier, *Decoding the Great Pyramid*, p.19.
18. See Friederich Ruhe on node sites (featured in *South African Archaeological Bulletin*, 1989).
19. For a fairly comprehensive study of the Bushmen paintings of this area, see Woodhouse, *The Rock Art of the Golden Gate*.

GLOSSARY

Afrikaans: South African language that developed from Dutch, spoken by white South Africans of Dutch descent and by many other South Africans.

Afrikaner: White South Africans of Dutch/Huguenot descent.

Archeoastronomy: Study of the alignments of sacred monuments to celestial bodies.

Biltong: Dried meat.

Boma: Protective circle of reeds and thorn bushes used for sheltering people and animals in the African bushveld.

"Brain explosion": The three-fold expansion in the size of the human brain corresponding to the evolutionary leap from *Australopithecus africanus* to *Homo erectus.* This leap is thought to be associated with the acquisition of language and hence social organization.

Dongas: Deep-etched soil erosion in Southern Africa.

Epigraphy: The study and classification of ancient inscriptions.

Equinox: Midspring and midautumn, when day and night are of equal length. Of mystical significance to Bushmen, the ancient Egyptians, and the lion priests of Africa.

Geodetic alignments: The alignment of archeological and mineral-bearing sites along the earth's key meridians.

Highveld: Highland savanna plateau of northern regions of South Africa into Zimbabwe.

Hottentots: Pejorative colonial name for nomadic pastoralist Khoikhoi tribes encountered by Dutch and English settlers in Southern South Africa.

Kaross: Cloak or wrap made of animal hide.

Ley lines: Geodetic lines of power.

Machairodontinae: Extinct huge saber-toothed cat.

Maroche: Spinach-like traditional African vegetable relish (also spelled *marogo*).

Mathimba or Matimba: Tsonga for "power," especially spiritual and ritual power.

Matsieng: Setswana name for the Orion constellation; according to Mutwa, Matsieng is the Eternal Wanderer, the Great Hunter.

Metacarpals: Foot or hand bones of wild animals; used in divination by *sangomas*.

Mopane: Bushveld trees, fruits eaten and used to make traditional beverages.

Muti: Traditional medicine, whether used for healing or the casting of spells.

WaNdau: Mythical ancient African lion priest of semi-divine origin, according to Mutwa's Great Knowledge.

Ndebele: African offshoot to the Zulu tribe who fled Shaka, led by their King Mzilikazi, to settle in Northern South Africa and Southern Zimbabwe after an epic journey of conquest.

Palaeoanthropology: The study of prehistoric man.

Precession of the equinoxes: The rotation of the constellations forming the starry backdrop behind the rising sun at each equinox through the ages. Hence, in the Age of Leo the constellation of Leo rises on the equinox just ahead of the rising sun precisely east. Precessionary theory of modern archeoastronomers (and geological weathering patterns) date the construction of the Sphinx to the Age of Leo in the Northern Hemisphere in 10,500 BC.

Rara avis: Rare species, literally a "rare bird."

Rondavel: Traditional rounded, thatched, wattle-and-daub African dwelling.

Sangoma: African healer/diviner/priest. The highest *sangoma* initiates are known as *izanusi* (singular: *isanusi*) in the Zulu tradition.

Sanusi: Initiate into the ranks of the *sangomas* (plural: *izanusi*). The *i* is dropped when an article is present. I have decided to treat this word in the same way as *sangoma,* which has been absorbed into South African English.

Shangaan: Can be pejorative, more properly Tsonga, an African tribe living in South Africa, Zimbabwe, and Mozambique.

Sharpeville massacre: In 1960, apartheid police shot dead more than 60 people protesting outside a police station at having to carry "native passes" on pain of arrest.

Songlines: Walking pathways across Australia used by Aborigines to "sing" the world into creation.

Soweto uprising: In 1976 the youth of Soweto and later the rest of South Africa began a street revolt that became one of the great forces that succeeded in removing apartheid.

Sterk (Afrikaans): Strong.

Sustainable utilization: The notion that wildlife conservation must be self-funding to work, i.e., if animals have commercial value in the tourist and hunting markets they will be conserved. Official government policy in most Southern African countries.

Taphonomic: The study of cave *brecchia* (deposits) by paleoanthropologists.

Therianthrope, therianthropic: Combined human-animal figures in African rock art.

Tsonga: See *Shangaan* above. Tsonga is both a tribe and the name of their language.

Twasa: The sickness, which can take many forms of mental and physical disturbance, that indicates an ancestral calling to become a *sangoma,* also the initiation phase, resulting in the shaman's state of heightened consciousnesses, expanded awareness, or revelation.

uBaba: African term for *father* or *patriarch.*

Veld: Bush country, African wilderness.

Venda: African tribe of Northern South Africa and Southern Zimbabwe related to the Mashona and Karanga peoples and said to descend from the Rozvi culture that built Great Zimbabwe.

/Xam: Cape Bushman tribe made extinct through colonial genocide.

Xhosa: Xhosa-speaking tribes of Southeastern Africa. Strong Bushman influence on the language and spiritual culture of many Xhosa clans.

Zulu: Zulu-speaking tribes of Southeastern Africa. Famed military organizers; their *sangomas* are highly regarded as powerful shamans. The word *Zulu* is said by Mutwa to mean "interstellar space."

BIBLIOGRAPHY

Africa

Aschwanden, Herbert. *Karanga Mythology*. Translated by Ursula Cooper. Harare, Zimbabwe: Mambo Press, 1989.

Balandier, Georges, and Jacques Macquet. *Dictionary of Black African Civilization*. New York: Leon Arniel Publishers, 1974.

Bourdillon, Michael. *The Shona People*. Harare, Zimbabwe: Mambo Press, 1976.

Chidester, David. *Religions in South Africa*. London: Routledge, 1992.

Coetzee, P.H., and A.P.J. Roux, eds., *Philosophy from Africa: A Text with Readings*. London: International Thompsons, 1998.

Gelfand, Michael. *The Spiritual Beliefs of the Shona*. Harare, Zimbabwe: Mambo Press, 1982.

Grant, Michael, and John Hazel. *Gods and Mortals in Classical Mythology: A Dictionary*. New York: Dorset Press, 1979.

Green, Lawrence George. *Karoo*. Cape Town: Howard Timmins, 1955.

Griaule, Marcel. *Conversations with Ogotemelli: An Introduction to Dogon Religious Ideas*. Oxford: Oxford University Press, 1975.

Makele, Benison. "African Soul Still Held Captive in Europe." *City Press*, 22 December 1996.

Marsh, Rob. *Unsolved Mysteries of Southern Africa*. Cape Town: Struik, 1994.

Mutwa, Credo. *Indaba, My Children*. Johannesburg: Blue Crane Books, n.d.

———. *My People: The Incredible Writings of a Zulu Witchdoctor*. Johannesburg: Blue Crane Books, n.d.

———. *Indaba, My Children*. London: Kahn & Averill, 1985 and 1994.

———. *Isilwane, the Animal: Tales and Fables of Africa*. Cape Town: Struik, 1996.

———. *African Signs of the Zodiac*. Cape Town: Struik, 1997.

Parfitt, Tudor. *Journey to the Vanished Land: The Search for the Lost Tribe of Israel*. London: Hodder & Stoughton, 1992.

Tyrrell, Barbara. *Tribal Peoples of Southern Africa*. Cape Town: Books of Africa, 1971.

———. *Her African Quest*. Cape Town: Lindlife, 1996.

Ancient Mysteries

Aveni, Anthony F. *Archaeoastronomy in Pre-Columbian America*. Austin: University of Texas Press, 1975.

———. *Nazca: Eighth Wonder of the World*. British Museum, 2000.

Aveni, Anthony, ed. *The Lines of Nazca*. Philadelphia: American Philosophical Society, 1990.

Baigent, Michael. *Ancient Traces: Mysteries in Ancient and Early History*. Harmondsworth: Penguin, 1999.

Bailey, James. *The God Kings and the Titans: The New World Ascending in Ancient Times*. London: Hodder & Stoughton, 1973.

Coe, Michael D. "Native Astronomy in Mesoamerica." In *Archaeoastronomy in Pre-Columbia America*. Edited by Anthony F. Aveni. Austin: University of Texas, 1975.

Cotterell, Maurice, and Adrian Gilbert. *The Mayan Prophecies: Unlocking the Secrets of a Lost Civilization*. Shaftesbury: Element, 1995.

Drummond, William. *Oedipus Judaicus: Allegory in the Old Testament*. London: Bracken Books, 1996.

Elkington, David. *In the Name of the Gods: The Mystery of Resonance and the Prehistoric Messiah*. Sherbourne: Green Man Press, 2001.

Freke, Timothy, and Peter Gandy. *The Jesus Mysteries: Was the Original "Jesus" a Pagan God?* London: Thorsons, 1999.

Gardiner, Sir Alan. *Egyptian Grammar*. 3rd ed. Oxford: Griffith, 1978. First published in 1927.

Goetz, Delia, trans. *Popl Vuh: The Sacred Book of the Ancient Quiche Maya*. Norman: University of Oklahoma Press, 1991.

Hadington, Evan. *Lines to the Mountain Gods: Nazca and the Mysteries of Peru*. London: Harrap, 1987.

Knight, Christopher, and Robert Lomas. *The Hiram Key: Pharaohs, Freemasons and the Discovery of the Secret Scrolls of Jesus*. London: Arrow, 1997.

Moorehead, Alan. *The Blue Nile*. London: Hamish Hamilton, 1962.

Morrison, Tony. *Pathways to the Gods: The Mystery of the Andes Lines*. London: Michael Russell, 1978.

———. *The Mystery of the Nazca Lines*. Foreword by Maria Reiche. London: Nonesuch Expeditions Ltd, 1987.

Taube, Karl Andreas. "The Major Gods of Ancient Yucatan." In *Studies in Pre-Columbian Art and Archaeology*, no. 32. Cambridge, Mass: Harvard University Press, 1992.

Temple, Robert. *The Sirius Mystery*. New York: St Martin's Press, 1977.

Tompkins, Peter. *Secrets of the Great Pyramid*. Harmondsworth: Penguin, 1973.

Larousse Encyclopedia of Archaeology. London: Hamlyn, 1972.

Vanished Civilizations. Sydney: Reader's Digest, 1983.

The World's Last Mysteries. Sydney: Reader's Digest, 1977.

Astrology

Campion, Nicholas, and Steve Eddy. *The New Astrology: The Art and Science of the Stars*. London: Bloomsbury, 1999.

Ertel, Suitbert, and Kenneth Irving. *The Tenacious Mars Effect*. London: Urania, 1996.

Gauquelin, Michel. *Planetary Heredity*. San Diego: Astro Communications, 1966.

———. *Cosmic Influences on Human Behavior*. New York: Aurora, 1994.

Hodgson, Joan. *Astrology: The Sacred Science*. Liss: White Eagle Publishing Trust, 1978.

McDonald, Marianne. *Star Myths: Tales of the Constellations*. New York: Friedman Group, 1996.

Mutwa, Credo. *Song of the Stars: The Lore of a Zulu Shaman*. Edited by Stephen Larsen. New York: Barrytown Ltd, 1996.

———. "Born under African Skies." *Drum* 203 (November 1996).

———. *African Signs of the Zodiac*. Cape Town: Struik, 1997.

Oken, Alan. *Complete Astrology*. Rev. ed. London and New York: Bantam, 1988.

Parker, Derek, and Julia Parker. *A History of Astrology*. London: André Deutsch, 1983.

Reinhart, Melanie. *Chiron and the Healing Journey: An Astrological and Psychological Perspective*. London: Arkana, 1989.

Seymour, Percy. *Astrology: The Evidence of Science*. Harmondsworth: Penguin, 1988.

West, John Anthony. *The Case for Astrology*. London: Viking/Arkana, 1991.

Astronomy and Astrophysics

Baker, David. *Larousse Guide to Astronomy*. New York: Larousse, 1980.

Boslough, John. *Beyond the Black Hole: Stephen Hawking's Universe*. Glasgow: Collins Fontana, 1984.

Davies, Paul. *How Things Are: A Scientific Tool Kit for the Mind*. Edited by John Brockman and Katinka Matson. London: Weidenfeld & Nicolson, 1995.

———. *The Fifth Miracle: The Search for the Origin of Life*. London: Allen Lane, 1998.

Gribbin, John, and Stephen Plagemann. *The Jupiter Effect*. Glasgow: Collins Fontana, 1977.

———. *In Search of Schrodinger's Cat: Quantum Physics and Reality*. London: Black Swan/ Transworld, 1984.

———. *In Search of the Edge of Time*. Harmondsworth: Penguin, 1995

———. *Stardust: The Cosmic Recycling of Stars, Planets and People*. London: Allen Lane, 2000.

Krauss, Lawrence. *The Fifth Essence: The Search for Dark Matter in the Universe*. London: Vintage, 1989.

Moore, Patrick. *Countdown!: or, How Nigh is the End?* London: Michael Joseph, 1983.

Taylor, John. *Black Hole: The End of the Universe?* Glasgow: Collins Fontana, 1974.

Bushmen

Bleek, Dorothea F. *Customs and Beliefs of the Xam Bushmen.* Cape Town: University of Cape Town Bantu Studies, issues 5, 6, 7, 9, n.d.

——. *Report of Dr Bleek Concerning His Researches into the Bushman Language and Customs Presented to the Honorable the House of Assembly by Command of his Excellency, the Governor.* n.d.

——. *Mantis and his Friends: Bushman Folklore.* Cape Town: Maskew Miller, 1923.

——. *Lecture on the Bushmen.* Cape Town: University of Cape Town Press, 1924.

Bleek, W.H.I. *Researches into the Bushmen Language and Customs.* Unpublished manuscript, 1873.

Bleek, W.H.I., and L.C. Lloyd (collected by). *Specimens of Bushman Folklore.* London: Allen, 1911.

Deacon, H.J., and Jeanette Deacon. *Human Beginnings in South Africa: Uncovering the Secrets of the Stone Age.* Cape Town: David Philip, 1999.

Fourie, Coral. *Living Legends of a Dying Culture.* Hartebeespoort, South Africa: Ekogilde, 1994.

Garlake, Peter. *The Hunter's Vision: The Prehistoric Art of Zimbabwe.* Seattle: University of Washington Press, 1995.

Johnson, R. Townley. *Major Rock Paintings of Southern Africa.* Cape Town: David Philip, 1991.

Katz, Richard. *Boiling Energy: Community Healing among the Kalahari Kung.* Cambridge, Mass: Harvard University Press, 1982.

Lewis-Williams, David. *The Imprint of Man: The Rock Art of Southern Africa.* Cambridge: Cambridge University Press, 1983.

——. "Testing the Trance Explanation of Southern African Rock Art: Depictions of Felines." *Bolliteno del Centro Communo di Studi Preistorici* 22 (1995).

Lewis-Williams, David, and Thomas Dowson. *The Images of Power: Understanding Bushman Rock Art.* Johannesburg: Southern Book Publishers, 1989.

Liebenberg, Louis. *Art of Tracking, The Origin of Science.* Cape Town: David Philip, 1990.

Skotnes, Pippa. *Miscast: Negotiating the Presence of the Bushmen.* Cape Town: University of Cape Town, 1996.

Van der Post, Laurens. *The Lost World of the Kalahari.* Harmondsworth: Penguin, 1958.

Watson, Stephen. *Return of the Moon: Versions from the /Xam.* Cape Town: Carrefour Press, 1991.

Woodhouse, Bert. *The Rain and its Creatures: As the Bushmen Painted Them.* Johannesburg: William Waterman, 1992.

——. *The Rock Art of the Golden Gate.* Johannesburg: William Waterman, 1996.

Climatology

Brain, C.K. "The Evolution of Man in Africa: Was It a Consequence of Cainozoic Cooling?" Alex L. du Toit Commemorative Lecture presented to the Geological Society of South Africa, 1979.

Dawson, Alastair G. *Ice Age Earth: Late Quaternary Geology and Climate*. London: Routledge, 1992.

Goudie, Andrew. *Environmental Change: Contemporary Problems in Geography*. 3rd ed. Oxford: Clarendon Press, 1992.

Partridge, Timothy and R.R. Maud, eds. *The Cenozoic of Southern Africa*. Oxford and New York: Oxford University Press, 2000.

Schwarzacher, W. *Cyclostratigraphy and the Milankovitch Theory*. Amsterdam and New York: Elsevier, 1993.

Tyson, Peter. *Weather and Climate of Southern Africa*. Oxford: Oxford University Press, 2000.

van Andel, Tjeerd H. *New Views on an Old Planet: A History of Global Change*. 2nd ed., Cambridge: Cambridge University Press, 1994.

Cosmology

Gribbin, John. *Companion to the Cosmos*. London: Weidenfeld & Nicolson, 1996.

Hetherington, Norris S., ed. *Encyclopedia of Cosmology*. New York: Garland, 1993.

Velikovsky, Immanuel. *Worlds in Collision*. London: Victor Gollancz, 1951.

Egyptology and Archeoastronomy

Alford, Alan F. *When the Gods Came Down*. London: Hodder & Stoughton, 2000.

Bauval, Robert. *The Secret Chamber: The Quest for the Hall of Records*. London: Random House, 1999.

Bauval, Robert, and Adrian Gilbert. *The Orion Mystery: Unlocking the Secrets of the Pyramids*, Mandarin, London, 1997

Bauval, Robert, and Graham Hancock. *Keeper of Genesis: A Quest for the Hidden Legacy of Mankind*. London: Mandarin, 1997.

Flinders, W.M. *Personal Religion in Egypt before Christianity*. London: Harper & Bros., 1909.

Gardiner, Sir Alan. *Egyptian Grammar*. 3rd ed. Oxford: Griffith, 1978. First published in 1929.

Gilbert, Adrian. *Magi: The Quest for a Secret Tradition*. London: Bloomsbury, 1997.

——. *Signs in the Sky: Prophecies for the Birth of a New Age*. London: Bantam, 2000.

Hancock, Graham. *Fingerprints of the Gods: A Quest for the Beginning and the End*. London: Mandarin, 1995.

Hancock, Graham, and Santha Faiia. *Heaven's Mirror: Quest for the Lost Civilization*. London: Michael Joseph, 1998.

Hassan, Selim. *The Sphinx: Its History in the Light of Recent Excavations*. Cairo: Government Press, 1949.

Lawton, Ian, and Chris Ogilvie-Herald. *Giza: The Truth*. London: Virgin, 1999.

LeMesurier, Peter. *Decoding the Great Pyramid*. Shaftesbury: Element, 1999.

Parker, Richard A. *The Calendars of Ancient Egypt*. Chicago: University of Chicago, 1950.

Schwaller de Lubicz, R.A. *Sacred Science: The King of Pharaonic Theocracy*. New York: Inner Traditions International, 1961 and 1988.

Spence, Lewis. *Myths and Legends of Ancient Egypt*. London: Harrap, 1915.

Wallis Budge, E.A. *Egyptian Language*. New York: Dover, 1977.

——. *An Egyptian Hieroglyphic Dictionary*. Vol. 1. New York: Dover, 1978.

West, John Anthony. *Serpent in the Sky: The High Wisdom of Ancient Egypt*. London: Quest, 1993.

——. *The Traveller's Key to Ancient Egypt*. 2nd ed. London: Quest, 1995.

Wilson, Colin. *From Atlantis to the Sphinx, Recovering the Lost Wisdom of the Ancient World*. London: Virgin, 1996.

Zausich, Karl-Theodor. *Discovering Egyptian Hieroglyphs*. Translated by Ann Macy Roth. London: Thames & Hudson, 1992.

Esoteric

Berendt, Joachim-Ernst. *Nada Brahma: The World Is Sound – Music and the Landscape of Consciousness*. London: East West, 1988.

Blavatsky, Helena. *Isis Unveiled: A Master Key to the Mysteries of Ancient and Modern Science and Theology*. New York: Bouton, 1893.

——. *The Secret Doctrine: The Synthesis of Science, Religion and Philosophy*. 3rd ed. Point Loma, Calif: Aryan Theosophical Press, 1925.

Brennan, Barbara Ann. *Hands of Light: A Guide to Healing through the Human Energy Field*. New York: Bantam, 1987.

Chatwin, Bruce. *What Am I Doing Here?* London: Jonathan Cape, 1989.

Filotto, Guiseppe. *The Face on Mars*. Cape Town: Exact Print, 1995.

Hand Clow, Barbara. *Signet of Atlantis: War in Heaven Bypass*. Santa Fe, NM: Bear & Co., 1992.

——. *The Pleiadian Agenda: A New Cosmology for the Age of Light*. Santa Fe, NM: Bear & Co., 1995.

Hope, Murry. *The Sirius Connection: Unlocking the Mysteries of Ancient Egypt*. Shaftesbury: Element, 1990.

Kollerstrom, Nick, and Mike O'Neill. *The Eureka Effect: The Celestial Pattern in Scientific Discovery*. London: Urania Trust, 1996.

Masters, Robert. *The Goddess Sekhmet: Psycho-Spiritual Exercises of the Fifth Way.* Woodbury, Minn: Llewellyn Publications, 1991.

Morton, Chris, and Ceri Louise Thomas. *The Mystery of the Crystal Skulls.* London: Thorsons, 1997.

Musaios. *The Lion Path: You Can Take It with You.* Berkeley, Calif: Golden Sceptre, 1988.

Shackleton, Madgel. *Georgina and her Guardian Angels.* Cape Town: Kima Global, 2000.

Turkington, Kate. *There's More to Life Than Surface.* Johannesburg and London: Penguin, 1998.

Weiss, Brian L. *Many Lives, Many Masters.* New York: Simon & Schuster, 1988.

Wilbur, Ken. *Up from Eden.* London: Routledge & Kegan Paul, 1981.

Wilson, Colin. *Alien Dawn: An Investigation into the Contact Experience.* London: Virgin, 1996.

Evolutionary Theory

Ardrey, Robert. *African Genesis: A Personal Investigation into the Animal Origins and Nature of Man.* Glasgow: Collins Fontana, 1961.

——. *The Hunting Hypothesis: A Personal Conclusion Concerning the Evolutionary Nature of Man.* Glasgow: Collins Fontana, 1996.

Brain, C.K. "Hominid Evolution and Climactic Change." In *South African Journal of Science* 77 (1981).

——. *The Hunters or the Hunted?* Chicago: University of Chicago Press, 1981.

——. "Do We Owe Our Intelligence to a Predatory Past?" Lecture for the James Arthur Series on the Evolution of the Human Brain, New York, 2000.

Brain, C.K., ed. *Swartkrans: A Cave's Chronicle of Early Man.* Transvaal Museum Monograph, no. 8.

Brain, C.K., and V. Watson. "A Guide to the Swartkrans Hominid Cave Site." *Annals of the Transvaal Museum* 35 (1992): 343–365.

Bronowski, J. *The Ascent of Man.* London: BBC, 1981.

Coon, C.S. *The Hunting Peoples.* London: Jonathan Cape, 1971.

Gribbin, John, and Jeremy Cherfas. *The Monkey Puzzle: A Family Tree.* London: The Bodley Head, 1982.

Johanson, Donald, and Blake Edgar. *From Lucy to Language.* Johannesburg: Witwatersrand University Press, 1996.

Leakey, Richard E. *The Making of Mankind.* London: Michael Joseph, 1981.

Lee, R.B., and I. deVore, eds. *Man the Hunter.* Chicago: Aldine, 1968.

Lee-Thorp, Julia. "The Hunters or the Hunted Revisited." *Journal of Human Evolution* 39, no. 6 (December 2000).

Marshall Thomas, Elizabeth. "The Old Way." *The New Yorker*, 15 October 1990.

McKee, Jeffrey K. *The Riddled Chain.* Piscataway, NJ: Rutgers University Press, 2000.

Morris, Desmond. *The Naked Ape: A Zoologist's Study of the Human Animal.* London: Jonathan Cape, 1967.

Ruhe, Friedrich. "Node Sites." *South African Archaeological Bulletin* (1989).

Sheldrake, Rupert. *The Presence of the Past.* Glasgow: Collins Fontana, 1988.

Tobias, Phillip V. *The Brain in Hominid Evolution.* New York and London: Columbia University Press, 1971.

Wills, Christopher. *The Runaway Brain: The Evolution of Human Uniqueness.* London, Flamingo, 1995.

Geology

Edwards, Telford. "Gold Production in Matabeleland." *Bulawayo Chronicle*, 26 June 1897.

van Royen, William. *Mineral Resources of the World.* London: Constable, 1952.

Woodhouse, H.C. *Archaeology in Southern Africa.* Cape Town: Purnell, 1971.

Minerals Yearbook. Washington, DC: International United States Government Printing Office, 1999.

Ore Genesis: The State of the Art. Special publication no. 2 of the Society for Geology Applied Mineral Deposits. Berlin: Springer-Verlag, 1982.

General

Chatwin, Bruce. *The Songlines.* London: Picador, 1987.

Fischbacker, Siegfried, and Roy Ludwig Horn. *Siegfried and Roy: Mastering the Impossible.* New York: William Morrow, 1992.

Knox-Shaw, Peter. "Unicorns on Rocks: The Expressionism of Olive Schriener." *English Studies in Africa* 40, no. 2 (2008): 13–32.

Marais, Eugène. *Soul of the Ape.* Cape Town: Human & Rousseau, 1969.

Mountford, Charles P. *Aboriginal Paintings.* Glasgow: Collins Fontana, 1964.

Sobel, Dana. *Longitude.* London: Fourth Estate, 1995.

Van der Post, Laurens. "The Other Side of Silence." Lecture delivered at the World Wilderness Congress, published under the title *Voices of the Wilderness.* Edited by Ian Player. Johannesburg: Jonathan Ball, 1979.

Watson, Lyall. *Supernature: The History of the Supernatural.* London: Coronet/Hodder, 1973.

——. *Lightning Bird.* London: Hodder & Stoughton, 1982.

Willock, Colin. *Africa's Rift Valley.* The World's Wild Places series. New York: Time-Life Books, 1974.

Oxford English Dictionary, Advanced Learners' Edition. 4th ed. Oxford: Oxford University Press, 1989.

The Shorter Oxford English Dictionary. Oxford: Clarendon Press, 1980.

The Shorter Oxford English Dictionary on Historical Principles. Vol. 1. London: Clarendon Press, 1973.

General Science

Gribbin, John. *The Hole in the Sky.* London: Corgi, 1988.

Leakey, Roger. *The Sixth Extinction.* London: Weidenfeld & Nicolson, 1996.

Needham, J. *Science and Civilization in China.* Cambridge: Cambridge University Press, 1962.

Schnell, Jonathan. *The Fate of the Earth.* London: Picador, 1982.

Singer, Charles. *A Short History of Scientific Ideas to 1900.* Oxford: Oxford University Press, 1959.

Thompson, Damian. *End of Time.* London: Sinclair-Stevenson, 1996.

Great Zimbabwe

Beach, D.N. *Zimbabwe Before 1900.* Harare: Mambo Press, 1984.

———. *War and Politics in Zimbabwe 1840–1900.* Harare: Mambo Press, 1986.

Garlake, Peter. *Great Zimbabwe Described and Explained.* Harare: Zimbabwe Publishing House, 1982.

Hall, R.N., and W.G. Neal. *The Ancient Ruins of Rhodesia.* London: Methuen, 1906.

Jones, Neville, ed. *Guide to the Zimbabwe Ruins.* Harare: Secretary, 1949. Reprinted in 1960.

Keane, A.H. *The Gold of Ophir.* London: Edward Stanford, 1901.

Mallows, Wilfrid. *The Mystery of Great Zimbabwe: The Key to a Major Archaeological Enigma.* London: Robert Hale, 1985.

Mufuka, Ken. *Dzimbahwe: Life and Politics in the Golden Age, 1100–1500 AD.* Harare: Harare Publishing House, 1983.

Summers, Roger. *Ancient Mining in Rhodesia and Adjacent Areas.* Salisbury: Trustees of the National Museums of Rhodesia, 1969.

Walker, P.J., and J.G. Dickens. *An Engineering Study of Dry-Stone Monuments in Zimbabwe.* Harare: University of Zimbabwe, 1992.

Sacred Texts

Hermetica: The Writings Attributed to Hermes Trismegistus. Edited and translated by Walter Scott, with Foreword by Adrian Gilbert. Shaftesbury: Solos Press, 1993.

The Illustrated Bible Dictionary. Part 2. London: Hodder & Stoughton, 1962.

Shamanism

Castaneda, Carlos. *Tales of Power.* London: Arkana, 1974.
——. *The Fire from Within.* London: Black Swan, 1984.
Clottes, Jean, and David Lewis-Williams. *The Shamans of Prehistory: Trance and Magic in the Painted Caves.* New York: Harry N. Abrams, 1996.
Halifax, Joan. *Shaman: The Wounded Healer.* London: Thames & Hudson, 1982.
Krige, E. Jensen, and J.D. Krige. *The Realm of a Rain Queen: A Study of the Pattern of Lovedu Society.* Oxford: Oxford University Press, 1996.
Santillana, Giorgio de, and Hertha von Dechend. *Hamlet's Mill: An Essay on Myth and the Frame of Time.* London: Macmillan, 1969.

Symbolism and Mythology

Bailey, Adrian. *The Caves of the Sun: The Origins of Mythology.* London and New York: Random House, 1977.
Campbell, Joseph. *Primitive Mythology: The Masks of God.* London: Arkana, 1991.
Chevalier, Jean. *Penguin Dictionary of Symbols.* Translated by John Buchanan-Brown. London: Penguin, 1996.
Chevalier, Jean, and Alain Gheerbront. *Dictionnaire des Symboles.* Paris: Seghers, 1991.
Cirlot, J.E. *Dictionary of Symbols.* London: Routledge & Kegan Paul, 1962 and 1971.
Felgg, Graham. *Numbers: Their History and Meaning.* Harmondsworth: Penguin, 1983.
Fontana, David. *The Secret Language of Symbols: A Visual Key to Symbols and their Meanings.* San Francisco: Chronicle Books, 1993.
Frazer, Sir James. *The Golden Bough: A Study in Magic and Religion.* London: Macmillan, 1963.
Goodman, Frederick. *Magic Symbols.* London: Brian Trodd, 1989.
Grimal, Pierre, ed. *Larousse World Mythology.* London: Hamlyn, 1965 and 1973.
Hartner, W. "The Earliest History of the Constellation in the Near East and the Motif of the Lion-Bull Combat." *Journal of Near Eastern Studies* 24 (1965).
Herberger, Charles, F. *The Riddle of the Sphinx: Calendric Symbolism in Myth and Icon.* New York: Vantage, 1979.
Liungman, Carl G. *Dictionary of Symbols.* New York: W.W. Norton, 1991.
Saunders, Nicholas J. *Animal Spirits: the Shared World of Sacrifice, Ritual and Myth, Animal Souls and Symbols.* Living Wisdom Series. London: Macmillan, 1995.
Singh, Madanjeet. *The Sun in Myth and Art.* London: Thames & Hudson, 1993.
Tresidder, Jack. *Dictionary of Symbols: An Illustrated Guide to Traditional Images, Icons and Emblems.* London: Duncan Baird, 1997.
Wasserman, James. *The Art and Symbols of the Occult.* London: Tiger Books, 1993.
Willis, Roy. *World Mythology.* New York: Henry Holt, 1993.

The White Lions

McBride, Christopher. *The White Lions of Timbavati*. London: Ernest Stanton, 1977.
——. *Operation White Lion*. New York: St Martin's Press, 1981.
Morpurgo, Michael. *The Butterfly Lion*. London: Collins Children's Books, 1996.

LIST OF APPENDICES

Appendices can be found at the website **www.whitelions.org** when you become a member of the Global White Lion Protection Trust.

Appendix A – Hunting Hypothesis
Archeological and anthropological evidence relating to feline predators, hominid hunting techniques, and the shamanic notion of "hunting magic."

Appendix B – Lion Priests and Warriors
Notions of lion heroism and lion priesthood in Africa and Bushman beliefs regarding humans who change into lions.

Appendix C – Social Man, Social Cats
Lion–human myths: Hercules, Nemean Lion riddle, Androcles. How these relate to the evolutionary development of our species. Humans as social animals and lions as social cats – possible interspecies communication and parallel evolutionary development.

Appendix D – Leylines
Some examples of earth-line drawings. How the notion of leylines ("Songlines," or elements of geomancy) may relate to the energy line defined by the Nilotic Meridian.

Appendix E – The Word
Background on the Lion as Solar Logos – the Word of God. The use of the word *lion* among the world's early peoples.

Appendix F – Pentacle
Lion's sacred number-symbol: 5. World mythology corroborates Credo Mutwa's claim that the lion is intimately associated with the star symbol. The number-symbol 5 in relation to:

- Quintessence (fifth dimensionality), pentacle, pentagram
- Lion-star in hieroglyphics

- Fifth sun, fifth house, and quintessence
- Duat and quintessence

Appendix G – Quintessence and Physics

The mystic notion of the quintessence (fifth dimensionality) and how this may be reconciled with today's leading scientific theory. This survey covers the questions of the quintessence as star matter; "Fifth Force" and quantum physics; and the quintessence as a notion of singularity

Appendix H – Leonids and Hominids

Humankind's lion–human legacy in relation to archeological evidence as well as esoteric channeled material relating to leonine star beings from Sirius.

Appendix I – Astrology

Analysis of the specific day of the lion encounter in Timbavati (10 November 1991) using astronomical coordinates and astrological theory.

Appendix J – Fifth Sun

The notion of the Fifth Sun and how this relates the lion-star force. This survey covers the notions of:

- Four epochs, Four Suns
- Tezcatlipoca: the original state of black jaguar
- Quetzalcoatl: light out of blackness
- Pyramidal notion of the Fifth Sun
- Jaguar Sun – Quincunx
- Quintessence and the Fifth Sun
- Quaternary: our own epoch

Appendix K – Subterranean Sun

Shamanic notions of the "subterranean sun" in relation to recent astrophysical theory which links the activity of the sun with geomagnetic disturbances in the earth's liquid core. Hidden gold and Barberton mountain lands as gold site and site of earliest life forms.

- The correlation between sun and subterranean sun
- Polar reversal
- The lion as solar Logos: physical manifestation of solar power

Appendix L – Ice Ages and Snow Lions

Possible Ice Age antecedents for the White Lions. Possible connection between the White Lions and prehistoric sabertooths. Ice Age cave art as a means for verification of prior existence of the White Lions.

Appendix M – Ice Ages and Leo Ages

Leo Ages as possible determining factor in evolutionary Ice Age epochs. Based on a comparison between the Milankovitch Model of Ice Ages and the ancient astrological Ages of Man calendar. White Lions as heralds of the new Ice Age.

Appendix N – Egypt and Old Africa

Heroic solar lion gods identified with the Orion constellation, dealing with modern archeoastronomy and inherited knowledge of Old Africa.

ABOUT THE AUTHOR

Linda Tucker was educated at the universities of Cape Town and Cambridge, where she specialized in Jungian dream psychology and medieval symbolism. She began her research into the White Lion mysteries after being rescued from lions in the Timbavati region of South Africa in 1991 by a Shangaan shaman woman named Maria Khosa. Maria became her teacher and introduced her to other African lion shamans, who informed Linda that she carried the anciet shamanic title "Keeper of the White Lions." In 2002, Tucker founded the **Global White Lion Protection Trust** to ensure the protection of not only the White Lions, which were being kept in captivity and hunted as trophies, but also the indigenous African culture that holds them sacred.

INDEX

313

Hay House Titles of Related Interest

YOU CAN HEAL YOUR LIFE, the movie, starring Louise L. Hay & Friends
(available as a 1-DVD program and an expanded 2-DVD set)
Watch the trailer at: **www.LouiseHayMovie.com**

THE SHIFT, the movie,
starring Dr. Wayne W. Dyer
(available as a 1-DVD program and an expanded 2-DVD set)
Watch the trailer at: **www.DyerMovie.com**

ILLUMINATION: The Shaman's Way of Healing,
by Alberto Villoldo, Ph.D.

*SOUL ON FIRE: A Transformational Journey from
Priest to Shaman,* by Peter Calhoun

*SUPERCHARGED TAOIST: An Amazing True Story to
Inspire You on Your Own Adventure,* by The Barefoot Doctor

*THE THREE SISTERS OF THE TAO: Essential Conversations with
Chinese Medicine, I Ching, and Feng Shui,* by Terah Kathryn Collins

VISIONSEEKER: Shared Wisdom from the Place of Refuge,
by Hank Wesselman, Ph.D.

We hope you enjoyed this Hay House book. If you'd like to receive our online catalog featuring additional information on Hay House books and products, or if you'd like to find out more about the Hay Foundation, please contact:

Hay House, Inc., P.O. Box 5100, Carlsbad, CA 92018-5100

(760) 431-7695 or (800) 654-5126
(760) 431-6948 (fax) or (800) 650-5115 (fax)
www.hayhouse.com® • www.hayfoundation.org

Published and distributed in Australia by: Hay House Australia Pty. Ltd., 18/36 Ralph St., Alexandria NSW 2015 • *Phone:* 612-9669-4299 *Fax:* 612-9669-4144 • www.hayhouse.com.au

Published and distributed in the United Kingdom by: Hay House UK, Ltd., 292B Kensal Rd., London W10 5BE • *Phone:* 44-20-8962-1230 *Fax:* 44-20-8962-1239 • www.hayhouse.co.uk

Published and distributed in the Republic of South Africa by: Hay House SA (Pty), Ltd., P.O. Box 990, Witkoppen 2068 *Phone/Fax:* 27-11-467-8904 • info@hayhouse.co.za • www.hayhouse.co.za

Published in India by: Hay House Publishers India, Muskaan Complex, Plot No. 3, B-2, Vasant Kunj, New Delhi 110 070 • *Phone:* 91-11-4176-1620 *Fax:* 91-11-4176-1630 • www.hayhouse.co.in

Distributed in Canada by: Raincoast, 9050 Shaughnessy St., Vancouver, B.C. V6P 6E5 • *Phone:* (604) 323-7100 *Fax:* (604) 323-2600 • www.raincoast.com

Take Your Soul on a Vacation

Visit **www.HealYourLife.com**® to regroup, recharge, and reconnect with your own magnificence. Featuring blogs, mind-body-spirit news, nd life-changing wisdom from Louise Hay and friends.

Visit **www.HealYourLife.com** today!